MAR

MW01253527

MARGARET McEVOY, RN, MS, PNP

PAIN IN CHILDREN

Pain in Children

Nature, Assessment, and Treatment

Patricia A. McGrath, PhD
Child Health Research Institute
Children's Hospital of Western Ontario

Foreword by Patrick D. Wall

THE GUILFORD PRESS
New York   London

To all the children who have taught me about their pain and their pain relief—especially to Jennifer, Lisa, Nathan, Paul, Daryl, Bradley, and Lori.

© 1990 The Guilford Press
A Division of Guilford Publications, Inc.
72 Spring Street, New York, NY 10012

All rights reserved

No part of this book may be reproduced, stored in a retrieval system, or transmitted, in any form or by any means, electronic, mechanical, photocopying, microfilming, recording, or otherwise, without written permission from the Publisher.

Printed in the United States of America

This book is printed on acid-free paper.

Last digit is print number: 9 8 7 6 5 4 3 2 1

Library of Congress Cataloging-in-Publication Data
McGrath, Patricia A.
    Pain in children / Patricia A. McGrath.
        p. cm.
    Bibliography: p.
    Includes index.
    ISBN 0-89862-390-1
    1. Pain in children. I. Title.
    [DNLM: 1. Pain—in adolescence. 2. Pain—in infancy & childhood.
    3. Pain—therapy.   WL 704 M479p]
    RJ365.M37   1990
    616'.0472'083—dc20
    DNLM/DLC
    for Library of Congress   89-11009
                                                                     CIP

Acknowledgments

First and foremost, I would like to express my sincere appreciation to our child patients and their families, without whose assistance this book could not have been written. They patiently completed forms and answered many questions about their pain experiences to enable us to refine treatments and adapt adult pain control interventions for them. Children with arthritis, cancer, diabetes, growth hormone deficiency, phantom limb pain, recurrent headaches, and recurrent abdominal pain have led us to develop more effective programs for alleviating children's pain, distress, and anxiety. Pseudonyms have been used in presenting case material to protect the confidentiality of the children and their families.

I am indebted to my colleagues in the Department of Paediatrics at the University of Western Ontario and the Children's Hospital of Western Ontario (CHWO). In 1982, they supported the concept of an integrated research and service program for childhood pain. This concept evolved into a reality when a formal Paediatric Pain Programme and Children's Pain Clinic were established a year later. The knowledge that we have gained through the pain program has evolved from many multidisciplinary and interdisciplinary collaborative studies. Various research studies on pain in infants, children, and adolescents have been supported by the Ontario Ministry of Health, the National Health Research and Development Program of Health and Welfare Canada, and the CHWO Foundation. I am especially grateful to the Ontario Ministry of Health, which has granted me a Career Scientist Award, enabling me to devote the majority of my time to research on childhood pain. I am also particularly indebted to the CHWO Foundation for recognizing the importance of pain research for children, well before the topic was recognized as a priority by the scientific and medical communities. The Foundation provided critical bridge support to the Pain Programme between external operating grants and, through the Child Health Research Institute, enables us to provide cohesive service, integrated with research for all children's pain problems.

I would particularly like to thank Loretta Hillier, for sharing the development of the Children's Pain Clinic and Paediatric Pain Programme; Margaret Brigham, for her valuable assistance in directing the program, which enabled me to complete this book; Nan Fraser, for her extraordinary secretarial assistance; and Esther Wines, for her efforts in locating difficult research sources. My gratitude also goes to Peggy Cook, Farah Ahmed, Laura Marshall, and Mary-Ellen Brewster for their assistance in the research studies described in this book. My graduate students, Heather Cake, Deborah Glebe, and Manon Houle, shared in various aspects of the research programs described in this book. I thank my family, John, Dan, Donna, Patrick, and Kathleen, for their support and encouragement, as well as my friends for their constant enthusiasm. Finally, I would especially like to thank my editor, Sharon Panulla, for her consistent encouragement, warmth, tact, friendship, and sense of humor.

Foreword

The study of pain, particularly chronic pain, in adults is relatively recent. It is therefore not surprising that this is one of the early books on the problem of pain in children. The reasons for the neglect of pain by doctors were mistaken but honorable. Since the early 19th century, there has been an obsessive search by doctors and patients for specific diagnoses and cures. In the course of that search, symptoms such as pain or fever were regarded as mere signposts. To attack the signposts was condemned as bad medicine. This neglect of pain was aided by two factors. One was the marvelous ability of the anesthetists to control acute pain. The other was the trivialization of pain mechanisms by scientists who insisted on a single simple brain mechanism that took no account of the evolution of pains, their subjective individuality, or their interweaving with suffering as expressed to other people.

Animals may be treated with neglect or, almost as bad, they may be treated anthropomorphically as though they were people. Children suffer similar problems when they are either neglected or treated as little grownups. The problem gets even worse when they begin to speak and their speech is taken to have precise adult meanings. Those who care for babies have also tended to get the subject of pain wrong in two ways. One is to believe that the nervous system is so poorly formed at birth that the apparatus for the perception of pain has not yet formed. There is not a scrap of evidence for this common belief. It is undoubtedly true that a child does not have an adult's sophisticated perception of the significance of a pain, but that may make it all the worse. Evidence grows that pain, or at least the arriving nerve impulses that trigger pain, is bad at any age. It disturbs sleep, feeding, movement, and the endocrine system, which are at least as important for the child as the adult if not more so. The other error, which is contradictory to the first, is to regard the child as particularly fragile and therefore to hesitate or underuse analgesic treatments.

We are in a very exciting time when the whole issue is being explored by skilled people with open minds. Patricia McGrath is one of those who have opened up this subject for special study. May the children find a little ease while the readers find a disturbing intellectual challenge to their humanity.

Patrick D. Wall, FRS, DM, FRCP

Preface

Interest in the assessment and management of children's pain has increased dramatically during the past few years; this increase is concurrent with incredible advances in our understanding of the plasticity and complexity of pain processing. New information about internal pain-inhibitory systems and the factors that trigger them has revolutionized traditional approaches to pain control. The concept that guided much of the past management of children's pain—namely, that pain is simply and directly proportional to the nature and extent of an injury—is no longer tenable. Instead, we now realize that children's pain is plastic and that there are many ways in which we can alleviate their suffering.

This book presents some of the new information on how to assess and control acute, recurrent, and chronic pain in children. It focuses on the practical aspects of treating childhood pain from a multidimensional perspective, consistent with the neural and psychological mechanisms that mediate pain. The purpose is to provide readers with a cohesive rationale for designing and evaluating flexible interventions to reduce pain for infants, children, and adolescents.

Contents

PAIN IN CHILDREN

1

The Multidimensional Nature of Children's Pain Experiences

Both the experience and the alleviation of pain have been regarded successively as a mystery, a puzzle, and a challenge. The mystery of pain—why people may differ in their perceptions of pain, why pain can develop and persist without physical injury, and why pain is sometimes not felt despite major injury—has intrigued people in all cultures throughout recorded history. The diverse aspects of pain perception have perplexed not only the sufferers, but also the healers who have attempted to understand the nature of pain to provide effective treatments.

Pain is a common and a ubiquitous sensation for children and adults. The vast majority of people will experience many different pains throughout their lives. Pain may develop in most parts of the body—internally in muscles, bones, joints, teeth, and viscera, as well as externally on the surface of the skin. Pain can be caused by a diverse variety of mechanical, thermal, chemical, and electrical stimuli. Pain varies extensively in quality (aching, burning, tearing, gnawing, stinging, throbbing, sharp, or dull), intensity (weak to strong), duration (a few seconds to years), frequency (constant or episodic), and unpleasantness (a mild annoyance to an intolerable discomfort). Pain may be well localized in one body region or diffusely spread across several areas.

Children and adults may experience different pains from the same pain-inducing stimulus and may react differently, depending on their personalities, learning, expectations, and previous pain experience. Pain is not an immediate and inevitable consequence of an injury. There are numerous examples of athletes who sustain serious injuries during sports competition, but who do not feel pain until after their participation. People in many cultures can undergo presumably painful initiation rites and yet they do not feel pain. In fact, most people can recall an

1

incident in which they did not feel the sting of a small cut until after they had noticed some slight bleeding. In contrast, some people experience debilitating pain in the absence of any apparent bodily injury. People may experience pain in a body site that is different from the location where the pain actually originates. A familiar example of this type of referred pain is pain produced by a heart attack, which is often localized in the left arm rather than in the heart.

Although less familiar, several mysterious pains or pain-free conditions may afflict adults or children. Adults may develop abnormal conditions such as tabes dorsalis and causalgia, in which they experience excruciating pain from usually nonpainful stimuli, such as light pressure or warmth. After an amputation, both children and adults may develop phantom limb pains, in which they feel vivid pain sensations in the limb that was amputated. A few infants have been born without the capacity to feel any pain, regardless of the severity of an injury. Thus, although people may assume that there is a simple and direct relationship between an injury and pain, there are many circumstances in which this relationship is neither simple nor direct.

The dual challenge of pain is to understand the diverse and puzzling aspects of pain perception, and subsequently to provide adequate relief for all types of pain. The external and internal factors that cause pain and the physiological mechanisms that convey pain messages must be understood for both the normal circumstances in which healthy individuals perceive or fail to perceive pain, and the exceptional circumstances in which individuals develop abnormal pathological pains. Accurate knowledge about pain perception and the factors that modifiy pain provides a framework for designing methods to relieve pain.

A recognition of the multidimensional nature of the cures for pain, as well as the multidimensional nature of the causes and manifestations of pain, can be traced throughout the early writings of different cultures. Seemingly inexplicable pains that were not related to apparent physical injuries were generally regarded as afflictions caused by offended gods or as bodily invasions from evil spirits. Pain relief then required supplicating the offended deities or exorcising the evil spirits. The more explicable pains, those related to obvious bodily injury, were treated with a variety of pharmacological and physical methods. In the 10th century A.D., Avicenna summarized the available remedies for reducing pain related to sickness and injury. Several drugs, herbal preparations, therapeutic physical treatments, and mental relaxation techniques are listed in his *Canon of Medicine* (discussed by Gruner, 1930). Opium, seeds and root of mandrake, poppy, hemlock, white and black hyoscyamus, deadly nightshade, lettuce seed, snow, and ice water are listed as stupefacients that produce an insensibility to pain. Other means of alleviating pain are dry or hot cupping, poultices made with flour of orobs boiled in vinegar, walking about gently for a considerable time to relax the tissues, agreeable music, and being occupied with something very engrossing. Many of these therapeutic remedies are similar to those prescribed for pain relief today, 10 centuries later. Although much progress has been made since Avicenna summarized the medical knowledge on pain, many puzzling questions still remain about the diverse causes, the subjective perceptions, and the various cures for pain.

In spite of our enduring interest in understanding and controlling pain, the formal study of pain as a distinct sensation is relatively new. The International Association for the Study of Pain (IASP) was founded in 1973 to integrate the multiple disciplines essential for solving the puzzle of pain (the anatomy, physiology, and chemistry of the nervous system; the psychology of human pain perception; and the various approaches to pain control), so that all aspects of pain perception and pain management could be studied in a more cohesive manner. In 1975, the IASP journal *Pain* was established to provide a forum for the scientific exchange of information about pain from all disciplines. Today, three journals are exclusively devoted to research on pain perception and on the clinical management of painful conditions: *Pain*, the *Journal of Pain and Symptom Management*, and the *Clinical Journal of Pain*. Two other books on various aspects of children's pain have been published recently (McGrath & Unruh, 1987; Ross & Ross, 1988).

During the past 15 years, a vast amount of information has been obtained about the sensory system responsible for our pain perception, with the result that there have been dramatic changes in our understanding of how pain is experienced and how pain may be modified. Traditionally, the sensory system for pain was regarded as a relatively rigid and straightforward arrangement of nerve pathways; it was believed that pain is inevitably produced when a noxious stimulus (any stimulus that produces tissue damage) activates the system. The strength and quality of the resulting pain sensation were thought to be simply and directly related to the intensity and nature of the noxious stimulus. According to this concept, pain is produced in a manner similar to pulling a cord to ring a bell—an analogy used by Descartes in 1664. In his *Treatise on Man*, Descartes (1664/1972) described his theory that minute particles of fire activated nerves, which then transmitted the energy along the nerves to the brain in a cord-like fashion to produce burning pain.

The concept that there is a fixed, direct pathway from a noxious stimulus to the brain implies that human pain perception is only determined by the extent of tissue damage. However, we now have learned that the sensory system for pain is complex and that there are many places in the nociceptive system where the signals initiated by a noxious stimulus can be modified to alter pain perception. There are endogenous (internal) opioid or morphine-like systems that can be activated by environmental factors and by psychological factors to suppress pain. The traditional concept of a relatively rigid system is no longer tenable. Pain is not simply and directly related to the nature or extent of tissue damage. Because pain may be altered by many factors, the nociceptive system (the sensory system for pain) is regarded as plastic and complex. (The plasticity and complexity of the nociceptive system, and the different historical theories and attitudes about pain, are described in Chapter 3.)

The recognition that the body's responses to a noxious stimulus may be changed by many environmental and psychological factors has led to a renewed interest in the use of nonpharmacological methods (nondrug techniques), such as hypnosis, biofeedback, acupuncture, and relaxation training, for reducing many pain conditions. However, the recent advances in the management of pain that have originated from our increased understanding of the plasticity and complexity of the nociceptive system have been confined almost exclusively to adults. Consequently, our understanding of pain perception in infants, children, and adolescents; of the prevalence of different pain problems for children; and of the effectiveness of various pain control methods is limited.

The current lack of objective knowledge about pain in children is understandable in light of the evolution of the scientific study of pain. The major multidisciplinary investigation of pain is relatively young; in addition, initial research studies were conducted with adults, who could communicate their subjective experience of pain, or in animals, in which nerve pathways could be directly monitored. It was implicitly assumed either that children were unable to communicate their experiences of pain in a reliable manner or that they did not perceive pain in the same manner as adults. Also, much information on the development of valid methods for measuring pain, as well as on the effectiveness of different techniques for controlling pain, has been obtained in studies in which controlled levels of noxious stimuli were administered to healthy volunteers. Since ethical concerns limit the use of children in these experimental studies, there has been a lack of basic research on pediatric pain.

Finally, the clinical studies on pain control in children that were conducted were often misleading, because the investigators did not use objective and consistent criteria for assessing chlidren's pain or because they assumed that the strength of pain was directly and only determined by the type of pain-producing stimulus. They failed to recognize that the same noxious stimulus (e.g., an injection) could actually produce different strengths of pain for children, and that the pains were not simply related to how much tissue damage was produced by the injection.

Fortunately, research on pain measurement and pain control in children has increased dramatically during the past few years. New attention is focusing on how pain perception, pain behavior, and pain attitudes vary throughout childhood and how they may be influenced by sex, age, learning, and previous pain experiences. Also, more clinical research is being conducted on how to relieve pain in infants and children who require invasive medical procedures, who experience pain after surgery, or who suffer from painful diseases.

What Is Pain to Children?

Like that of adults, children's pain is an unpleasant sensory and emotional experience. Their pain perceptions are subjective, similar to their perceptions of color, sound, smell, and taste. Their pain perceptions are also like their other perceptions in that it is impossible to know exactly what a child's pain experience is like—even though there are methods to measure different aspects of pain, similar to those used to measure the color, brightness, or purity of a light. Children describe their pain according to both its unpleasantness (i.e., its aversive dimension) and its sensory attributes—the strength, quality (e.g., aching, sharp, pounding), location, and duration. At a very early age, they recognize the multidimensional and ubiquitous nature of pain.

Children's understanding about pain and their descriptions of pain naturally depend on their age, cognitive level, and previous pain experience. They judge the strength and unpleasantness of their pains in relation to the types of pains that they have already experienced. Children learn specific words to describe the various aspects of all their perceptions—words to denote different sounds, colors, shapes, and tastes. Similarly, they learn a vocabulary to use to describe their pains. Their understanding about pain and their ability to communicate their understanding are dependent on their developmental level and the nature and diversity of their pain experiences. My colleagues and I are currently conducting a study to evaluate differences in children's pain perceptions according to their age, sex, and health status (healthy children vs. children with cancer, headaches, or arthritis). The study includes asking children to define pain, to describe their most and least painful experiences, and to use a pain diary to rate the intensity and unpleasantness of all pains that they experience during a 1-month period. A sample of the responses obtained thus far from healthy children illustrates how their age, sex, and previous pain experience can affect their understanding and perceptions of pain.

A 9-year-old girl defined pain as "hurt—it gives you bad feelings." Her most intense pain occurred when her brother punched her in the stomach. Her least strong pain was "a pinch on my back from a friend at school for fun." On her pain diary, she listed "a pinch on the hand, the need to have a bowel movement during a track meet, a sore on my thumb that is aggravated when I play the piano, my mother cut my nails with a clipper, and the doctor pricked my finger for blood tests." A 14-year-old girl described pain as "a feeling of hurt physically or mentally by someone or something." Her strongest pain occurred at age 4, when she cut her foot and received 10 stitches to close the wound. Her smallest pain was when she was bitten by an ant. On her pain diary, she listed "a rash on my legs, a cut while shaving, sunburn, a bang on my leg when I hit the table, and terrible stomach-aches." A 16-year-old girl defined pain as "when you have a hurt in part of your body by doing something with it that it cannot handle doing." Her most intense pain was when "I smashed my face against the dashboard in a truck accident"; her least strong pain was when she "cut her knee during baseball." On her pain diary, she listed "a scraped knee, headache, cut finger with knife, and emotional pain because my boyfriend left."

A 7-year-old boy described pain as "something very bad and unuseful." His most intense pain was when he broke his leg; his least strong pain was when his brother pinched him. He listed "leg aches, a hurt foot, and stomach cramps" on his diary. A 10-year-old boy defined pain as "a feeling, but what I don't understand is why it is so bad and why sometimes you cry. It's just like any other feeling. I think the reason why you cry is because it looks bad and it's mostly all in your head." His most intense pain was when he fell from his bike and required stitches in his knee; his weakest pain was when he was hit in the stomach with a soccer ball. His pain diary included "alcohol on a blister, a fall in a soccer game, and a bump on the head when I hit the wall." An 11-year-old boy defined pain simply as "it hurts." His strongest pain was when he stepped on a nail; his weakest pain was when his sister punched him in the arm. On his diary, he listed "a broken blood vessel in my thumb, a twisted ankle, my hand collided with a dog's teeth, hit in head with stone, riding bike without shoes uphill, stubbed toe on rock while swimming, walking on gravel with bare feet, stone hitting my leg while I was mowing the lawn, and a burnt marshmallow fell on me." A 16-year-old boy described pain as "a feeling of hurt to an area of your body when tissue has been damaged and there are nerves. It ranges from sharp to dull, to strong to weak." His strongest pain occurred when he had pins removed from his hand; he listed a paper cut as his minimum pain experience. He experienced no pains during the month he kept the diary.

In contrast to the bumps, scrapes, burns, and dog bites recorded by these children on their pain diaries, the pain diary shown in Figure 1.1 lists predominantly vague body aches. This diary was completed by a 7-year-old girl who experienced recurrent stomachaches. She defined pain as "hurting and it doesn't feel that good, you wouldn't like it." Her most intense pain occurred when she had measles on her hand; her weakest pain occurred when her brother pinched her on the arm. As shown on her diary, only 1 of her 18 pains ("fall down") was related to a typical childhood complaint. She rated most of her pains as quite strong (the heavy pencil mark drawn on the right extreme of the visual analog scale). Clearly, her pain experiences were quite different from those of the children described previously. She may have reported more pains because she had learned to interpret a variety of somatic sensations as pain, or simply because she experienced a diverse variety of aches.

Although the language that they use, the ingenuity of their pain descriptions, and the quality and diversity of their pains are different, it is clear that all these children understand the concept of pain and the multidimensional nature of pain experiences. Naturally, their concepts differ according to their age, cognitive level, sex, and pain experience. They begin to understand pain through their own experiences, and they describe pain in the language that represents those experiences. Even if they lack the language, children can still communicate an accurate concept of pain. For example, a 5-year-old boy at first seemed unable to respond to the question "What is pain?" When prompted by "Imagine that you have a friend who has never felt pain; how would you tell him what it was like?" he thought for a moment and then quickly and eagerly responded, "I'd kick him in the leg."

Even very young children describe the emotional and suffering aspects of pain, as well as the physical aspects. Many children describe teasing as a painful experience. A 7-year-old girl reported "My dad was sick with cancer" as a painful event on her diary. A 6-year-old boy described his grandfather's death as his most

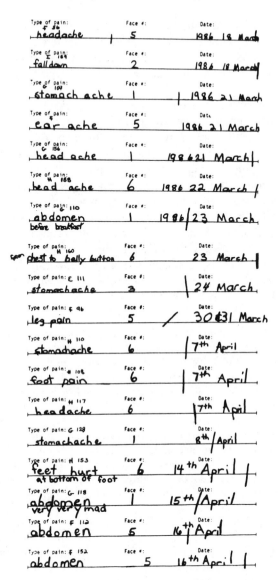

FIGURE 1.1. Pain diary completed by a 7-year-old girl with recurrent abdominal pains. She listed the type of all pains that she experienced during a 1-month period. She rated the strength of her pains on the visual analog scales; the left endpoints of the 160-mm lines represent no pain, while the right endpoints represent the strongest pain imaginable. The numerical values shown on the left are determined by measuring the length of the line from the left endpoint to her mark. She rated the unpleasantness of her pain by selecting a face from nine faces on an affective interval facial scale. The alphabetical letter denotes her face choice: face A is the most positive face and face I is the most negative. The faces were shown on a card in random order with number codes. The visual analog and affective interval facial scales are described in more detail in Chapter 2. From "The Enigma of Pain in Children: An Overview" by P. A. McGrath and L. M. Hillier, 1989, *Pediatrician*, 16, p. 8. Copyright 1989 by S. Karger. Reprinted by permission.

intense pain experience. As children mature, they are able to describe both the physical and emotional aspects of pain in more abstract terms with more sophisticated terminology, and they rely less on concrete analogies from their own lives. However, all children feel the physical and emotional aspects of pain when they first experience pain.

Almost every feeling person knows what pain is, and yet it is difficult to define pain precisely and comprehensively. In spite of the general sophistication of their vocabularies, even adults have difficulty in defining pain. Adults' descriptions convey their awareness of the diverse qualities of pain and an appreciation of its unpleasant aspects. But the major theme common to all their definitions is the same as that expressed by a young child: "Pain is what hurts." From both a scientific and an experiential view, the hurting aspect of pain may be the only salient feature that is common to an extremely wide variety of pain phenomena. A Subcommittee on Taxonomy was formed by the IASP to construct concise descriptions for different types of pain and to define the term "pain" (IASP, 1979). The definition for "pain" consists of a single sentence, followed by a lengthy note to elaborate and to clarify the diverse experiences encompassed by the term ("Classification of Chronic Pain," p. S217):

> Pain: An unpleasant sensory and emotional experience associated with actual or potential tissue damage, or described in terms of such damage.
>
> Note: Pain is always subjective. Each individual learns the application of the word through experiences related to injury in early life. Biologists recognize that those stimuli which cause pain are liable to damage tissue. Accordingly, pain is that experience which we associate with actual or potential tissue damage. It is unquestionably a sensation in a part or parts of the body, but it is also always unpleasant and therefore also an emotional experience. Experiences which resemble pain, e.g. pricking, but are not unpleasant should not be called pain. Unpleasant abnormal experiences (dysaesthesiae) may also be pain but are not necessarily so because, subjectively, they may not have the usual sensory qualities of pain.
>
> Many people report pain in the absence of tissue damage or any likely pathophysiological reasons; usually this happens for psychological reasons. There is usually no way to distinguish their experience from that due to tissue damage if we take the subjective report. If they regard their experience as pain and if they report it in the same ways as pain caused by tissue damage, it should be accepted as pain. This definition avoids tying the pain to the stimulus. Activity induced in the nociceptor and nociceptive pathways by a noxious stimulus is not pain, which is always a psychological state, even though we may well appreciate that pain most often has a proximate physical cause.

As is illustrated by the formal IASP definition, pain is a difficult sensation to describe in a simple and cohesive manner. It is a complex perception because many factors, such as expectations, beliefs, emotions, past experience, culture, familial history, and learning, can modify the strength or unpleasantness of pain. The same noxious stimulus may produce different pains for children or for the same child at different times. Figure 1.2 shows the strength of pain evoked by the same noxious stimulus (intramuscular injections) for two girls, both during and after the children participated in a pain management program to learn some techniques to reduce their pain (described in Chapters 6 and 7). Clearly, the pains children feel as the result of these injections are not simply and directly related to the amount of tissue damage.

What Types of Pain Do Children Experience?

Like adults, most children experience a wide variety of pains that differ in strength, quality, location, duration, and affective components. However, a few infants have been born without the ability to perceive pain—a condition described as "congenital insensitivity to pain." These children lack the warning signals that pain usually provides when they hurt themselves, the signals that motivate them to stop harmful

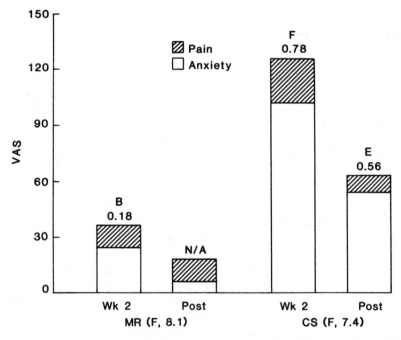

FIGURE 1.2. Pain intensity evoked by intramuscular injections of growth hormones for two children during the second week of their pain management program and postintervention. Each histogram represents the strength of pain (from baseline to top of hatched area) and preinjection anxiety (from baseline to top of open area) measured on visual analog scales (0–160 mm). The letters above the histograms indicate the faces selected by children to depict their affect; the numerical values below each letter denote the affective value (0 to 1, where 1 represents maximum distress).

activities. Without the protective warning signals of pain, children with congenital insensitivity to pain often sustain serious injuries when they are young. Common injuries include skin burns when they touch a hot surface, tongue lacerations when they bite their tongues while eating, and bone fractures during rough physical play. These children must learn to rely on their other senses to signal them about possible injury, such as to look for tissue damage rather than to feel it.

Merskey (1975) described two children with congenital pain insensitivity. A 2-year-old girl's foot became swollen after a callus developed around a fractured metatarsal bone. She had walked normally after the break without noticing the injury. The fracture was identified later only because of the swelling. Other injuries that she sustained were chewing the end of one finger; lacerating her tongue; fracturing her skull; and skinning the palmar surfaces of her hands raw while circling around on a climbing frame at school. After her initial examination, she became capable of experiencing some noxious stimuli as painful. It is not known what changed to enable her to begin to perceive pain. Another child did not report pain during injections or spankings. He hit his head many times, pulled fingernails until they bled, and did not complain about cuts and bruises unless attention was drawn to them. Yet when he was 5 years old he showed normal threshold and tolerance levels to noxious stimulation.

Scientists have studied individuals who are congenitally insensitive to pain, in order to identify any physiological abnormalities that underlie the selective absence of their pain sensation (Baxter & Olszewski, 1960). Some studies have shown that there is a selective loss of particular nerve fibers (presumably the "pain nerves") or that specific brain areas are destroyed, whereas other studies have reported no physical abnormalities. Consequently, it is not yet known which physiological mechanisms are responsible for congenital insensitivity to pain or whether the same mechanisms are responsible for all cases.

An inability to perceive pain afflicts only a few rare children. Instead, most children will experience a diverse array of pains from bruises, cuts, scrapes, broken bones, stomachaches, headaches, toothaches, burns, and injections. Some children will also experience pain produced by major injuries and accidents; pain after surgery; and pain associated with such diseases as arthritis, hemophilia, or cancer. In addition, children can develop referred pain (pain felt in one body region but originating from an injury in another body site), causalgia pains (intense pain sensations produced by normally nonpainful stimuli), and phantom limb pain (pain felt in a limb that has been amputated). In fact, the phantom sensations or pains that may develop for children after amputations are so real that children (and adults) can find it difficult to believe that an arm or leg has actually been removed. Figures 1.3 and 1.4 illustrate the phantom tingling and itching sensations experienced by a 15-year-old girl after her right leg was amputated above the knee. As shown, her phantom sensations were so vivid that she was easily able to describe their strength, quality, duration, and gradual spread from her toes to her stump.

Children's pain experiences can range from an inability to feel any pain, regardless of the intensity of the noxious stimulus, to the real perception of pain in a limb that is no longer there. The same mysterious pains, which are difficult to explain because the physical causes are not apparent, that afflict adults can also afflict children. Some neuralgias, medical conditions caused by inflammations of nerves, constitute special pain problems. Causalgia, a syndrome of burning pain that may develop after a traumatic nerve lesion, is a condition in which non-noxious stimuli (e.g. warmth and touch, rather than noxious heat or intense

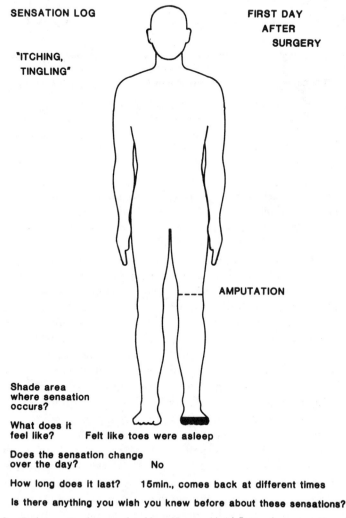

FIGURE 1.3.   Daily sensation log completed by a 15-year-old girl, Betty, after amputation of her right leg. She completed this record for 28 days after surgery to show how her phantom sensations changed. From "The Enigma of Pain in Children: An Overview" by P. A. McGrath and L. M. Hillier, 1989, *Pediatrician, 16*, p. 9. Copyright 1989 by S. Karger. Reprinted by permission.

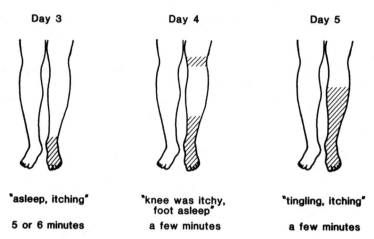

FIGURE 1.4. Temporal changes in the location, duration, and quality of phantom limb sensations after amputation. Betty completed a daily sensation log after her right leg was amputated above the knee.

pressure) can evoke severe pain. Although children experience fewer neuralgias and unusual pain problems than adults, they clearly can experience a wide variety of pains. Table 1.1 lists the common types of pain referrals made to the Pain Clinic at the Children's Hospital of Western Ontario.

All children's diverse pain experiences may be categorized generally as "acute," "chronic," or "recurrent" pains. Acute pain is produced by a well-defined noxious or tissue-damaging stimulus (e.g., an injection or a bee sting). Acute pain has a relatively short duration and usually provides an important biological warning signal that something is wrong. Most of the bumps and scrapes that children experience during their normal daily activities constitute different types of acute pain. Chronic pain is a persistent pain that is produced by a prolonged disease, such as arthritis, or an injury. Chronic pain may also be any pain that lasts beyond the usual time period required for healing or that persists without clear evidence of injury or tissue damage. Chronic pain often does not provide a warning signal, even when it is associated with an underlying disease process. Although chronic debilitating pain is a serious problem for adults, the incidence of chronic pain in children is generally low, particularly chronic pain that is not associated with a specific disease or injury. Instead, chronic-like recurrent pain syndromes are more common problems for children and adolescents. Recurrent pain syndromes are defined as frequently occurring episodes of headaches, abdominal pains, or limb pains in otherwise healthy and pain-free children. The episodes persist beyond a 3-month period and are not symptomatic of an underlying physical disease requiring medical treatment. Although these recurrent syndromes do not represent classic chronic pain states because of their episodic nature, they represent

TABLE 1.1. Types of Referrals to the Children's Pain Clinic

Acute pain
    Management of pain related to medical procedures
        Cancer treatments
        Diabetic blood-sampling and injections
        Growth hormone injections
        Surgical procedures
    Management of pain evoked by injury or disease
        Burns
        Phantom limb pain
Recurrent pain syndromes
    Assessment and management of recurrent
        Headaches
        Abdominal pain
        Limb pain
Chronic pain
    Management of pain associated with disease or injury
        Hemophilia
        Arthritis
        Neuralgia
        Accidents
    Management of pain associated with a psychological etiology
        Masked depression
        Conversion reaction syndrome

chronic conditions in which the primary concern of syndrome management is to decrease the frequency and intensity of painful episodes.

Acute Pain

Acute pain, produced by the tissue damage caused by a noxious stimulus, is the most common type of pain that infants and children experience. Although the strength of pain is generally proportional to the intensity of the noxious stimulus, the pain produced by an injury is modified by many factors in addition to the nature and extent of the wound. As described previously, children's pain perceptions are influenced by situational, emotional, and familial factors, so that even their perceptions of acute pain produced by a certain amount of tissue damage (e.g., an intramuscular injection) also depend on the situation in which they experience the noxious stimulus.

    In general, children experience two forms of acute pain: pain caused by accidents that occur during their normal activities, or pain caused by invasive procedures required during medical or dental treatments. These forms may be considered as special categories of acute pain because of the different situational and emotional factors unique to each context. Pain that occurs during children's daily lives in their play activities generally does not cause serious anxiety or fear, but is accepted as a normal part of their lives. Children perceive these acute pains more as the occasionally inevitable result of falls, sports, and rough play than as something to fear. Yet children can perceive the acute pains evoked during medical treatments quite differently. They often feel that they have no control in a medical or dental situation; they may be uncertain about what to expect; they may not understand the need for a treatment that will hurt, particularly if they do not feel sick; and they may not know any simple tools to use to help them cope with their anxiety and pain. In fact, a child may be told how to cope during a painful treatment in a manner that makes the procedure easier for the adult administering the treatment, but that does not necessarily make it better for the child.

These situational factors can lead to increased fear and anxiety for children, so that the same noxious stimulus can produce stronger levels of pain. A young girl who is anxious and afraid is shown during a finger prick in Figure 1.5. Her anxiety and distress may have contributed to her experiencing stronger pain during this procedure than is usually experienced by other children at the same age. Children's concepts of their illness, whether it is a potentially life-threatening condition such as cancer or a chronic but non-life-threatening disease, will also affect their perceptions of acute pain associated with their treatments. The anxiety a 5-year-old who has had diabetes for 2 years experiences when she pricks her finger for a blood sample is probably much less than the anxiety another 5-year-old experiences during the same procedure when she has relapsed with leukemia and her parents are overtly anxious about new test results. Although the noxious stimuli that cause tissue damage to evoke acute pain may be similar, the pains that children experience are not always the same.

The management of all acute pains in infants and children requires an evaluation of the context in which each pain occurs and of the pain's emotional effects on the child and family, not simply knowledge of the source of noxious stimulation. Relatively simple and straightforward principles of pain control can be used with children of all ages to reduce the acute pain evoked both by the normal injuries that they sustain and by the medical or dental treatments that they may require. However, the optimal control of children's acute pain must begin with a consideration of the pain in relation to the individual child experiencing it, and not only the source or type of noxious stimulus that initiates the pain. (The management of acute pain is presented in Chapter 7.)

Recurrent Pain Syndromes

Many children suffer from relatively unpredictable episodes of severe headaches, abdominal pains, or limb pains. In fact, approximately 30% of children and adolescents may experience recurrent headaches or abdominal pains. Several features are common to all recurrent pain syndromes: Children experience severely

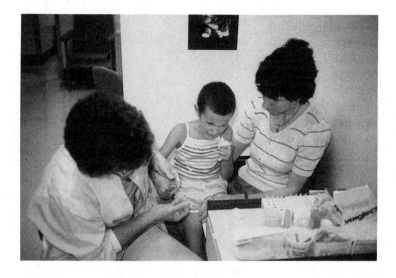

Are you now afraid (or anxious) about this procedure?   Yes ✓ No___

If yes, how much?

69
Not at all   Most afraid possible

How much did it hurt during the procedure?

94
Not at all   Very much

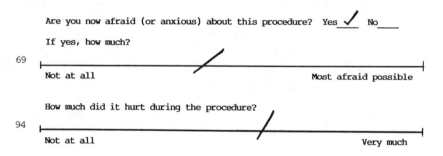

Which face looks like you felt deep down inside when you had the procedure?

FACE   G   =   .75

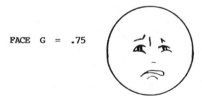

FIGURE 1.5.   A 7-year-old girl is shown immediately before receiving a finger prick. She rated her fear or anxiety before the procedure on a visual analog scale; she rated pain intensity and affect after the procedure using visual analog and affective interval facial scales. The numerical estimates of anxiety, pain strength, and affect are shown beside her marks.

painful episodes in the absence of a well-defined organic etiology; the pain episodes may be triggered by a variety of external and internal factors, particularly events that provoke stress; children are usually healthy and pain-free between episodes; and there is frequently a history of similar pain for one of the children's parents. The absence of a well-defined organic etiology in children who suffer recurrent pains does not necessarily indicate a psychological etiology, in the same manner that the initial inability to provide a logical physiological explanation for phantom limb pain did not indicate emotional disturbances in the individuals who suffered from phantom sensations.

At present, the specific etiology of recurrent pain syndrome is not known. Some confusion inevitably exists about the probable causes and treatments for the syndrome, because the syndrome is often evaluated by examining only the sensory aspects of children's pain (quality, intensity, frequency, location, duration). This may be quite misleading, since many children with a recurrent pain syndrome may have similar pain episodes (e.g., a 6-year-old girl may have migraine headaches that are qualitatively similar in pain symptomatology to those of an 8-year-old boy), but the causative factors for their headaches and therefore their optimal treatments may be quite different. A study of 200 children from 5 to 17 years old with recurrent headaches (described in detail in Chapters 6 and 8) indicates that many different situational, emotional, and familial factors can initiate recurrent pain episodes and that these factors cannot be identified by only examining sensory aspects of the headache pain symptomatology. Some factors are common to all children with recurrent headaches, but other factors are unique to particular children.

The incidence of children who continue to experience recurrent pain or who develop new pains has been estimated at 33% for abdominal pain (Apley, 1958, 1975; Apley, MacKeith, & Meadow, 1978; Barr, 1983b) and 40–60% for headaches (Bille, 1982; Jay & Tomasi, 1981). However, there have been few scientific studies on the incidence or prognosis of recurrent pain syndromes, so there is a lack of accurate, objective information about the true time course of these pain syndromes and about the efficacy of various methods of pain control for these children. Definitive longitudinal studies are needed to determine a realistic prognosis for children with recurrent pain syndromes, as a function of their age at pain onset, sex, the contributing situational or emotional factors, and the treatments they receive.

Clinical evidence suggests that the longer children endure relatively unpredictable episodes of severe pain, the more likely they are to develop emotional and psychological difficulties, particularly when they are unable to receive an age-appropriate explanation of the syndrome and some methods for coping with both the painful episodes and the factors that initiate the recurrent episodes. Also, children who have one type of recurrent pain when they are young often develop another type as they reach adolescence.

Many questions remain to be answered about the etiology and control of recurrent pains in childhood. A major question relates to the effects of the frequent painful episodes on children's development. How does the pain syndrome affect their pain perceptions and coping abilities as adults? Do a subset of the large group of children with recurrent pains become adults with debilitating chronic pains that are often resistant to effective treatment? If so, would it be possible to reduce the proportion of adults with chronic pain if these syndromes were identified and managed in childhood? Although definitive answers to these questions require further research, initial clinical studies indicate that effective pain management is possible for children with recurrent pains. However, the first step in the control of the syndrome is an objective and comprehensive assessment of the relevant situational, emotional, and familial factors associated with the syndrome, as well as an assessment of the sensory aspects of the painful episodes. The various techniques available for reducing the strength and frequency of painful headaches, abdominal pains and limb pains are presented in Chapter 8, along with a review of the probable causative factors.

Chronic Pain

Chronic pain, in which pain persists beyond the usual time course for healing an injury or persists in the absence of an obvious injury, is a major health problem for adults. Although children may experience less chronic pain than adults, they can develop many of the same chronic pains. Children and adolescents may experience chronic pain that is evoked by an injury or by disease. In addition, children may develop chronic pain that is evoked primarily by psychological factors.

The most common chronic pains for children are those associated with disease, such as arthritis, hemophilia, and sickle cell anemia. Unlike adults, the vast majority of children with cancer do not experience chronic pain. Most adult cancers are solid tumors, whereas most pediatric cancers are acute leukemias. Leukemias and lymphomas are not extremely painful diseases for children, although they can produce joint aches during periods of active disease. (Cancer pain, however, is discussed with other types of childhood chronic pain in Chapter 9.) Juvenile rheumatoid arthritis is the most prevalent of the arthritic diseases in children. There is no medical cure for the disease; the goals of treatment are the preservation of joint function and the control of pain. Children with hemophilia, a congenital hereditary disorder of blood coagulation, suffer from recurrent unpredictable internal hemorrhaging. Repeated bleeding into the joint areas can cause degenerative hemophilic arthropathy and chronic arthritic pain. Children with sickle cell anemia may develop painful sickling crises from vasoconstriction, which impairs oxygenation of the blood. Crises may last from several days to several weeks.

Children with nerve damage may develop painful conditions that persist beyond the apparent healing time of their injuries. Children who have been in accidents or have suffered serious infections may experience recurrent painful episodes or develop constant pains. Children who sustain serious burns will experience acute pain during burn treatments and experience prolonged pain as their skin heals.

Children can develop a variety of disease- and injury-related chronic pains. The management of chronic pains associated with disease or injury begins with an understanding of the source of tissue damage, but must include an understanding of children's perceptions of their illness and the relevant factors that can intensify their pain. These factors will necessarily differ in each case, in relation to the type of disease and the child's and family's response to the diagnosis and prognosis. Reliance on information about the psychological, situational, and emotional factors that exist for a particular child, rather than sole reliance on the nature and severity of the phsyical disorder, is important for the provision of comprehensive pain control.

Children may also develop chronic pain as a consequence of psychological factors, such as anxiety or depression. In essence, their pain may become the somatic expression of their emotional distress. Usually these children are unable to identify their true emotional reactions to events, but attempt to accept disappointments or frustrations without allowing themselves to feel hurt, frustrated, or sad. They keep their emotions "bottled up" while they present an apparently calm disposition to the world. Their emotions surface in the form of a pain complaint, as more stress affects them and they are unable to cope with it. Often children's failure to recognize true stress-inducing situations (school, peers, family) means that it is not possible for them to respond appropriately in these situations to reduce the stress. Their attempts to deny the stress associated with common childhood situations prevents them from learning how to resolve conflicts and solve problems effectively, so that each new conflict or problem adds progressively to their underlying anxiety. The pain that they develop as a result of their anxiety is real, not imagined, and helps to remove them from the situation or source of anxiety. The pain can eventually become a method for coping with stress because it temporarily removes these children from an aversive situation, and perhaps provides emotional support through the attention of parents, teachers, and friends.

Children can develop additional chronic pain from their anxiety about a disease. Some referrals to our pain clinic have included children who begin to develop various pains that are seemingly unrelated to their illness. For example, a 6-year-old girl who required regular growth hormone injections complained of a constant ache throughout her body. Pain assessment indicated that her ache was related to her concerns about being small, despite the injections she regularly received, rather than to her condition per se. After a brief period of counseling about her condition to provide her with more accurate expectations about the results of treatment, her aches disappeared. Children with chronic pain associated with a disease can also experience increases in their pain because of fears about the possibility of dying, anxiety about necessary treatments, or frustrations about living their lives differently from other children. These factors can exacerbate the pain accompanying their disorder. Also, the anxiety that children may perceive in their parents' reactions to their disorder can cause them to feel guilty, upset, and frustrated, so that the pain increases or becomes more unpleasant for them.

Summary

Children do suffer from chronic pain, both pain associated with disease and injury and pain associated with psychological factors. However, their perceptions of chronic pain, like their perceptions of acute and recurrent pain, are not simply and directly related to the extent of their physical injuries or to the severity of their diseases. Children perceive pain in relationship to a certain context. The context is defined by their frame of reference—that is, their age and cognitive level; their previous pain experience against which they evaluate each new pain; the significance of the pain-producing stimulus or disease to their lives; their expectations for obtaining eventual pain relief; and their ability to control the pain by themselves. Children's emotional responses to pain are also not determined solely by the intensity or quality of the noxious stimulus, but are determined by the context in which they experience that pain. Several emotions, such as anger, fear, frustration, depression, or anxiety, may result from the same pain experienced in different contexts. Certain emotions, such as fear or anxiety regarding the outcome of an amputation to prevent metastases of a tumor, may subsequently alter children's perceptions so that any pain after amputation is exacerbated. Consequently, it is essential to evaluate the contextual factors and emotional responses that may modify pain in children.

In summary, children experience many different acute, chronic, and recurrent pains. However, their pain experiences have not been well studied, so that many questions remain unanswered. Descriptive studies on the incidence and prevalence of different types of pains in infants and children have often consisted of retrospective surveys, in which information is inferred from medical charts, rather than prospective surveys using objective criteria for describing and measuring pain. As yet, the true extent to which children experience different types of acute pains; recurrent headaches, abdominal pains, or limb pains; and chronic pains related to disease, injury, or psychological factors is not known.

Factors That Modify Children's Pain Perceptions and Behaviors

Children can experience pain without injury or apparent injury, and they can sustain injury without experiencing pain. Although pain is often initiated by tissue damage caused by a noxious stimulus, the consequent pain is neither simply nor directly related to the amount of tissue damage. As described previously, the pain produced by a relatively constant noxious stimulus can be different for children, depending on their expectations, their perceived control, and the significance that they attach to the painful procedure. In fact, the same child may feel quantitatively different pains when the same noxious stimulus is experienced in different situations. A noxious stimulus is described in terms of its physical attributes: quality, the type of stimulus (thermal, electrical, mechanical, chemical), intensity, location, and duration of application. Differences in these attributes will naturally produce differences in the nature and extent of tissue damage, and presumably some corresponding differences in the quality, strength, location, and duration of pain. However, the final pain that children experience is not solely related to the physical attributes of the noxious stimulus. The pain depends on the noxious stimulus in relation to the child experiencing it (sex, age, cognitive level, family, culture, previous pain experience, and emotions) and the situation in which it is experienced.

The effect that the situation in which a noxious stimulus is experienced can have on a child's pain is illustrated in Figure 1.6, in which the impact of the visual background on the perceived brightness of two identical visual stimuli is shown. Two grey circles are surrounded by different backgrounds, a black one and a lighter grey one. Although the inner grey circles are the same physical intensity, the circle on the left is perceived as lighter than the one on the right. The two greys look different because our eyes see the brightness of the inner circles in relation to the context in which they are presented. The inner circles and their backgrounds together represent the visual stimulus, not simply the two inner circles in isolation. Similarly, a noxious stimulus is not experienced in isolation, but is experienced by an individual in a particular context. If the inner circles represent a noxious stimulus, it is simple to visualize the dramatic difference in intensity that can be produced by merely changing the context or background. Although the nociceptive system does not parallel the visual system with respect to how contextual factors may alter pain intensity, the net effect is the same. The same noxious stimulus can produce different pains, depending on the context in which it is administered.

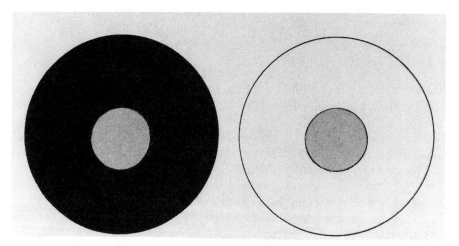

FIGURE 1.6. Concentric circles illustrate brightness contrast. The two inner circles are the same shade of grey, but are perceived differently because of the contrasting backgrounds. The circle on the left is perceived as brighter.

Much research has been conducted to identify the critical features of the background for human pain perceptions—the diverse factors that modify these perceptions (Barrell & Price, 1975, 1977; Beecher, 1956, 1959; Boehncke, 1970; Collins, 1965; Craig, 1980, 1984; Dworkin, Chen, Schubert, & Clark, 1984; Dworkin, Schubert, Chen, & Clark, 1986; Hilgard, 1969; Johnson, Dabbs, & Leventhal, 1970; Johnson, Leventhal, & Dabbs, 1971; Lewis, 1942; Melzack, 1961, 1973, 1976; Merskey, 1968; Price 1984b; Thompson, 1981; von Graffenried, Adler, Abt, Nuesch, & Spiegel, 1978; Weisenberg, 1977, 1984; Weisenberg & Tursky, 1976; Zborowski, 1962). The model shown in Figure 1.7 depicts the factors that influence children's pain perceptions. The pain sensation produced by a noxious stimulus depends not only on the tissue damage produced by the stimulus, but also on many situational and emotional factors, as well as on a child's age, sex, cognitive level, family, pain history, learning, and culture. In designing programs for managing pain in infants and children, it is essential to recognize the role of developmental, familial, situational, and emotional factors in determining their pains. Several factors must be investigated in order to provide optimal management for any type of pain that children experience. Although the causal relationship between an injury and a consequent pain sensation seems direct and obvious, the pain from even such a cause is modified by a variety of factors.

Developmental Factors

The assessment and management of pain in children are complicated by a lack of information about possible developmental differences in their ability to perceive pain, their ability to understand pain, their ability to communicate meaningful information about their pain experiences, their ability to cope during a painful situation, and their behavioral responses to pain.

Age and the Ability to Perceive Pain

Many health professionals disagree about the age at which infants are able to perceive pain. Some assume that neonates (infants younger than a month) and infants are relatively insensitive to pain, whereas others believe that pain sensitivity is present at birth. The lack of agreement about when infants perceive pain has led to some inconsistency in prescribing and administering medications for pain relief to infants. Clinical surveys indicate that neonates and infants may receive invasive procedures without analgesia or may have surgery without anesthesia or postoperative analgesics. In 1976, Poznanski reported that many anesthesiologists did not use general anesthesia for children until they were about 3 months of age. More recently, Purcell-Jones, Dorman, and Sumner (1988) surveyed the attitudes and practices of pediatric anesthetists in regard to infants' pain. Although most anesthetists believed that even neonates feel pain, they were generally reluctant to

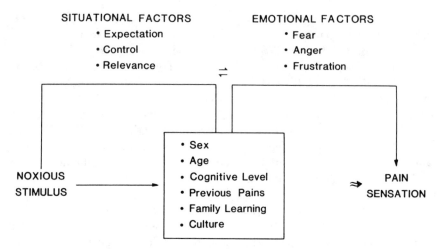

SITUATIONAL FACTORS
- Expectation
- Control
- Relevance

EMOTIONAL FACTORS
- Fear
- Anger
- Frustration

NOXIOUS STIMULUS

- Sex
- Age
- Cognitive Level
- Previous Pains
- Family Learning
- Culture

PAIN SENSATION

FIGURE 1.7. A model depicting the factors that modify children's pain perceptions. Pain produced by a noxious stimulus depends on relevant situational and emotional factors, which are influenced by a child's sex, age, cognitive level, previous pain experience, learning, and culture.

prescribe analgesics. Opioid analgesics were seldom administered to infants younger than 3 months, whereas these analgesics were administered to older infants.

The reluctance to administer analgesics or anesthetics to neonates and infants is presumably based on an assumption that pain sensitivity is not fully present at birth because of infants' immature nervous systems. Although cortical development is not complete at birth and pain sensitivity may be reduced in immature nerve pathways, clinical studies indicate that neonates and infants do experience pain. In fact, most people who observe infants during blood-sampling procedures or during unanesthetized circumcisions are convinced that they feel pain. Poznanski (1976) described how neonates react by crying, screaming, and overt body movements when the foreskin is clamped during circumcisions. Apley (1976) reported that infants with meningitis cry shrilly but then stop suddenly, presumably because crying increases the cranial pressure and produces severe pain in the head. Similarly, Dunn and Jannetta (1973) noted that neonates with hydrocephalus exhibit gross irritability, probably because of their pain, and that this irritability is reduced by proper shunting that reduces intracranial pressure. Infants who receive dorsal penile blocks show less behavioral and physiological distress than infants circumcised without anesthetic (Williamson & Williamson, 1983). Both clinical observations and objective assessments of infants' behavioral responses, crying, and physiological changes indicate that neonates experience pain. (The measures for assessing pain in infants are described in Chapter 2.) Fortunately, a dramatic and pervasive commitment to alleviating infants' pain is now occurring throughout health care systems (American Academy of Pediatrics, Committee on Fetus and Newborn, 1987; D'Apolito, 1984; Downes & Betts, 1977; Gottfried & Gaiter, 1985; Hain & Mason, 1986). More information on infant pain management is presented in Chapters 4, 6, and 7.

Several studies of infants' and young children's behavioral responses to painful stimuli have led to a general understanding of their distress behaviors. Infants' reactions to a noxious stimulus change as they develop, from a general body distress response to a more specific response localized to the site of stimulation. Toddlers communicate pain nonverbally by clenching their lips, rocking, rubbing, opening their eyes widely, and showing agitated or aggressive behaviors (e.g., kicking, hitting, or biting) (Gildea & Quirk, 1977). Hospitalized toddlers may hide under the bed or covers or run away at the sight of an approaching nurse or physician with a syringe. As children mature, they develop a wider variety of verbal and nonverbal behaviors to respond to pain. Although children are able to perceive pain at birth, the nature of their responses and their abilities to communicate pain perceptions caused by a noxious stimulus clearly depend on their age.

Laboratory and clinical studies have been conducted to evaluate how children's actual pain perceptions may change as they mature. In the laboratory research, pain is induced experimentally by applying controlled levels of pressure, heat, or electrical stimulation and determining the minimal level of noxious stimulation at which children first report pain ("pain threshold") or the maximal level of noxious stimulation that they are willing to tolerate ("tolerance threshold" or "pain tolerance"). Clinical research examines how a child's responses in a more naturally occurring pain situation may vary according to the child's age.

Many laboratory studies have reported that thresholds to noxious stimuli increase with age, indicating that pain sensitivity decreases with age (Chapman & Jones, 1944; Hall & Stride, 1954; Haslam, 1969; Schludermann & Zubek, 1962; Sherman & Robillard, 1960; Wolff & Jarvik, 1965). The various noxious stimuli that were used in these studies included: heat applied to the skin, a balloon distended in the lower esophagus, pressure applied to the tibia, pressure applied to the styloid process, and a grater apparatus applied steadily to the forearm. Yet similar studies of pain thresholds in adults and children have reported that there are no age-related differences (Hardy, Wolff, & Goodell, 1952; Sherman, 1943). It is difficult to interpret the results of many threshold studies that have been conducted to investigate the effects of age on pain perception, because although they have focused on chronological age, they have ignored the powerful contribution of learning and previous experience on children's pain perceptions.

Investigations of pain thresholds alone, whether for mechanical, electrical, thermal, or chemical stimuli, can provide only partial information about the effects of age on pain perception. Thresholds for reporting pain represent children's criteria for labeling a stimulus as painful or nonpainful. Their thresholds do not provide information about the strength or unpleasantness of their pain sensations. Since thresholds are defined as the minimal amount of stimulation that can evoke pain, pain at threshold is assumed to be felt as mild or weak. While this assumption is true for adults, it has not been examined for children. Children may rate a steadily increasing and unfamiliar noxious stimulus as painful more quickly than adults because they are afraid of the unusual sensation, because the sensation is stronger, or simply because their previous pain experience is quite limited. A young child who has limited pain experience may be more likely to label a strong sensation as painful, even when the experience is identical to that of an older child or an adult, who may report that it is a strong but nonpainful sensation.

Children's criteria for interpreting pain from their sensations evolve as they develop. Children may not experience noxious stimuli any differently because of their age per se. Rather, they may experience different pains because of differences in their understanding of the noxious stimuli, the diversity and intensity of their previous pains, and their attitudes and expectations. None of the threshold studies have controlled for the effects of these important variables. In order to elucidate the nature of the perceptual differences in pain that may occur with age, it is necessary to match children of different ages according to their cognitive level, previous pain experience, and relevant familial, situational, and emotional factors.

Clearly, differences in children's pain experiences, pain expressions, and pain behaviors exist (Barr, 1983a, 1983b; Beyer & Byers, 1985; Craig, Grunau, & Branson, 1988; Flannery, Sos, & McGovern, 1981; Frodi & Lamb, 1978; Gelfand, 1963; Jerrett, 1985; Jerrett & Evans, 1986; McGrath & Hillier, 1989; Merskey, 1970; Notermans & Tophoff, 1967; Richards, Bernal, & Brackbill, 1976; Ross & Ross, 1982, 1988; Woodrow, Friedman, Siegelaub, & Collen, 1972). However, such differences are probably related more to developmental–experiential differences than simply to age differences. Although there are general age-related differences in children's behavioral responses to pain, there is no clear information available as to whether there are specific age-related differences in children's sensitivity to pain.

Cognitive Level

The ability to understand the sensation that is triggered by tissue damage is related to a child's level of cognitive or intellectual development. Consequently, children's cognitive levels may be more indicative of their perception, expression, and behavioral responses to pain than their actual chronological ages may be. Piaget's sequence of cognitive levels through which children acquire information about the world and eventually develop logical thinking (Piaget & Inhelder, 1969) provides an appropriate framework for describing children's concepts about illness (Bibace & Walsh, 1979; Caradang, Folkins, Hines, & Steward, 1979; Kalnins & Love, 1982; Perrin & Gerrity, 1981) and may provide a framework for describing children's concepts about pain (Gaffney, 1988; Gaffney & Dunne, 1986, 1987). According to Piagetian theory, children progress from a "sensorimotor" level of cognitive development (birth to 2 years) to a "preoperational" level (ages 2–7) to a level of "concrete operations" (ages 8–10) and then to a level of "early formal operations" (ages 11–14) (Flavell, 1963; Piaget & Inhelder, 1969).

During the sensorimotor level of cognitive development, infants and toddlers become gradually aware of the environment through sensory exploration. Infants are active and seek contact with their environment. During the preoperational period, children are not able to distance themselves from their environment. Their explanations for illness consist of a simple cause-and-effect relationship, based on the specific spatial and temporal cues in children's environments. The major developmental shift into the concrete operational period occurs when children begin to differentiate between themselves and others. Children begin to distinguish their internal from their external states and to distinguish between the cause of illness and its effects. The cause is viewed as a person, object, or action that is external to the child and that has an aspect or quality that is bad or harmful to the body. The final stage of cognitive development is the formal operational stage, during which children begin to think about and understand the world in more abstract terms. Children may attribute illness to physiological or psychological causes. Since effective alleviation of children's pain requires an understanding of how they perceive pain, it is important to evaluate their developmental level to provide an appropriate course of therapy or pain management.

Several developmental trends have been reported in studies on children's ideas and beliefs about pain (Gaffney & Dunne, 1986; Jeans & Gordon, 1981; Schultz, 1971). Schultz (1971) reported that younger children were more likely to attribute color and shape to different types of pain than older children. Jeans and Gordon (1981) reported a definite development trend in their analysis of pain drawings and interviews conducted with 54 children from 5 to 13 years old. Children's concepts of pain changed from a primarily physical understanding to a more abstract understanding, comprised of both physical and psychological aspects.

Lollar, Smits, and Patterson (1982) interviewed 240 children and adolescents from 4 to 19 years old, in order to evaluate their pain perceptions and their beliefs about causes and coping strategies for pain. Children rated the pains depicted in 24 pictures that included familiar usual pain experiences and medical pain experiences. They compared the children's responses in the pictures according to the level of their own pain experiences. Children with little pain experience rated all situations as more painful than children with extensive pain experience. Savedra, Gibbons, Tesler, Ward, and Wegner (1982) interviewed 214 children aged from 9 to 12 about their attitudes about pain. Children's responses did not differ according to their age, but children who were hospitalized described pain differently. Hospitalized children listed causes of pain that were related to illness and medical procedures more often than did nonhospitalized children. Boys differed from girls in their selection of words to describe pain and in their emotional response to pain. As an example, significantly more girls chose the words "sad" and "miserable" to describe pain than boys. Similarly, significantly more girls felt "sick to my stomach," "like crying," "embarrassed," and "nervous" when they had pain than boys. Only 34% of the sample recognized the positive significance of pain as a warning signal that something was wrong. Although developmental differences were not shown in the analysis of children's responses, they may not have been detected simply because of the relatively restricted age sample in the study.

Ross and Ross (1984a) interviewed 994 children from 5 to 12 years old about their specific pain experiences, pain language, reactions to pain, and coping strategies. They asked open-ended questions to determine the extent of children's knowledge and understanding of pain. The majority of pain definitions were unidimensional, with 80.9% of the sample emphasizing general discomfort and 12.2% emphasizing specific pain events. Children attributed pains to specific causes such as accidents, environmental factors, illness, surgery, and aggressive actions of others. There was rarely evidence that children attributed pain as a punishment. Fewer than 5% of the children knew about the "warning signal" aspect of pain, and fewer than 20% used any type of self-initiated cognitive coping strategies. Some maladaptive pain behavior was evident in the sample. Approximately 20% of children indicated that they had used pain complaints to avoid school or other responsibilities, or to earn special attention, at least once; another 15.7% of children reported that they had used pain for these secondary gains more than once. Although children were able to clearly communicate their understanding of pain, their responses were not consistently related to their sex or age.

Gaffney (1984) interviewed 600 Irish school children from 5 to 14 years of age about their understanding of pain. She asked them to complete 10 statements:

- Pain is _____ .
- A person gets pain because _____ .
- A pain sometimes is _____ .
- A pain can make you _____ .
- The worst thing about pain is _____ .
- When I have pain _____ makes me feel better.
- A pain can feel like _____ .
- I had a pain in _____ .
- People who get pains are _____ .
- You can get pains in _____ .

Gaffney was investigating children's definitions of pain and their ideas about the causes, consequences, possible cures, and the specific locations of pain. According to Piaget's theory of cognitive development, the responses of younger children (those aged 5, 6 and 7, in the preoperational stage of cognitive development) should be perceptually dominated and very concrete. Responses for progressively older children should shift from perceptual to conceptual functioning, showing an increasing abstraction as children develop an awareness of the psychological and emotional concomitants of pain.

Children's responses were analyzed for three age groups: 5–7, 8–10, and 11–14, corresponding to the preoperational, concrete operational, and early formal operational levels of cognitive development, respectively. Gaffney and Dunne (1986) classified three types of definitions in the children's responses; these are listed in

TABLE 1.2.   Children's Definitions of Pain

Definition 1: Concrete definitions. Pain is "a thing," "something," "it"; pain is defined by a location in the body or by its unpleasant physical properties; something that hurts, or the association with illness or trauma.

Definition 2: Semiabstract definitions. Pain is described in terms of feeling or sensation, without specific elaboration to a body part. Pain is not a thing that hurts, but is a hurting feeling or sensation. Children use synonyms to describe qualities of pain, such as "ache" or "cramp," or describe pain associated with sickness.

Definition 3: Abstract definitions. Pain is described in physiological, psychological, or psychophysiological terms. Children refer to the physiological substrate or purpose of pain—pain as damage that sets off nerves. Pain is also emotional, such as worry, anxiety, or depression.

Note. Summarized from Gaffney and Dunne (1986, p. 109).

Table 1.2. Children's use of concrete definitions of pain gradually decreased with age, whereas semiabstract and abstract definitions increased with age, as shown in Table 1.3. Similarly, the number of different themes used by children to define pain increased with age, as shown in Figure 1.8. As an example, 5-year-old boys used seven themes in their definitions of pain: location in stomach (or a synonym); unpleasant physical qualities; aversive nature; direct identification with sickness; mention of other body parts as locations; association with eating; or association with transgression. Boys used a total of 38 themes in their definitions of pain, and girls used a total of 36 themes.

TABLE 1.3.   Results of a Chi-Square Analysis for Significant Differences between Age Groups in the Use of Category Variables

Category variable	χ^2 ($df = 2$)								p		
Def. 1: Concrete	64.33								$< .0001$		
Def. 2: Semiabstract	44.97								$< .0001$		
Def. 3: Abstract	82.13								$< .0001$		
Theme	CA = 5	6	7	8	9	10	11	12	13	14
Psychophysiological							———————			
Physiological							————————————			
Psychological					———————————————————					
Semiabstract, feeling			———————————————————————							
Concrete, unpleasant physical		———————————————————————————————————								—
Concrete, in tummy		———————————								

Note. CA, chronological age. From "Developmental Aspects of Children's Definitions of Pain" by A. Gaffney and E. A. Dunne, 1986, *Pain, 26*, p. 110. Copyright 1986 by Elsevier Science Publishers. Reprinted by permission.

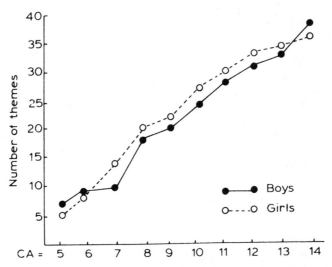

FIGURE 1.8. The increase with age in the repertoire of themes used by children in their pain definitions. From "Developmental Aspects of Children's Definitions of Pain" by A. Gaffney and E. A. Dunne, 1986, *Pain, 26*, p. 110. Copyright 1986 by Elsevier Science Publishers.

The appearance of new themes in children's data reflected an increasing understanding of the biological purpose of pain and its causal relationship with illness and trauma, as well as a developing awareness of the more abstract psychological and psychosocial aspects of pain. Younger children had a more passive perspective about pain, which gradually shifted with age to a perspective that included a degree of perceived control. The pattern of children's responses showed significant differences among the three age groups, supporting Gaffney's hypothesis that the acquisition of a concept of pain follows a developmental sequence, congruent with Piaget's theory of cognitive development. Children's definitions shifted from concrete, perceptually dominated perspectives in the younger children to more abstract, generalized, and psychologically oriented views for older children.

The responses of children at the preoperational level were characterized by a tendency to focus on perceptually dominant features and to connect events without understanding or describing the relationships between them. As children began to conceptualize pain in a more generalized and less passive way, they used analogies to describe pain and provided more vivid qualitative descriptions. Children developed an awareness of the psychological aspects of pain. Responses such as "Pain is something that hurts you; you feel miserable and unhappy and you start crying" were characteristic of children at the concrete operational level. During the formal operational period, children became introspective and began to think about the purely abstract in terms of their conceptualizations of pain. They defined pain as having both physical and psychological components. They also began to recognize pain as a biological warning signal. The pattern of understanding pain observed for these school children in Ireland parallels the developmental pattern observed in our preliminary analysis of responses from 300 Canadian school children (current developmental study described earlier). The Canadian sample consists of both healthy children and children with various pain problems. Children's responses will be analyzed with the methodology used by Gaffney and Dunne to provide a cross-cultural comparison of the development of children's concepts of pain.

Previous studies that have not reported definite developmental patterns do not necessarily contradict this recent research. Gaffney and Dunne (1986) cite two methodological differences between their study and earlier studies. First, children were grouped by cognitive age (roughly indicated by age and grade in school); second, a higher age ceiling of 14 years (compared to 12) was used, which allowed the responses of children at the formal operational level to become evident. The authors also used a coding system that included multiple responses. In this way, they could demonstrate that all children may respond "Pain is something that hurts," but could also demonstrate that some children, who were at a higher cognitive level, could use more sophisticated themes and responses in addition to the basic "hurting" one.

Children's level of cognitive development determines how they are able to understand pain, which has an important effect on how they perceive pain. The recognition that children's concepts of pain follow a developmental pattern provides a framework not only for evaluating their understanding of pain, but also for designing interventions to reduce their pain. The methods that are available to assist children with painful diseases or procedures must be selected according to the children's ability to understand and use them. Toddlers, who are in the preoperational stage of cognitive development, may perceive and respond to painful situations with much more fear than is seen in younger infants or older children (Jeans, 1983a). Younger children are less able to understand the significance of the pain (e.g., the rationale for invasive medical procedures), or they may be less able to develop or to consistently use pain-coping strategies. Hypnotic suggestions, desensitization, visual imagery, and behavioral management programs may be more effective pain interventions for younger children, whereas cognitive coping strategies should be more effective for older children. (These techniques are described in Chapters 5 and 6; the applications of these techniques to different childhood pain problems are described in Chapters 7, 8, and 9.)

Katz, Kellerman, and Siegel (1980) and Jay, Ozolins, Elliott, and Caldwell (1983) provide further evidence for the importance of cognitive development in children's reactions to pain. They have shown that younger children exhibit more behavioral distress during invasive medical procedures than older children. Overt distress behaviors (e.g., crying, flailing, withdrawal) decreased dramatically when children were approximately 7 years old—an age that corresponds in Piagetian theory to the typical onset of concrete operational thinking. The increased sophistication in children's thinking at this point allows them to acquire a more logical and realistic understanding of the need for performing medical procedures. An accurate understanding of the noxious stimulus alters the relevance of the situation for a child and reduces anxiety and fear, with the result that the procedures will produce less distress and pain.

Previous Pain Experience

The nature and diversity of children's pain experiences provides the basis by which they learn about all aspects of pain: its sensory qualities, its emotional effects, its significance, and methods of reducing pain. They interpret each new pain according to a frame of reference defined by the number and variety of pains that they have already encountered. As children mature, they generally experience a wider variety of pains that differ in quality, intensity, location, duration, and unpleasantness. They also learn new methods for coping with their pains, and gradually develop a repertoire of strategies to alleviate different types of pain. Consequently, they evaluate the strength and unpleasantness of any new pains in reference to an ever-changing background of their previous pains. Thus, common pains related to mild tissue damage, such as bruises, cuts, or scrapes, may be rated as less strong or less unpleasant as children develop. In fact, our preliminary analysis of the pain diaries of 54 healthy children suggests that the strength and unpleasantness of children's normal pain experiences decrease with age, as shown in Table 1.4. However, children at the same chronological age or cognitive level who differ extensively in pain experience may perceive certain pains differently. As an exam-

TABLE 1.4. Mean Number, Pain Intensity, and Pain Affect for All Pains Reported on Pain Diary

Group	Number of pains		Pain intensity		Pain affect	
All ($n = 54$)	4.9	(4)	77.7	(30)	.79	(.1)
Girls ($n = 33$)	5.7	(5)	74.4	(34)	.78	(.1)
Boys ($n = 21$)	3.9	(3)	82.8	(25)	.81	(.1)
< 8 yr ($n = 16$)	4.0	(4)	88.9	(26)	.84	(.1)*
> 8 yr ($n = 38$)	5.3	(4)	73.0	(31)	.77	(.1)*
< 6.5 yr ($n = 8$)	3.2	(2)	97.4	(29)	.85	(.1)
6.6–8.5 yr ($n = 10$)	4.3	(4)	84.9	(22)	.78	(.1)
8.6–12.5 yr ($n = 23$)	5.4	(4)	75.8	(32)	.78	(.1)
> 12.6 yr ($n = 13$)	5.4	(4)	63.2	(29)	.73	(.1)

Note. Pain intensity was rated on a visual analog scale, with endpoints of 0 and 160 mm; pain affect was rated on an affective interval facial scale, with endpoints of 0 and 1 (1 = "saddest feeling possible"). Numbers in parentheses are standard deviations.
   * $p < .05$.

ple, children who have routinely experienced many intramuscular injections may perceive these injections as less painful than children who have only experienced a few medical procedures.

Children's frames of reference for evaluating their pains change as they mature and experience new pains that vary in quality, intensity, and affect. Table 1.5 lists the most frequent responses to the questions "What is the least and most pain that you have experienced?" for 142 healthy children. As shown, the diversity of responses changes with children's ages. The age at which children experience an intense physical or emotional pain will influence their perceptions of pain produced by more common and less severe injuries. Table 1.6 lists samples of the maximum and minimum pains that children have experienced. Forty-four children were interviewed again 2 years after their initial assessment; only 30% reported the same "strongest" pain. As shown by some of their answers in the top portion of Table 1.6, the children whose maximum pains remained the same were those whose pain had been related to serious injury and only rarely to a common occurrence, such as a headache. More often, children's maximum pains changed to pains associated with more serious physical injuries, as shown in the bottom portion of Table 1.6. The effects of age, cognitive level, and previous experience interact with children's emotional response to a painful stimulus, so that their perception or behavioral response to pain cannot be determined by a consideration of only one of these factors.

Familial and Cultural Factors

Although hereditary factors are responsible for the development of certain painful diseases in childhood or for familial predispositions to various physical conditions, the role of families in influencing children's pain perceptions is not limited solely to genetic factors. Instead, family members' responses to children when they experience pain inevitably affects the nature of the children's pain expressions, their pain perceptions, and perhaps the type of pains that they will experience. In

TABLE 1.5. Modal Responses to Maximum and Minimum Pain Experiences

Age	Maximum	Minimum
< 6.5 yr (n = 16)	Finger pinched in door; fall on hard surface	Finger prick; scraped knee
6.6–9.5 yr (n = 45)	Fall off bike; fall down stairs; needle; injection; intravenous procedure	Bruise; pinch; scraped knee
9.6–12.5 (n = 37)	Needles; injections, broken or sprained limb; headache	Bruise; scraped knee; needles
> 12.6 yr (n = 44)	Injury from major fall or accident; broken or sprained limb; needles; headache	Bruise; scratch or scrape; finger prick; light punch or injury

TABLE 1.6. Children's Maximum and Minimum Pain Experiences at Initial Interview and 2 Years Later

Child	Sex	Age	Maximum	Minimum
			Children whose maximum pains remained the same	
J. I.	F	4.9	Cracked head	Hurt knee
		6.9	Cracking my head	Cut finger
J. D.	F	8.8	Appendix operation	Bruise
		10.7	Appendix operation	Broke toe
L. K.	F	9.5	Cut chin open	Bruise
		11.5	Cracked chin	Burned hand
R. C.	F	11.6	Migraine headaches	Finger prick
		13.7	Migraine headache	Hangnail
I. O.	F	11.8	Broke wrist	Bruise
		13.8	Broke my wrist	Hit on nose
D. C.	F	14.7	Breaking head open	Gerbil bite, getting teased
		15.9	Breaking my head open	Ripping finger nail
J. M.	M	7.4	Stitches on my face	Door hit foot
		9.5	Head cut open	Stitches in my ankle
D. L.	M	8.2	Falling off bike on knee	Drop book on foot
		10.4	Fell off bike on knee	Hit in stomach
			Children whose maximum pains changed	
Q. V.	F	4.4	Scraped knee	Tummyache
		6.2	Fell off bike, knee bled	Fell down, little scab
J. O.	F	10.0	Saw mom in hospital with tubes	When I get tickled I get stomachache
		12.0	Big headaches	A mosquito
F. F.	F	12.8	Shut car door on finger	Cut my knee
		14.8	Wire pulled in braces	Pinch nerve in foot
A. D.	M	10.8	Broke my finger	Scraped my knee
		12.8	Bit tongue right through	Hitting a ball with my hand
C. M.	M	11.6	Finger caught in Cuisinart	Hit by small stick
		13.6	Breaking ankle	Given a needle
S. L.	M	13.9	Fell off bike onto face on tarmac	Stubbing my toe
		16.0	Having pins removed from hand	Receiving a paper cut

addition, children observe their parents' and siblings' own pain experiences, pain behaviors, and methods for coping with pain. Family members' attitudes and responses will necessarily influence how children's attitudes about pain develop and how they learn to cope with different types of pain.

Children learn from their parents how to express pain through their behaviors and language. They learn to cope with pain initially by seeking parental reassurance and often by receiving special hugs and kisses to alleviate their discomfort. They evaluate the significance or relevance of a pain by their parents' reactions. Parental reactions vary widely—from telling toddlers to get up and not complain after a small fall because they are not hurt, to smothering children with attention whenever they complain about any aches or pains.

Age, Sex, and Birth Order

Parents often respond differently in the same situation, depending on the age, sex, and birth order of a child. Younger children may require more reassurance and support, while older children may be encouraged to cope more independently. Boys may be encouraged to suppress their verbal pain complaints and to develop active pain-coping methods, such as sports and physical activities. Girls may be subtly reinforced for their pain complaints, particularly if they develop pains similar to those experienced by a mother or grandmother (as is often the case for girls who suffer from migraine headaches; see Chapter 8). Girls may also be encouraged to rely on more passive pain-coping methods, such as resting and taking medication. Parents often respond differently to the same pain complaints, depending on whether the child is their first-born or a later-born child. They tend to be more anxious, overtly protective, and concerned about the routine bumps and scrapes of childhood for their first child than for later-born children. Parents gradually become more accustomed to the types of injuries and pains that infants and children sustain, so that they can evaluate the significance of their children's pain complaints and respond to those complaints in a more confident manner as children mature. Differences in parental responses may account for the higher pain sensitivity reported for first-born children (Johnson et al., 1970; Schachter, 1959; Vernon, 1974).

Secondary Gains

Children will naturally learn from their parents how to express and respond to pain. If they perceive that their pains enable them to receive special attention that they do not receive in other family interactions, they may begin to use their pain complaints to gain attention. Some of the children who have been referred to our pain clinic for excessive pain complaints in the absence of an underlying physical disorder are quite astute, in that they have developed an increasingly severe repertoire of physical symptoms to convince their parents that they are unable to attend school. Common questions asked by these children are "How much does it have to hurt before I can stay home?" and "How sick do I have to be?" All children can develop exaggerated somatic complaints and various aches and pains to avoid difficult responsibilities, particularly if parents inadvertently reinforce their pain behaviors. But most children do not develop excessive pain behaviors, because their pain complaints are evaluated and managed thoroughly, but without paren-tal overreaction. Parents who encourage their children to rely on them alone for pain relief, instead of encouraging their children to rely on them as necessary but also to learn to cope independently, increase the likelihood of the children's developing exaggerated pain complaints and behaviors. Children must learn to interpret the warning signals provided by pain to minimize their body injuries. However, they must also learn some simple tools for coping with pain so that their pains can be minimized. Children's excessive reliance on parents, physicians, or medication for all pain relief will prevent them from using their own natural ability to suppress pain.

Attitudes and Expectations Regarding Prognosis and Pain Control

Familial attitudes and expectations about the prognosis for a child's painful condi-tion may also influence the intensity or duration of the pain. Parents who expect children to live as normally as possible despite a chronic pain condition, such as arthritis, may actually help their children to experience less severe and less disabling pains. Children's participation in peer activities, school functions, and sports (when possible) provides a relatively normal context that should enhance their physical and mental health and promote their natural ability to reduce pain by distraction, mental concentration, and relaxation (reviewed in Chapters 5 and 6).

The stress of living with a chronic disorder is compounded when parental and familial attitudes restrict children's ability to participate in usual childhood activi-ties even more stringently than the disorder per se does. The added stress and the consequent lack of enjoyment can increase children's pain. Similarly, the stress that parents experience as they begin to adjust when a child has been newly diagnosed with a chronic condition can exacerbate the child's stress, anxiety, and subsequent pain. Parents may have difficulty in accepting the diagnosis, yet must cope maturely in front of the child and reassure him/her. Parents also require support and realistic reassurance. When parents do not receive support, when they are unable to understand and accept the situation, or when they somehow feel responsible, their emotional distress may be communicated to the child.

In addition, families may profoundly influence the prognosis for some pain problems. The duration of childhood recurrent pain syndromes may be affected by familial expectations about the eventuality of obtaining adequate pain relief. As an example, girls with migraine headaches are often informed that they will probably continue to have headaches, whereas many boys are informed that they will outgrow their headaches. Mothers may inadvertently reinforce the belief that headaches will persist for their daughters, because they themselves have had headaches since they were teenagers and their mothers also suffered from headaches.

In addition, parental beliefs about the efficacy of available pain control methods may affect how well these methods reduce their children's pain. If parents communicate to their children, either verbally or nonverbally, that nonpharmacological methods cannot reduce the pain of a migraine headache, then these methods will generally not reduce pain for their children. Consequently, a family's attitudes toward a pain management program must be neutral or positive for successful pain control. (The common family factors that affect specific childhood pains are described in Chapters 7, 8, and 9; the integration of the family into a general program for the optimal management of children's pain is summarized in Chapter 6.)

Clearly, families exert a powerful influence on how children learn to express and cope with pain. The major question, though, is this: To what extent do familial responses and familial pain experiences (parents, siblings, and extended family) affect the nature and severity of children's actual pain experiences? As an example, parents whose children suffer from recurrent pain syndromes frequently had similar pain complaints when they were children. Some parents may continue to experience several pain complaints. Do parents' own experiences contribute to the development of similar pain problems in their children? If so, are hereditary or environmental factors responsible? Unfortunately, the respective contributions of genetic predispositions and family learning to various painful childhood conditions are not yet known. Clinical studies suggest that both heredity and environment not only modify children's pain expressions, but also may modify their predisposition to certain painful conditions that develop in the absence of organic disease (described more fully in Chapter 8).

Learning

Pain produced by an injury teaches children about potentially dangerous objects or actions. Children associate a painful injury with a particular action, such as a burn with touching a hot stove. However, they can also learn by association or contiguity that relatively neutral actions or events (i.e., non-tissue-damaging actions) produce pain, simply because these neutral events are temporally or physically connected with the actual noxious stimulus. Children learn quite quickly about the cues that signal pain, as can be readily evidenced from observing the reactions of hospitalized children to an approaching adult in a white coat.

A difficulty may arise, though, when children believe that the neutral cues are the actual causes of their pain. This situation develops for many children with recurrent pain syndromes. When there seems to be no specific external cause for the relatively unpredictable episodes of severe pain, parents often search for an environmental trigger. They investigate foods, weather conditions, sports activities, noise, light, and many of their children's normal activities in a logical attempt to identify and avoid the responsible trigger. However, as they naturally evaluate the situational factors that occurred together with or prior to their children's painful episodes, they tentatively identify many neutral events or actions as causes. Children can become anxious that these neutral events may cause episodes of pain.

The previously neutral events then become conditioned or learned pain triggers. The actual cause for pain is the anxiety about such an event, not the event itself. It is important to teach parents of children with recurrent pain syndromes that there are probably both natural and learned triggers for painful episodes, but that for many children the conditioned pain-inducing events represent the major factors responsible for their pains (see Chapter 8).

Children learn how to express their pain. They learn from their parents, their siblings, their peers, and characters depicted in books, television, and in movies. They may be taught to behave differently because of their age or sex. The developmental studies described previously indicate that girls and boys differ in their emotional responses to pain. Girls may express more fear and anxiety, whereas boys express the need to be stoic and brave. Similarly, girls and boys may be taught to cope with pain differently, so that girls learn to rely on parents for reassurance while boys learn to rely more on themselves.

Society and Culture

Parents teach their children to conform to their personal expectations of how to behave when in pain or during an illness. Diverse family and cultural beliefs lead to significant variations in how children are raised, so that there are many differences in what children learn about pain and how to behave when in pain. Cultural variations and patterns of pain expression reflect a process of observational learning by repeated exposure to consistent patterns of distress in other members of the family, peer groups, and the community. Familial and cultural behaviors provide the framework in which children learn how to interpret somatic signs, how to avoid injury or disease, and how to relieve pain. The cultural precepts are immediately available and are supported by powerful social sanctions to conform. Weisenberg (1980) has proposed a theoretical framework for ethnocultural variations in pain expression. Pain is characterized as a private, ambiguous experience that requires definition and structure. The sufferer turns toward others in the social environment to determine what reactions are appropriate and how pain is best communicated. Is it permissible to cry, or does one have to grin and bear it? When is it permissible to ask for help? When is it appropriate to mask the pain with analgesics? People learn to express their reactions by observing the reactions of others.

The importance of observation and modeling for modifying pain thresholds in adults and for modifying fear, anxiety, and distress behaviors in children has been well documented (Craig, 1975; Craig & Best, 1977; Melamed & Siegel, 1980). The family and society are the primary models for children's development of pain behaviors and pain attitudes. The observational learning that occurs within the family reflects the attitudes and beliefs of the relevant community and culture to which the family belongs. Parents also actively teach their children to conform to their own personal expectations of how they should react to somatic symptoms and pain.

Situational and Emotional Factors

Recently, more attention has been focused on the role of situation-specific variables as important modifiers of pain. The term "situational variables" refers to the specific combination of psychological and contextual factors that exist in a particular pain situation, such as a child's expectations for obtaining pain relief, a child's ability to use a simple coping strategy, a child's perceived control in the situation, a child's understanding about the pain-producing stimulus, the relevance of the pain to the child's life, parental behaviors, and parental expectations for the child's behavior. These situational variables exert a profound effect on children's pains.

As an example, a 3-year-old girl with leukemia required regular lumbar punctures (LPs), but had developed an allergic reaction to the drugs normally used for sedation. She participated in a brief multistrategy pain management program (described in Chapter 7), in which the situational factors that affected her pain were identified and modified. Although she had received several LPs, she did not understand what happened during the procedure. She was extremely frightened when ethyl chloride was sprayed on her back prior to the insertion of the anesthetic needle, and very upset by the need to be held in the fetal position throughout the procedure. Her pain program included an age-appropriate educational component, to improve her understanding of the purpose and technical aspects of the procedure and to teach her some simple tools to reduce pain and improve her control during the procedure. The predictability of each sensory component (the sounds, smells, and tactile stimulation) in the procedure, from the first swab of alcohol on her back to the capping of the test tube in which her cerebrospinal fluid dripped, improved as she understood more fully what was happening behind her back. She learned some relaxation techniques to maintain the necessary curled position without restraint, and she became more positive about the LP. As her expectations about the procedure became more realistic and as her control increased, her fear and anxiety decreased. The goal of her pain management program was to modify the situational and emotional factors that exacerbated the pain evoked by the LP. During her first LP without sedation, she used her pain-coping strategies with her parents' assistance, described what was happening at different times, did not cry or move, and reported afterwards that "it was a piece of cake." Although not all children show such immediate and dramatic reductions in pain, anxiety, and distress behavior, the relatively straightforward approach of identifying and modifying the situational factors that affect children's pain can profoundly alter their perceptions.

Children who require regular invasive medical procedures may develop fear and anxiety about future appointments. Parents may inadvertently increase their anxiety by not preparing them for these appointments. The resulting lack of predictability and control can greatly increase children's fear and behavioral distress, so that their pains are actually increased. Although parents may believe that it is easier for children not to know ahead of time which appointments will involve painful procedures, it is usually better for the children to prepare for these appointments. When children are not informed in an accurate but reassuring manner about what may happen, fear and anxiety may become generalized to all hospital personnel and all medical procedures, even noninvasive procedures. Difficulties may also arise because children begin to distrust their parents, thus increasing parental anxiety and distress that will adversely affect the children's ability to cope with treatments. In general, children will experience less pain when they are prepared in an age-appropriate manner for a potentially pain-inducing stimulus.

Parents may place undue stress on their children by expecting them to cope with painful medical procedures like "little adults." However, children are not little adults and must be assisted to cope in an age-appropriate manner, if they are to minimize the situational and emotional factors that can increase their pain. In our pain program for children with cancer, children complete brief forms to rate the strength and unpleasantness of all painful procedures, so that we can objectively evaluate the efficacy of our interventions. Children are encouraged to respond honestly so that we can develop the best program for each child. Although we attempt to interview children separately, parents are occasionally present when children complete their forms. Parents have expressed opinions about their children's answers, such as "That didn't hurt that much, did it?" "You're not really that scared, are you?" or "You want me to be here, don't you?" These statements can create much emotional stress for children, who may be learning to cope on their own rather than to depend on a particular physician, nurse, parent, or treatment room to make procedures less painful or anxiety-producing. Parents often underestimate the powerful situational cues that they provide to children; these cues can adversely affect their children's pains and their ability to cope with those pains.

Although the specific situational factors that influence different types of pain are described in Chapters 7, 8, and 9, it is essential to recognize the power of often-overlooked situational factors in modifying children's pains. When parents dim the lights in a child's treatment room prior to a certain treatment and begin to whisper, whereas lights remain at regular intensity and the parents speak normally for all other weekly treatments, they are conveying to the child that this treatment has a special and usually aversive significance compared to other treatments. How much does this situation, rather than the procedure itself, contribute to the child's anxiety? Since the relevance of pain-inducing procedures affects how much pain will be perceived, it is essential to reassure children that all the procedures that are required for the management of their medical condition are normal for the treatment of that condition and that the children themselves can learn techniques to reduce their anxiety and pain.

Animal behavioral studies in which the physiological responses activated by a noxious stimulus are directly recorded have demonstrated that certain situational variables, such as attention, predictability, and relevance, can directly modify the physiological responses evoked by a constant noxious stimulus (Dubner, Hoffman, & Hayes, 1981; Hayes, Dubner, & Hoffman, 1981; Hoffman, Dubner, Hayes, & Medlin, 1981). Human psychophysical experiments in which adults rate the painfulness of noxious stimuli in different contexts have investigated situational factors and demonstrated that it is possible to control and evaluate their pain-reducing effects (Craig & Best, 1977; Dworkin & Chen, 1981; Johnson, 1973; P. A. McGrath, 1983; McGrath, Brooke, & Varkey, 1981; Price, Barrell, & Gracely, 1980). Situational variables may modify pain by activating descending pain-suppressing systems, which modulate neuronal activity at spinal cord and medullary levels (see Chapter 3). Although the precise mechanisms by which these factors affect nociceptive processing are unknown, it is important to begin to identify and evaluate their influence in pediatrics, particularly in order to refine techniques for pain management in infants and children.

Summary

Pain for infants, children, and adolescents is a complex multidimensional perception that varies in quality, strength, duration, location, and unpleasantness. The strength and unpleasantness of their pains are neither simply nor directly related to the nature or extent of tissue damage produced by a noxious stimulus. Instead, children's pain is modified by many situational, emotional, familial/cultural, and developmental factors. Even newborn infants may experience different pains from the same noxious stimulus, because of differences in the situation in which it is administered. Infants' cries, facial expressions, overt distress behaviors, and physiological reactions in response to a noxious stimulus indicate that they can experience pain at birth. Although children's understanding of pain and their descriptions of pain naturally depend on their age, cognitive level, previous pain experiences, and familial learning, very young children recognize the unpleasant sensory and emotional aspects of pain.

Children's pain experiences can range from an inability to perceive pain, regardless of the intensity of noxious stimulation, to the actual perception of pain in a limb that has been amputated. The same mysterious pains that adults experience, in which there are no apparent physical causes, can also afflict children. Children can experience a diverse variety of acute, recurrent, and chronic pains, related to injury, disease, or psychological factors. However, children's pain experiences have not been well studied until recently, so that the true incidence of specific pediatric pain problems is not yet known. Similarly, the extent to which children's pain experiences affect their pain perceptions and behaviors as adults is not known.

Children's perceptions, expressions, and reactions to pain are influenced by genetic, developmental, familial, psychological, social, and cultural variables. Children's concepts of pain follow a consistent developmental pattern that provides a framework for our design of interventions for children at different developmental levels. Children learn about pain and about how to cope with pain through the diverse nature of their own pain experiences and the reactions of their parents and families. As children mature, they generally experience a wider variety of pains that differ in quality, strength, location, duration, and unpleasantness, and they gradually develop a repertoire of strategies to reduce pain. Children learn from their parents how to express pain through their behaviors and language. Parents may naturally respond differently when their children are in pain, depending on the age, sex, and birth order of a child, in addition to the nature of the pain-producing injury. Consequently, children in the same family may be taught differently how to express or cope with pain. Such differences may persist as the children mature into adults. The family and society, in addition to being the primary models for the treatment of children's development of pain attitudes and pain behaviors, can also exert a powerful influence on children's actual pain perceptions.

Psychological factors, such as the situational and emotional factors that exist when children experience pain, may profoundly alter their pain perceptions. Children's attention, understanding, perceived control, and expectations, as well as the aversive significance of the pain for them, will affect their perceptions. Emotions such as anxiety, fear, or depression can increase the strength of acute pain produced by a noxious stimulus, can evoke episodes of recurrent pain, or can exacerbate chronic pain related to disease or injury. Consequently, the control of pain in infants, children, and adolescents requires recognition of and management of the many developmental, familial, situational, and emotional factors that modify their pain perceptions.

2

Pain Assessment in Infants and Children

The objective assessment of the intensity or quality of pain in infants and children constitutes a challenge for parents and health professionals. Reliable descriptions of children's pain experiences are necessary not only to facilitate a precise medical diagnosis, but also to determine which treatments are most effective for reducing different types of pain and which treatments are most beneficial for which children. Moreover, since pain is not always a correlating symptom of disease or injury—that is, it may not diminish progressively as the disease is treated or as the injury heals—it is necessary to objectively assess and modify the situational factors that can exacerbate children's acute pain or that can contribute to the development or maintenance of recurrent or chronic pediatric pains. An evaluation of the factors that affect children's pain, in addition to the measurement of their pain experience, is an essential prerequisite for the design of effective pain management programs.

Basically, children's pain is measured on a qualitative (categorical) or quantitative (numerical) scale that provides meaningful information about the strength, unpleasantness, location, duration, and quality of their pains. Research on the utility of different scales and techniques for measuring acute, recurrent, and chronic pain in infants and children has dramatically increased during the past 5 years; as a result, a variety of methods and instruments are now available. Like adult pain measures, children's pain measures may be classified as behavioral, physiological, or psychological, depending on the nature of the pain response that is measured. Behavioral measures include several observational procedures in which independent raters record the type of behaviors that children exhibit when they are in pain, as well as the frequency of their occurrence (e.g., the number of

41

minutes children cry during an injection). Presumably, an objective evaluation of
the nature and frequency of children's pain behaviors provides an accurate estimate of the strength of their pain experiences. Physiological pain measures include
a variety of techniques that monitor the body's responses to a noxious stimulus,
such as increased heart rate or respiration rate. A description of the nature and
extent of the body's natural pain responses might constitute an objective index for
children's pain experiences. Both behavioral and physiological measures provide
indirect estimates of pain, however, since the presence or strength of children's pain
is inferred solely from the type and magnitude of their behavioral and physiological responses to a noxious stimulus. Psychological measures, which evaluate children's perceptions of pain from their own perspective, can provide direct estimates
for many different dimensions of pain. Several projective and self-report methods
are available in which children describe their understanding of pain or their
subjective experiences of pain. Table 2.1 lists the primary methods for assessing
children's pain within the behavioral, physiological, and psychological categories.
However, not all methods are equally appropriate for all children or for all pain
conditions. Selection of an appropriate method for measuring pediatric pain
requires a careful consideration of the accuracy of the available measures in
relation to the age, sex, and cognitive level of children and to the nature of their
pain problems.

The criteria for an accurate pain measure for children are generally consistent
with those that have been described for adults. (For a review of pain measures in
adults, see Chapman, 1980; Gracely, 1980; Hukisson, 1974; Melzack, 1983.) A pain
measure must be reliable; that is, it must provide consistent pain scores when
children have the same pain, regardless of the time of testing or the children's sex,
age, and cognitive level. The method must also be valid. That is, it must unequivocally measure a specific dimension of a child's pain (e.g., intensity, duration,
quality), and not the various emotional responses that may occur as a consequence
of the pain; in addition, changes in children's responses or scores should accurately
reflect changes in their pain experiences. Third, the method should be relatively
bias-free, providing the same information regardless of the biases of the person who

TABLE 2.1. Methods for Assessing Pain in Infants and Children

Behavioral–observational	Physiological	Psychological	
		Projective	Self-report
General body position	Reflexes	Colors	Interviews
Specific distress behaviors	Heart rate	Shapes	Questionnaires
Facial expression	Respiration rate	Cartoons	Thermometers
Vocalization or cry pattern	Sweat index	Drawings	Facial scales
	Beta-endorphin level		Visual analog scales

administers it or the response biases of the children who use it. Finally, a pain measure should be versatile—practical for assessing acute, chronic, or recurrent pain, and applicable for use in a variety of medical, dental, and familial situations. Although these criteria are identical to those required for any measuring instrument, special problems arise in pediatric pain measurement because the influence of developmental factors on children's perceptions and expressions of pain is not yet known. Consequently, current research is necessarily focused on the adequacy of a pain measure according to children's age, sex, cognitive level, and previous pain experience. The validity and reliability of a pain measure should be demonstrated prior to using the method to evaluate the efficacy of various treatments for reducing children's clinical pain.

Although many behavioral, physiological, and psychological measures are available for assessing pain in infants and children, a major practical question is this: Which method will provide the most accurate and objective information about a child's pain experience, so that health professionals can understand the source of the pain and provide an effective treatment? This question represents the crucial issue in pediatric pain assessment. Consequently, this chapter reviews the recent advances in the measurement of pain in infants and children, with special emphasis on the methods that satisfy the criteria for reliability and validity; the methods that can be used to assess multiple dimensions of pain; and the methods that may be appropriate for assessing all acute, recurrent, and chronic pediatric pains. In addition, a model is introduced that can be used to determine the reliability and validity of a proposed pain measure for children. This chapter also presents some practical strategies for minimizing the common difficulties that may develop when children's pain is measured in clinical situations.

Behavioral Pain Measures

Assessing children's pain by objectively recording the occurrence and frequency of their pain-related behaviors evolved as a scientific approach from the more common practice of inferring children's emotions by observing their overt behavioral responses. From birth, infants communicate their physical and emotional needs through their behaviors. They communicate when they are in pain by their cries, facial expressions, and torso and limb movements in reaction to a pain-inducing stimulus. Observations of infants' behavioral responses to a noxious stimulus provide an accessible and practical method for inferring that they are experiencing pain. In fact, since infants and young children are unable to communicate information directly about the quality and intensity of their pain experiences, health professionals and parents must rely on either infants' behaviors or their bodies' physiological changes in order to assess their pain.

Although older children can communicate more directly about their pain experiences, their pain vocabularies will evolve gradually as they mature and as they experience different types and different intensities of pain. Children learn to describe the temporal, spatial, and qualitative aspects of all their sensations, not just their pain sensations. The language that they learn to describe their own pains develops from the language that is used by their families, by their peers, and by characters depicted in books, on television, and in movies. Children naturally differ in the words that they use to describe their pains because of differences in their backgrounds, previous pain experiences, and learning. Since children's pain vocabularies vary among one another and are generally quite different from those of adults, research investigators and health professionals have often been reluctant to rely on even older children's verbal descriptions as reliable indices of their pain. Instead, there has been an almost implicit assumption that children's pain behaviors are less subject than children's pain language to change as a result of maturation, learning, or previous pain experience. Older children's nonverbal behaviors have often been regarded as more reliable and more objective indices of their pain than their verbal descriptions.

Unfortunately, several problems can develop when children's behaviors are used to infer their pain in a clinical situation. Health professionals may interpret children's behaviors differently; for example, behaviors that represent pain to one individual may represent anxiety or emotional arousal to another. As a result, the same behaviors may be rated differently, and this will produce conflicting pain scores for a child. When a child's pain and analgesic requirements are reviewed with parents, nurses, and physicians, it is not unusual for each person to have inferred a different level of pain for the child. Their different pain estimates presumably result from differences either in their criteria for which behaviors represent pain or in the time periods during which they have observed the child. Children's behavioral responses also change over time, so that it is necessary to monitor their behaviors at successive time periods. The selection of well-defined pain behaviors, and the choice of an appropriate time period during which children's behaviors are observed, are critical for the proper use of behavioral measures. Clearly, in addition to the criteria for pain behaviors, the selection of sampling times for observing children's behaviors will influence the final estimates of children's pain. Even when uniform criteria are established for defining children's pain behaviors and frequent sampling periods are used to ensure accurate data, a major question remains unanswered: Are children's pain-related behaviors valid indices of their pain?

Children's behaviors are not simple and direct expressions of the quality or intensity of their pains. As described in Chapter 1, their behavioral responses to a noxious stimulus are influenced by learning and may also reflect their emotional states, rather than their pain experience alone. As an example, two children who are in the hospital recovering from similar surgical procedures may behave differently, even though they are experiencing equivalent levels of pain. A child with extensive pain experience who has learned to cope with his/her pain may not exhibit the same overt distress behaviors as a child with less pain experience. The second child may show more overt distress to the same level of pain, while not necessarily perceiving more pain. In order to select the appropriate analgesic drug to relieve both children's postsurgical pain, it is necessary to assess their pain. If the children's presumed pain behaviors are different, although their pain experiences may be equivalent, they may not receive equivalent analgesics. Observation of children's behaviors alone as indices of their pain, without information about their usual pain behaviors and their previous pain experience, may lead to inappropriate analgesic administration, particularly when more than one person assumes responsibility for drug selection and dosing regimens. Although physicians and nurses must rely on children's behavioral and physiological responses when they administer medication to children who lack verbal communication skills, consistent criteria should be applied for identifying and recording children's pain-related behaviors according to their age, sex, and cognitive level. Also, valuable information can be obtained from parents in an initial interview about a child's usual manner of expressing pain. Such information can be noted on each child's medical chart to provide a framework for evaluating subsequent behavioral responses.

Because of the potential difficulties inherent in the use of behavioral pain measures, the emphasis in much of the recent research in pediatrics has been on identifying the behaviors that are primarily associated with infants' and children's pain, so that consistent criteria may be developed for children of different ages and pain experiences. In addition, research has been conducted to determine the optimal sampling periods for observing children and to evaluate the reliability and validity of behavioral scales completed by trained observers. The majority of these behavioral studies on pediatric pain are clinical studies in which observers record children's natural responses during medical procedures that evoke acute pain (e.g., blood-sampling procedures or injections). Children's behaviors prior to, during, and after noxious stimulation are noted in order to define distinct behaviors that may represent different qualities or intensities of pain.

These studies have shown that children's repertoire of pain-related and distress-related behaviors change as they develop. Infants' responses to acute pain may include general body movements, specific facial expressions, and crying patterns. Toddlers' and young children's responses to acute pain usually include specific body reactions that are more precisely localized to the painful body region, accompanied by verbalizations of their discomfort. Older children display more subtle behavioral responses to acute pain from invasive medical procedures, usually slight facial grimaces and brief pain reports. Children's responses to recurrent or chronic pain are usually not characterized by their specific behaviors at any one time period, but rather by the overall pattern of their behaviors. Young children respond to recurrent headaches by withdrawing from their physical activities in order to seek a quiet and restful environment. In addition to withdrawing from physical activities and activities requiring mental concentration, older children and adolescents may respond to recurrent or chronic pain through school absences, sleep disturbances, eating difficulties, and personality changes.

Infants' Pain Behaviors

Body Movements

General body movements (torso and limb), facial expressions, and cry patterns have been investigated as behavioral measures of infant pain. Several studies have monitored infants' body movements after noxious stimulation in order to identify the motor behaviors that constitute a pain response (for reviews, see Johnston & Strada, 1986; McGrath, 1987c; Owens, 1984, 1986; Pratt, 1954). McGraw (1941, 1945) studied developmental differences in the behavioral reactions of 75 children (neonates to 4-year-olds) after they received a noxious stimulus, a pin prick. Infants from birth to 10 days of age either did not respond or made only diffuse body movements in response to the pin prick; they rarely made specific reflex withdrawals to the stimulus. Diffuse body movements in response to the pin prick increased as infants developed during their first month, and later decreased during their second month. Infants aged 6–12 months began to withdraw their limbs consistently from the stimulus, often looking at the stimulated body region. At approximately 12 months of age, they began to touch the painful area after the pin was withdrawn. McGraw described a further developmental shift at 2–3 years when infants exhibited protective behavioral responses in anticipation of the approaching pin and showed an ability to cope with the situation.

However, subsequent research on the nature and intensity of infants' motor responses after noxious stimulation has resulted in contradictory findings. Some studies have shown that newborns do not respond to noxious stimulation (Pratt, 1954); other studies have reported that diffuse body movements are newborns' characteristic pain responses (Graham, 1956; Graham, Matarazzo, & Caldwell, 1956). In addition, still other investigators have reported that neonates produce specific reflex withdrawal in response to noxious stimulation (Lipton, Steinschneider, & Richmond, 1965). The discrepancies in these reports about infants' characteristic motor behaviors in reaction to noxious stimuli may only be the results of differences in the studies' experimental designs. Experiments were not standardized according to the time of testing, the nature of the pain-inducing stimulus, and the extent to which observers were trained to recognize individual motor behaviors in infants. Or these contradictions may provide evidence that there are no specific motor behaviors that constitute pure pain behaviors in neonates. Individual differences in reactions to pain-inducing stimuli may exist at birth.

In fact, a recent study (Craig, McMahon, Morison, & Zaskow, 1984) assessed developmental changes in the facial expressions and behaviors of 30 infants (2–24 months of age) in response to immunization injections. Trained raters used a behavior rating scale to score the frequency of infants' general motor responses, vocal actions (e.g., crying, screaming), facial expressions (e.g., distortion, eye orientation), torso positions (e.g., rigid, withdrawing), and limb positions (e.g., protecting, thrashing). The raters observed the infants prior to, during, and after their immunization injections, to determine how their behaviors changed throughout the procedure. The behaviors of the infants' mothers and attending nurses were also rated, to evaluate changes in infants' behaviors that could be attributed to the mothers' soothing actions during the immunization. Although crying and other vocalizations were the most common and salient reactions to the injections, there were variations in infants' responses and some infants showed idiosyncratic pain behaviors, even at this early stage of life. In general, infants from 12 to 24 months of age responded differently than did younger infants. They cried and screamed for a shorter time period, oriented toward the painful body sites, visually followed the nurses and their mothers to a greater extent, protected and touched their limbs more often, and displayed less torso rigidity in response to the injections than the younger infants. The investigators' standardized observations of infants' behaviors, which provided reliable and valid indices of infants' reactions to noxious stimulation, indicated that infants' pain behaviors were influenced by their orienting behavior, ongoing activity, and situational constraints, rather than being exclusively related to the injection.

Johnston and Strada (1986) described the body responses of 14 infants (2 and 4 months old) before, during, and after receiving diphtheria–pertussis–tetanus (DPT) injections. Prior to the injection, 12 infants had torso, arms, and legs at rest. During the injection, all infants had rigid body positions, either in only the torso and arms or in all three body regions. Immediately after the injection, half the infants had rigid torsos. Twelve had arms and legs that were withdrawn or thrashing, while the other two returned to the at-rest position. Approximately 2½ minutes after the injection, none of the infants had rigid torsos, arms, or legs. Although the three categories (at rest, rigid, and thrashing) do not constitute a specific pain measure, they provide a reliable and valid method by which to qualitatively categorize infants' overt distress reactions to noxious stimuli.

An almost continuous monitoring of infants' behaviors is possible in clinical situations when immunizations are videotaped. The qualitative behavioral changes observed in infants at different ages could yield valuable information about developmental differences in pain responses. More research must be conducted to determine how infants' pain responses change with repeated exposure to noxious stimulation, such as when they require prolonged medical care. Similarly, more research must be conducted to identify which components of infants' behaviors represent pain intensity and which represent their emotional responses in a potentially aversive situation. Although infants' overt distress behaviors are not pure pain measures, because they reflect both their pain experience and their emotional responses to their pain, behavioral assessments may be useful for evaluating the efficacy of different physical methods (e.g., rubbing the intended pain site or a contralateral site vigorously prior to an injection) for reducing infants' pain reactions, their emotional distress, and presumably their pain.

Facial Expressions

Facial expressions have been investigated extensively in order to identify the expressions uniquely associated with different human emotions. Studies have focused on the ability of human observers to recognize the emotions depicted in the facial expressions of infants, children, and adults, in order to understand how facial expressions change developmentally and vary among different cultures. The belief that certain facial expressions may represent an innate response to an individual's emotional state led to the more recent studies on infants' facial expressions in response to noxious stimulation (Charlesworth 1982). Ekman and Oster (1979) were able to distinguish between facial expressions associated with pain and sadness in infants. Later, Izard (1982) developed a coding system (the Maximally Discriminative Facial Movement Coding System, or MAX) to classify human emotions in infants. Infants' facial expressions are photographed for subsequent analysis by raters trained in MAX. Three regions on infants' faces are analyzed separately: their forehead and brow regions, their eyes and nose ridges, and their mouth regions. This system was used to characterize the facial expressions that occurred in newborns in response to heel lance procedures (Izard & Dougherty, 1982; Izard, Huebner, Risser, McGinnes, & Dougherty, 1980). Their brows were lowered and together, their nasal roots broadened and bulged, and their eyes were tightly closed with angular and square mouths. Since facial expressions in infants should be less subject to the influences of learning and previous pain experience, their analysis by trained observers may provide a valid and reliable manner to study pain naturally. Another study evaluated the facial expressions of 2- to 19-month-old infants in response to immunization injections (Izard, Hembree, Dougherty, & Spizzirri, 1983). Infants showed a distinct distress expression and an anger expression, but the four different age groups (2.1, 4.2, 8.1, and 19.2 months) responded differentially with distress and anger expressions. The duration of a physical distress expression decreased with age, whereas the duration of an anger expression increased with age. It is not clear, though, whether these differences were due to developmental factors in how infants responded to the same noxious stimulus or to experiential factors. The four age groups also corresponded to the four stages in the immunization sequence (first, second, third, and fourth injections), so that older infants had experienced more injections.

In a recent study on pain expression in infants, Grunau and Craig (1987) evaluated the facial expressions and vocalizations evoked by heel rub and heel lance procedures. They observed the responses of 140 infants to these procedures during different physical activity and alert states: quiet and sleeping, active but sleeping, quiet and awake, and actively awake. The investigators were interested in how infants' behavioral responses to discomfort (the presumed sensation associated with heel rub) differed from their responses to pain (the presumed sensation evoked by heel lance) and how their responses differed according to their levels of activity and alertness. The authors used a coding system for facial movement based on the Facial Action Coding System (FACS) approach (Ekman & Friesen, 1969) in which trained raters scored nine facial movements: brow bulge, eye squeeze, naso-labial furrow, open lips, vertical stretch mouth, horizontal stretch mouth, lip purse, taut tongue, and chin quiver. The infants were videotaped during the entire heel rub, heel lance, and blood collection procedures. Neonates (second day of life) showed a constellation of facial changes after heel lance that differed substantially from the quality and extent of facial movement evoked by heel rub. Eyes squeezed, brows contracted, the naso-labial furrows deepened, tongues were taut with open mouths and a cry response occurred after heel lance. However, infants' reactions were not determined solely by the noxious stimulation, but also by their alertness. Alert infants in both the quiet and awake states responded initially to the invasive procedures with significantly more facial movements than sleeping infants. Vertical stretch mouth and taut tongue occurred after heel lance with the highest frequency for alert infants and with the lowest frequency for sleeping infants. (Vertical stretch mouth is characterized by a tautness at the lip corners, coupled with a pronounced downward pull on the jaw. Stretch mouth is often noted when an already wide open mouth is opened a fraction further by an extra pull at the jaw. Taut tongue is characterized by a raised, cupped tongue with sharp, tensed edges. The first occurrence of taut tongue is usually easy to see, often occurring with a wide open mouth. After this first occurrence, the mouth may close slightly.)

Grunau and Craig (1987) showed that pain expressions in newborns occur in relation to their ongoing behavioral state, thus reflecting early differences in their inherent capacity for pain responsivity or pain modulation. Although it is not possible to determine the extent to which infants' facial expressions are direct representations of their pain experience, it is probable that they are relatively bias-free representations of their emotional distress. The major disadvantage in relying on facial expressions as indices of pain is that infants' expressions may reflect their initial reactions to a relatively short-duration noxious stimulus, and therefore may indicate only the presence of acute pain. It is important to begin to evaluate how infants' facial expressions change after repeated noxious stimulation, such as may occur in intensive care units, and how their expressions vary for different health problems. As yet facial expressions alone do not provide sufficient information about the intensity or quality of infants' pain experiences. However, future research may reveal more subtle changes in infants' facial expressions that are correlated with quantitative or qualitative differences in their pain perceptions.

Cry Patterns

The intensity, duration, and frequency or pitch of infant cries have been evaluated as possible pain indices (Fisichelli, Karelitz, & Haber, 1969; Fisichelli, Karelitz, Fisichelli, & Cooper, 1974; Johnston, 1987; Johnston & O'Shaugnessy, 1988; Levine & Gordon, 1982; Michelsson, Jarvenpaa, & Rinne, 1983; Porter, Porges, & Marshall, 1988). Infant cries are defined as intense, penetrating noises that are ideally designed to alert, to arouse, and to maintain a listener's attention (Ostwald, 1972). Studies of infants' cries include analyses by sound spectrography to identify characteristic physical patterns, and listener analyses to evaluate the ability of adults to recognize the nature of infant cries (e.g., birth, hunger, or pain). The newborn cry consists of an expiratory cry that lasts from 0.6 to 1.4 seconds, followed sometimes by a brief inspiratory whistle (0.1–0.2 seconds) and by another period of rest (about 0.2 seconds) prior to the onset of the next expiratory cry (Murray, 1979; Sedlackova, 1964; Truby & Lind, 1965; Wolff, 1969). There is often a rising–falling change in the pitch of the cry, as the auditory frequency of the expiratory cry increases and decreases. The loudness of the cry is about 80 dB when measured 12 inches from the infant's mouth (Ringel & Kluppel, 1964). Infant cries for hunger, anger, and pain have been classified generally according to the acoustical properties of the cries. The pain cry is either a sudden onset of loud crying without preliminary moaning, or an initial long cry followed by an extended period of breath-holding (Wolff, 1969). Pain cries eventually settle to a rhythm that is indistinguishable from other cries.

Wasz-Hockert, Lind, Vuorenkoski, Partanen, and Valanne (1968) identified 11 acoustical attributes of infant cries, such as the length of the expiratory cry, the phonation, the pitch, and the melody type (rising–falling, rising, falling, flat, and no melody). However, only two attributes, the length of the cry and the phonation, were predictive of the type of cry. Phonation, dysphonation, and hyperphonation are three auditory patterns determined by sound-spectrographic analysis of the cries recorded from 1- to 12-day-old infants, who had been pinched to provide a standard stimulus to cry (Truby & Lind, 1965). Phonation represented the basic auditory pattern, with a harmonic structure and a smooth, symmetrical spectrogram. Dysphonation represented the pattern when the harmonics of the basic cry were obscured by noise, caused by overloading at the infant's larynx. Hyperphonation represented an abrupt shift in the auditory pattern either from or to a high frequency of 2,000 Hz, producing a whistle-like noise caused by the strain and constriction of the infants' vocal apparatus. The three types of phonation seem to reflect an increasing amount of effort. Murray's (1979) analysis of infants' cries showed that pain cries were often dysphonated or hyperphonated, lacked a rising–falling melody, and lasted longer than other cries. She postulated that infants' cries are not uniquely different according to what causes them, but rather differ in intensity according to the degree of discomfort experienced by the infant.

Owens and Todt (1984) studied crying in response to noninvasive tactile stimulation (alcohol-swabbing) and to noxious heel lance in twenty 2-day-old infants. Crying began consistently after heel lance, and the percentage of time crying after heel lance was significantly greater than that after tactile stimulation. Grunau and Craig (1987) evaluated the latency, duration, number of cry cycles, and frequency of infants' cries in response to heel lance and reported some differences due to sex and state (quiet or active and alert or sleeping). Boys cried sooner than girls, and they cried significantly more cycles than girls. Infants who were quietly sleeping cried less quickly than other infants. The fundamental cry frequency, the primary pitch, rose over the first 300 milliseconds for all infants' independent of their sex or state. Johnston and Strada (1986) evaluated infants' cries in response to medical injections. Audiotaped recordings of cries were analyzed to determine the fundamental frequency, latency, duration, phonation, and melody patterns of the cries. Despite an extremely wide variability in infants' cries, some common patterns emerged. The initial cry (3–6 seconds after injection) was high-pitched and phonated, with a flat or slightly falling melody. The second cry (16.5–17.5 seconds) was dysphonated, whereas the last cry (at 55–60 seconds) was phonated and lower-pitched with a rhythmic rising–falling melody.

The studies reviewed indicate clearly that some characteristic cry patterns have been identified when infants receive invasive medical procedures. As yet, though, no one cry pattern has been shown to be consistently related to a pain-inducing stimulus. There is also conflicting evidence about the existence of unique pain cries from research studies on listener analysis (the identification of the type of cry by observers). Some studies have shown that mothers and experienced caregivers are more accurate than inexperienced caregivers in distinguishing among infants' cries of hunger, pain, birth, and pleasure (Petrovich-Bartell, Cowan, & Morse, 1982; Sagi, 1981; Wasz-Hockert, Partanen, Vuorenkoski, Valanne, & Michelsson, 1964). Other studies have failed to demonstrate maternal identification of infant cries (Muller, Hollien, & Murry, 1974; Murry, Amundson, & Hollien, 1977). In general, the acoustical properties of infants' cries may provide insufficient information about the nature of the cry. Instead, listeners may need to rely on the length of the cry and contextual cues in order to determine the source for the cry (Muller et al., 1974). Both spectrographic analysis and listener analysis indicate that the intensity, latency, and duration of an infant's cry may provide the salient cues that signal an infant's distress.

In summary, body movements, facial expressions, and cries in response to both experimentally induced pain and clinical pain have been monitored in infants in order to identify a characteristic pain behavior. As yet, no one single behavior constitutes an unequivocal measure of an infant's pain. However, characteristic patterns of distress behavior have emerged from the analysis of infants' facial expressions and cries. More research must be conducted to evaluate the nature of infants' facial expressions and cries in relation to differences in the quality, intensity, and duration of their pain, so as to understand how these behaviors may reflect their perceptions. Although analysis of videotapes of infants' behaviors and sound-spectrographic analysis of infants' vocalizations can provide reliable and valid measures of their responses to noxious stimulus, at present they are not practical methods for spontaneous clinical evaluations of infants' pain. Their use has been limited to acute pain situations.

It is essential to begin to monitor infants' behaviors throughout longer time periods during hospitalization for various medical treatments. Infants recovering from surgery would presumably exhibit more restricted body movements and may exhibit different facial expressions and vocalization patterns than those identified for acute pain induced by blood-sampling techniques or injections. In order to assess infants' pain by observing their behaviors, it is necessary to extend the research on acute pain to other clinical populations. If behavioral indices vary according to the nature of the pain and the age, sex, and activity state of the infant, then it should be possible to develop normative standards for infants' behaviors that are appropriate for different diseases, ages, and activity levels. These norms could facilitate the development of brief standardized behavioral pain measures for infants that could be used conveniently in the clinic.

Research on infants' responses during noxious stimulation has shown that infants' responses are not simple and consistent reflexes to a tissue-damaging stimulus. Their reactions represent complex responses dependent on their age and behavioral state. Although not yet wholly proven to be objective pain measures, infants' facial expressions and vocalizations show promise as reliable and valid methods to assess infants' distress. Future research should provide a framework for understanding their behaviors and developing scales that are practical and convenient for clinical use and versatile for a variety of painful conditions.

Children's Pain Behaviors

Behavioral measures of pain in children consist primarily of observation scales or checklists in which a trained observer watches a child throughout a pain-inducing situation and records the occurrence of certain pain-related behaviors, such as crying, refusing treatment, or stalling. Several behavioral scales have been developed to objectively evaluate children's overt responses to acute pain produced by invasive medical procedures. The frequency and duration of distress behaviors that occur prior to and during the medical procedure are scored to produce a numerical value that represents a child's overt distress. Although this value is an integrated index of children's anxiety, fear, distress, and pain, children's behavioral scores have been interpreted as their pain scores (Katz, Varni, & Jay, 1984; Shacham & Daut, 1981). Two observational distress scales—the Procedural Behavior Rating Scale-revised (PBRS-r; Katz, Kellerman, & Siegel, 1980, 1981) and the Observational Scale of Behavioral Distress (OSBD; Jay, Ozolins, Elliott, & Caldwell, 1983)—have been developed for pediatric oncology patients during their lumbar punctures and bone marrow aspirations. The term "behavioral distress" refers to both children's anxiety and their pain because of the difficulty in distinguishing between them by observing children in clinical situations. The PBSR-r records the occurrence of 11 behaviors during three time periods within the medical procedure, whereas the OSBD continually samples the same 11 behaviors throughout the procedure. The behaviors are weighed according to the amount of anxiety or distress that they indicate. Intensity ratings vary along a scale of 1–4, in which 4 indicates maximal anxiety or pain. The behaviors and their respective weights are cry (1.5), scream (4), physical restraint (4), verbal resistance (2.5), requests for emotional support (2), muscular rigidity (2.5), verbal pain (2.5), flail (4), nervous behavior (1), and information-seeking (1.5). Both the OSBD and PBRS-r are reliable and valid scales for assessing children's distress behavior. There is evidence that the distress behaviors are correlated with children's pain or anxiety, since both children's self-reports of pain and their anxiety ratings on a standardized anxiety measure were correlated with their scores on the OSBD (Jay et al., 1983).

A behavioral scale—the Children's Hospital of Eastern Ontario Pain Scale (CHEOPS; P. J. McGrath et al., 1985)—was developed to assess postoperative pain. Six behaviors (crying, facial expression, verbal expression, torso position, touch behavior, and leg position) are rated every 30 seconds by a trained observer. Numerical values are assigned according to whether the child's behavior is regarded as positive (0); neutral, representing no pain (1); or representing mild (2), moderate (3), or severe pain (4). The investigators used the scale to assess pain behavior in 30 boys (1–7 years old) during the hour immediately after their circumcisions. Children's pain scores on the behavioral scales correlated with nurses' pain ratings. However, this correlation would be expected if nurses based their pain estimates on knowledge of the children's surgical procedure, the time since surgery, and the children's postoperative behaviors. If both CHEOPS pain scores and the nurses' estimates of children's pain were based on the same overt behaviors, then the two pain scores should correlate with each other. A more precise method of determining the reliability of the scale would be to ask nurses to score children's pain without prior knowledge of the children's condition and to score children in different health and pain states. The behavioral pain scores on the CHEOPS decreased after children received intravenous administration of a short-acting narcotic, fentanyl. Again, however, the reduced scores may reflect primarily a restriction in the children's overt distress behaviors because of the depressive effects of a narcotic on their motor responses, and may not necessarily reflect their subjective experience of pain. Although it is a promising tool for assessing children's behavioral responses when in pain, the CHEOPS requires further validation as an accurate and sensitive pain measure.

Behavioral scales may be most valuable as part of a comprehensive pain management program for individual children. As an example, Frank, a 10-year-old boy with acute myelogenous leukemia, was scheduled for intravenous chemotherapy to be administered throughout a 3- to 4-hour period in an ambulatory outpatient area. He had been referred to the Children's Pain Clinic because of his excessive pain complaints during previous intravenous procedures and anticipatory nausea prior to his scheduled treatments. Frank's regular treatment was monitored as part of his pain assessment. Both his parents and the therapist completed brief behavioral scales outlining Frank's general activities for the 24 hours prior to his procedure and his specific behaviors during his appointment. The pain therapist noted that Frank's behaviors in the 24 hours preceding his appointment changed from his usual active play with others to more passive activities by himself (e.g., watching television). In the clinic, he seemed agitated and apprehensive, and was unable to concentrate in play activities or conversations with other children and staff. He attempted to stall the onset of the procedure. He reported more pain during the chemotherapy and was much sicker than most other children who received the same treatment.

Although Frank's pain management program included the same components as those used to reduce acute pain evoked by medical procedures for all children (described in Chapter 7), a behavioral assessment enabled him and his parents to understand how his physical activity and mental state prior to treatment could influence his anxiety and subsequently his pain and nausea. The situational factors that contributed to Frank's pain during chemotherapy were primarily increased fear and anxiety about pain and nausea, resulting from his inability to understand the need for treatment and to use some simple techniques to control any pain. He was also deprived of the relaxation and stress-reducing benefits of play, mental absorption, and interacting with other children. A cognitive-behavioral program was used to modify these factors. His family introduced apparently spontaneous, but actually well-planned, activities with other children the afternoon and evening before his treatment. The more active and absorbed Frank was in positive activities the evening before treatment, the less apprehensive he appeared in the morning. In order to help him concentrate on a positive activity, he was allowed to play video games only while he received treatment. He was encouraged to select a game a week before treatment, and he received a small reward for trying to concentrate on the game during his intravenous therapy.

Both Frank and his parents noted that as his preprocedure and in-clinic behavior became more active and positively oriented, he reported less pain, was sicker fewer times throughout the treatment, and felt less apprehensive in general. Assessing his behavior, as well as his reported pain and anxiety, made it possible to incorporate a behavioral component into his pain program; this allowed him to understand concretely that he could modify the context in which he received his treatment, so as to modify the quality and strength of his discomfort. He learned that the video games were not a magic solution, but simply one tool that helped him to focus his attention away from the needle and drugs.

An illustration of an abbreviated behavioral scale for children with cancer who require repeated invasive medical procedures is shown in Figure 2.1. Information is obtained from parental interviews and the pain therapist's observations. In our program, the scale is not quantified to produce a numerical score of children's distress or pain, but merely used as a qualitative estimate of children's global behaviors and their orientation toward others.

In summary, behavioral measures of pediatric pain have been generally restricted to assessments of children's distress in acute pain situations. Little research has been conducted on the utility of behavioral measures for recurrent or chronic pain. Although behavioral measures have been shown to be reliable and valid indices of children's overt distress, children's overt behaviors do not always constitute direct expressions of the intensity or quality of their pain experiences. Caution must be used in inferring children's pain solely from their behaviors during a pain-inducing situation. Children's behaviors in a medical or dental situation are influenced by the environmental cues (the sights and sounds asso-

Pre- and Postprocedure Behaviors

Behaviors	Usual for child	24 hours pre	Postprocedure
1. Affect	Y/N	pos. neu. neg.	pos. neu. neg.
2. Acting out physically	Y/N	nil. mod. ex.	nil. mod. ex.
3. Orientation	Y/N	self/others	self/others
4. Behavior	Y/N	pass./act.	pass./act.
5. Specific difficulties	Y/N	nau./eat./sleep/ other	nau./eat/sleep/ other

6. Specify major activity (e.g., TV)
   Pre _____
   Post _____

7. Specify unusual behaviors or difficulties
   Pre _____
   Post _____

8. Did the child do any of the following during the procedure?

	Yes	No
Cry	—	—
Stall	—	—
Refuse treatment	—	—
Converse normally	—	—
Use some pain control technique	—	—

FIGURE 2.1.   Behavioral checklist for children receiving invasive medical procedures in outpatient clinic.

ciated with invasive procedures), familial factors (parental responses and expectations), emotional factors (fear, anxiety, sadness), and situational factors (children's expectations, their control, the relevance of the scheduled medical or dental treatment). Parents exert a strong modifying influence on children's behaviors, particularly when children have a chronic or life-threatening disease. Parents may have difficulty adjusting to the illness and necessary medical treatments, with the result that they may place excessive demands on their children to be compliant and cope like "little adults" during invasive procedures. Children's natural responses (either verbal or nonverbal expressions of their emotions) may be restricted in stressful situations, so that their overt distress behaviors increase. Children's behaviors may then reflect their underlying emotions about a disease or medical procedure, rather than the strength or quality of the pain evoked by the procedure. Children's distress behaviors are not passive reflections of their pain. Their behaviors are complicated responses, dependent on the noxious stimulus in relation to the context in which it is perceived.

Although children's behaviors when they are experiencing acute pain do not constitute a precise measure of their pain, they can provide a quantitative index of their overt distress (Glennon & Weisz, 1978; LeBaron & Zeltzer, 1984; Piquard-Gauvain, Rodary, Rezvani, & Lemerle, 1984). For some children, their overt distress may be proportional to the perceived strength of the pain; for the majority of children, however, their overt distress is influenced by many other factors. Children's overt behaviors must be considered when evaluating their pain, because they provide valuable information about their responses in a stressful and pain-inducing situation and because certain behaviors can contribute to increased pain and emotional distress. However, when standardized behavioral scales are used to provide a numerical pain score, it is necessary to evaluate the validity of the designated pain behaviors for the children being assessed. Some behaviors that may indicate pain in one situation are not appropriate pain indices in another situation. For example, children may request emotional support and seek information about a medical procedure as positive coping strategies (as described in Chapter 7) and not as anxiety-related or pain-related behaviors.

Physiological Pain Measures

Several physiological changes that occur in response to a noxious stimulus have been investigated as objective pain measures. These include determining the latency, duration, or size of a reflex; recording the frequency or intensity of neuronal activity; monitoring physical parameters (e.g., heart rate, respiration rate, and skin resistance); and describing the patterns of electrical activity in the brain. Basic research on physiological pain measures generally involves the application of a controlled noxious stimulus to a healthy adult volunteer. The body's natural responses to different intensities or durations of the stimulus are correlated with the volunteer's subjective reports of pain to determine whether there is a characteristic body response coincident with the experience of pain. However, many of these basic psychophysical studies have failed to demonstrate that changes in the recorded physiological responses are related unequivocally to changes in human pain experience. The physiological responses evoked by a noxious stimulus are obviously related to the parameters of that stimulus (intensity, location, and duration), but the physiological responses may be more or less independent of the quality and strength of the final sensation produced by the noxious stimulus. Although the physiological responses and pain sensations are both initiated by the same noxious stimulus, they do not necessarily correlate consistently with one another.

As an example, the masseter inhibitory period, a protective reflex in the masseter muscle (a jaw-closing muscle) that can be evoked by a tap on the tooth or an electrical stimulus applied to the tooth, had been proposed as a physiological measure for pain sensation. However, psychophysical experiments subsequently demonstrated that the latency, duration, and configuration of the masseter inhibitory periods produced by electrical pulses applied to the teeth, when electrical pulses were perceived as painful, were not significantly different from those recorded after subjects received a narcotic, even though subjects reported significant reductions in their pain. As shown in Figure 2.2, when 30 pulses at 80 micro-

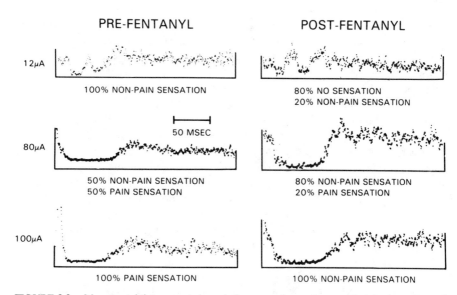

FIGURE 2.2. Masseter inhibitory periods and the type of sensations produced when electrical stimulation (a train of 30 pulses lasting 1 second each) was applied to the upper teeth of adult volunteers. Stimulus intensities of 12 μA, 80 μA, and 100 μA were applied before and after the intravenous administration of a short-acting narcotic, fentanyl. The percentages of the 30 pulses that were not detected, or that produced nonpainful or painful sensations, are shown below each trace. From "Masseter Inhibitory Periods and Sensations Evoked by Electrical Tooth Pulp Stimulation" by P. A. McGrath, Y. Sharav, R. Dubner, and R. H. Gracely, 1981, *Pain, 10*, p. 11. Copyright 1983 by Elsevier Science Publishers. Reprinted by permission.

amperes (μA) were administered to the teeth, the subjects reported that half the pulses produced pain sensations and the other half produced tingling nonpain sensations. When 30 pulses at 100 μA were administered, all pulses produced painful sensations. When the stimulation was repeated after the subjects received fentanyl, a short-acting narcotic, the 80-μA and 100-μA pulses produced predominantly nonpain sensations. However, the characteristics of the masseter reflex did not correlate with the change in pain perception. In this instance, the subjective reports of pain (shown below each reflex trace) provided a more accurate measure of pain than the masseter reflex (McGrath, Sharav, Dubner, & Gracely, 1981). When physiological responses are used as pain measures in children, it is essential to determine whether the responses reflect changes in children's pain experience or simply reflect some parameters of the noxious stimulus.

Infants

The physiological responses that have been studied in infants and children include heart rate, respiration rate, palmar sweating, cortisol and cortisone levels, transcutaneous oxygen pressure (PO_2) levels, and endorphin concentrations. Heart rate, the number of beats per unit of time, generally decreases when infants attend to or orient to a new stimulus and increases when they respond to a stressful or painful stimulus (Campos,1976; Campos, Emde, Gaensbauer, & Henderson, 1975; Wolff 1969). Several studies have indicated that the heart rate response to simple stimuli changes during the first few months of life (Clifton & Meyers, 1969; Clifton, Graham, & Hatton, 1968; Gray & Crowell, 1968; Lipton et al., 1965). Stimuli that produced accelerations in the heart rates of newborns produced decelerations in the heart rates of 2½- to 5-month-old infants, presumably as a result of the orienting responses of the older infants. Berg, Berg, and Graham (1971) showed that infants' heart rate responses to auditory stimuli depends on whether they were alert or sleeping, as well as on the intensity and rise time of the stimulus. Heart rate changes in response to a noxious stimulus would probably also depend on infants' alert states, their general orienting responses, and the stimulus intensity. Williamson and Williamson (1983) showed that heart rate was significantly lower for neonates who received penile nerve blocks for circumcision than for those who received no type of anesthesia, indicating that the infants were less stressed and presumably experienced less pain. Owens and Todt (1984) reported that infants' heart rates rose in response to heel lance during routine blood sampling procedures. Johnston and Strada (1986) found that infants initially responded to acute pain evoked by injections by a brief decrease in their heart rates (for about 6 seconds), with subsequent elevations to tachycardic levels. However, as infants recovered from the painful injections with a progressive return to their at-rest body position, their heart rates remained elevated. Heart rate acceleration alone is not a sufficient index of an infant's pain, since not all studies show the same positive relationship between heart rate and pain- or stress-inducing stimuli (Field, 1982; Obrist, Light, & Hastrup, 1982; Scarr & Salapatek, 1970; Scarr-Salapatek, 1976). Instead, heart rate may be most appropriate as part of an assessment battery in which physiological and behavioral methods are integrated for a multivariate approach to infant pain measurement.

The palmar sweating response increases significantly during heel prick in infants and decreases to prebaseline levels as infants recover from the noxious stimuli (Harpin & Rutter, 1982). This characteristic increase in palmar sweating led Harpin and Rutter to evaluate the painfulness associated with different methods of obtaining blood samples by heel pricks, in order to select the method that produced the lowest sweat increase and presumably the least distress in infants (Harpin & Rutter, 1983). Although palmar sweating has not been studied extensively as a specific pain measure in infants, this response can provide a useful correlate for assessing infants' distress states. Future research should examine how palmar sweating changes for the variety of noxious stimuli that infants may receive during hospitalization, as well as how palmar sweating changes for novel innocuous auditory, visual, and tactile stimuli that infants experience. These studies would provide valuable information as to whether the palmar response is related to their pain experience or to their general physiological arousal.

In a number of studies, the elevations in plasma cortisol that occurred in response to circumcision in newborns were positively correlated with their distress behaviors (Anders, Sachar, Kream, Roffwarg, & Hellman, 1971; Gunnar, Fisch, Korsvik, & Donhowe, 1981; Gunnar, Isensee, & Fust, 1987; Gunnar, Malone, Vance, & Fisch, 1985; Talbert, Kraybill, & Potter, 1976; Tennes & Carter, 1973). Similar positive correlations between plasma cortisol levels and overt distress were reported when infants received heel lance blood-sampling procedures (Gunnar, 1986; Gunnar, Wall, & DeBoer, 1985). The increased cortisol levels presumably reflected the effect of the stress or pain on the infants' systems. Gunnar and colleagues also measured cortisol levels when infants were soothed during circumcisions and during blood-sampling procedures. The soothing significantly reduced infants' behavioral distress, but did not reduce their cortisol levels (Gunnar, 1986; Gunnar, Fisch, & Malone, 1984). In fact, the magnitude of cortisol elevations that occurred in response to innocuous stimulation (e.g., weighing, measuring, or discharge examinations) in infants was similar to that induced by noxious stimulation (Gunnar, Wall, & DeBoer, 1985). Cortisol levels may have been interpreted inaccurately as physiological measures for arousal related to infants' pain experiences. Cortisol levels change in response to both external and internal events that create some demands for infants; infants may not be able to respond immediately to reduce the demands. The cortisol elevation may reflect the size of the mobilization of the infants' resources required to meet the demand. Since the ability to meet physical (e.g., from noxious stimuli) and psychological (e.g., from stress of handling) demands changes with infants' development, situations that seem to place similar external demands on infants and children may actually constitute very different internal demands for children at different levels of development (Gunnar, 1986).

The majority of research on physiological pain measures has been conducted in infants. As reviewed, the results of these studies indicate that no one physiological measure constitutes a pure pain measure in infants. Instead, the physiological parameters that have been studied represent complex body responses to stress-inducing stimulation. In order to determine which physiological parameters may represent pain responses, it is necessary to conduct research studies on infants' responses to novel or stressful non-pain-inducing stimuli, such as visual, auditory, or tactile stimuli, and to determine which physiological responses are specific to noxious stimuli and which responses may be common to all novel or stressful situations.

Children

Although fewer studies have been conducted to evaluate physiological measures of pain in children than in infants, research has been conducted to identify physiological measures of anxiety and distress. Melamed and Siegel (1975) demonstrated that the palmar sweat response was a useful measure of children's pre- and postoperative anxiety. Sweating increased proportional to children's anxiety level.

Later, Jay et al. (1983) found that increases in pulse rate and blood pressure were reliable indices of children's distress level prior to bone marrow aspirations. However, it is not yet known whether the physiological changes children experience prior to and during noxious stimulation are indicators of their general emotional distress or their pain experience.

The recent interest in endogenous pain-inhibitory systems has led to investigations of beta-endorphin immunoreactivity as possible correlates for children's pain experience. Katz et al. (1982) and my colleagues and I (McGrath, Hargreaves, Dionne, & deVeber, in preparation) measured beta-endorphin immunoreactivity in the spinal fluid of children with leukemia. Cerebrospinal fluid (CSF) samples were obtained during children's lumbar punctures, and the beta-endorphin values were compared with observational and self-report measures of children's pain. Katz et al. (1982) found that endorphin concentrations correlated moderately with the nurses' ratings of children's distress during the procedure, but were not consistently related to children's pain reports. Similarly, in our study, despite wide variability in endorphin concentrations (probably due to differences in children's ages, time on the cancer treatment protocol, and the number of previous lumbar punctures), there was a positive correlation between parental ratings of children's anxiety and children's endorphin concentrations. These results suggest that as children's anxiety increased (as measured by their overt distress behaviors), their endorphin concentration increased. In our study, children's endorphin concentrations were monitored at each of the lumbar punctures they received throughout a 36-month period. Their concentrations often changed consistently throughout this period, independently of changes in their pain reports. Although there is evidence for a positive relationship between children's overt behavioral distress (usually the basis for parental and nurses' ratings of children's anxiety) and endorphin concentrations in CSF, there is no firm evidence that a positive relationship exists between children's pain levels during lumbar punctures and their endorphin levels. In order to determine the possible nature of the relationsip betwen beta-endorphin concentration and acute pain, anxiety, and distress during lumbar punctures, it is necessary to collect and analyze CSF samples routinely throughout children's treatment and identify variations in endorphin levels that may be due to children's ages, weights, time on treatment, treatment protocols, and general stress levels. We noted that several children who relapsed while on treatment had significantly elevated endorphin levels during the months prior to their deaths. These increases were not systematically related to children's distress, anxiety, or pain; they probably reflected the general physiological effects of their disease.

Szyfelbein and colleagues (Szyfelbein & Osgood, 1984; Szyfelbein, Osgood, Atchison, & Carr, 1987; Szyfelbein, Osgood, & Carr, 1985) examined the relationship between plasma levels of beta-endorphin and pain reports in 15 acutely burned children during their necessary debridement procedures. They measured plasma levels at several intervals before and after the treatment. Children used the scale shown in Figure 2.3 to rate their pain at 1-minute intervals throughout the

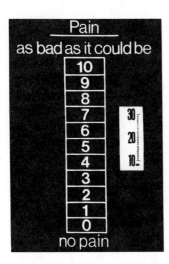

FIGURE 2.3. A pain thermometer used to assess pain in acutely burned children during dressing changes. The figures are white on a crimson background. From "The Assessment of Pain and Plasma β-Endorphin Immunoactivity in Burned Children" by S. K. Szyfelbein, P. F. Osgood, and D. B. Carr, 1985, *Pain*, 22, p. 175. Copyright 1985 by Elsevier Science Publishers. Reprinted by permission.

procedure. Children's mean pain scores were inversely related to their plasma levels of beta-endorphin immunoreactivity, indicating that their pain decreased as their plasma endorphin levels increased. It is still not clear, however, whether the plasma endorphin level represented children's distress and pain during the debridement procedure or represented a conditioned physiological response that occurred in advance of the painful procedure. In order to conclude unequivocally that plasma endorphin levels constitute objective pain measures, it is necessary to demonstrate that they change when analgesics are administered and that they are not elevated prior to the painful procedure. The results of these studies on beta-endorphins in plasma and CSF are not necessarily contradictory. Changes in beta-endorphin level in one fluid system are not always reflected by similar changes in other systems. Szyfelbein et al. (1985) suggest that circulating plasma levels of beta-endorphin may reflect a concurrent central response to stress that involves endogenous opioid systems and that may lead to stress-induced analgesia. This interpretation is consistent with their finding of an inverse relationship between endorphin level and pain.

In summary, several physiological responses have been studied in infants and children as potential pain measures. Evidence indicates that physiological responses mirror the state of the infant or child in a stressful and painful situation. Thus, physiological responses are often positively correlated with self-report indices of pain. However, there is insufficient evidence to conclude that physiological responses correlate directly with pain experience. Instead, some physiological changes occur in direct response to the quality, intensity, and duration of a noxious stimulus; other changes occur in response to the child's stress and reactions to that stimulus. Physiological responses do not passively reflect a child's perception of pain evoked by a noxious stimulus.

Psychological Pain Measures

Behavioral and physiological pain measures do not provide sufficient information about the nature of children's pain experiences. Information about the quality, intensity, location, duration, and affective dimensions of children's pain can only be obtained by objectively evaluating their subjective experiences. Psychological pain measures are methods that assess children's perceptions or their psychological experience of pain. These include a diverse array of projective methods, in which children's attitudes or perceptions of pain are inferred from their selections of colors, their drawings, and their interpretations of cartoons; they also include several self-report methods, in which children directly describe their attitudes and perceptions of pain (Abu-Saad & Holzmer, 1981; Beales, 1982; Beyer & Knapp, 1986; Eland, 1983; Jacox, 1980; Jeans, 1983b; Jerrett, 1985; Petrovich, 1957; Pothman & Goepel, 1984; Savedra, Tesler, Ward, Holzemer, & Wilkie, 1987; Savedra, Tesler, Ward, Wegner, & Gibbons, 1981; Tesler, Savedra, Ward, Holzemer, & Wilkie, 1988).

Projective Methods

Colors

Stewart (1977) developed a pain scale that initially consisted of all the colors in the visible spectrum, a linear continuum from yellow–orange to red–black. Subjects adjusted a pointer along the continuum to indicate the color that best represented pain. The color red was most often chosen by people to describe pain. Stewart later developed a projective technique in order to assess the emotional tone accompanying pain. The instrument consists of a set of six figures, each figure consisting of two concentric circles with varying diameters of red and black, to denote the intensity (red) and affective (black) dimensions for pain. This color scale represents the first projective tool for assessing two dimensions of pain. Stewart recognized the importance of assessing the emotional or suffering dimension of pain, particularly for pain associated with life-threatening diseases. The different proportions of intensity and affect depicted by the different proportions of red and black comprising the circles are more useful as a measure of clinical pain than the simple choice of one color. Stewart's development of a color scale provided the basis for later studies that examined children's use of colors to depict their pain.

   Eland (1974) examined children from 4 to 10 years of age with Stewart's first color scale. Red, black, and purple were the most common colors used by children to depict pain. She later constructed another color scale, the Eland Color Tool, in which children construct their own color scale from eight crayons, choosing which colors represent different levels of hurt from "no hurt at all" to "worst hurt." Children then use the crayons to color a body outline, differentiating different areas of pain (Eland, 1982; Eland & Anderson, 1977).

Drawings

Children's drawings can provide valuable information about the feelings associated with their pain, as well as information about their pain experiences. Jeans and Gordon (1981) asked 54 healthy children from 5 to 13 years old to draw pictures that showed pain. They used five markers in colors of blue, black, red, yellow, and green. Children were interviewed later to discuss their drawings and to obtain information about their previous pain experiences, their pain language, and their coping abilities. The investigators then coded the pictures according to their content; the colors used; and the type, source, and intention of the pain (Jeans, 1983a). The majority of children (88.9%) drew a person or part of a person as the subject of pain; the pains were generally localized in the limbs and head. Red and black were chosen most frequently to represent the pain. Physical pain was depicted in 88.7% of the drawings, whereas emotional pain was depicted in only 5.6%. The source of the pain was classified as self-inflicted (44.2%), other-inflicted (38.5%), or inflicted by a natural or unspecified source (17.3%). Pictures of self-inflicted pain decreased with age; pictures of other-inflicted pain increased with age. The intention of pain (accidental or purposeful) also varied with age, in that accidental pain was most prevalent in the pictures of younger children. Jeans and Gordon's research is the first study to interpret children's understanding of pain by relating their drawings to the relevant factors that can modify pain perceptions. Scoring systems were derived after consideration of children's pictures to provide practical and meaningful codes for analysis. This method and basic coding system could be easily incorporated in subsequent developmental and cross-cultural studies on children's pain perceptions.

Children's drawings of painful situations will parallel their actual painful experiences and their emotional responses in those situations, as well as the type of interventions that are used. Although drawings do not provide a quantitative measure for assessing children's pain level in the clinic, they provide a qualitative measure for assessing children's understanding and their frame of reference— that is, their previous pain experiences and their abilities to cope in painful situations. DiLeo (1977) found that children were able to communicate more openly through their drawings than through their conversations. More recently, a team of investigators (Kurylyszn, McGrath, Capelli, & Humphreys, 1986; Unruh, McGrath, Cunningham, & Humphreys, 1983) reported that the details shown in children's drawings of their migraine headaches provided a valuable clinical tool for understanding their pain experiences. However, no studies have specifically compared the nature, reliability, or validity of information about children's pain that is inferred from their drawings with that obtained from their direct self-reports in structured interviews and from their responses on standardized pain inventories.

Cartoons

Cartoon inventories have been designed as structured projective tools to evaluate children's pain attitudes and to compare pain perceptions among children of different ages or health groups. Scott (1978) used illustrative cartoons to measure the sensory, cognitive, and affective factors associated with children's pain perceptions. Children from 4 to 10 years old described the pain depicted in two cartoons according to color, texture, shape, pattern, and continuous or intermittent quality. Later, Lollar, Smits, and Patterson (1982) developed the Pediatric Pain Inventory, a set of 24 cartoon pictures depicting potentially painful situations in four settings: medical, recreational, common activities of daily living, and psychosocial. A total of 240 children and adolescents, ranging in age from 4 to 19, were first asked a series of forced-choice demographic questions in order to obtain information about number of hospitalizations, illnesses, and school attendance in relation to illness. Children then examined the figures depicted in the 24 pain situations. They were asked, first, who was responsible for the situation presented; second, whether the youngster depicted needed assistance; third, who would provide the assistance; and fourth, what would be done. After responding to these questions, each child rated the pictures according to the perceived intensity and duration of the pain. Intensity of pain was measured by sorting the pictures in terms of a three-color scale, with red, yellow, and green representing "much," "some," and "little" pain, respectively. Children also selected the pain intensity group that represented the most hurt that they had experienced, the most that their mothers had experienced, and the most that their fathers had experienced.

Lollar et al. (1982) examined the relationship between adults' perception of children's pain intensity and the children's own perceptions. Adults consistently underestimated the intensity of children's reactions. Children's pain ratings were also evaluated as a function of the intensity of their own previous pain experiences. Children who reported little pain experience rated all categories of pain as more painful than did children who had experienced much previous pain. These findings support the hypothesis that children's pain ratings of usual and common pain experiences decrease with maturation as they experience more frequent and diverse pain experiences. Each child evaluates a new pain against his/her previous pain experiences. As the diversity and intensity of pain experiences increase, then pains that are more common will tend to be perceived as less strong or less unpleasant. Although this structured inventory shows promise, numerical values were assigned to the different color responses to represent different pain scores. But these values may not accurately represent differences in children's pain perceptions, so that the specific quantitative differences among pain values derived from this pain scale may be ambiguous.

Eland (1974) developed a set of five cartoons as a projective tool for assessing pain in hospitalized children. The cartoons depicted a dog in various painful situations (resting, being bumped in the nose by a swing, falling off its doghouse, bumping its head, having a paw slammed in a car door, and in a medical situation analogous to that of the hospitalized child). Twenty-five children with varying medical problems rank-ordered the pictures according to the intensity of pain depicted by each situation. Although all children were able to recognize that the dog was in pain, they did not rank-order the pictures in the same sequence, suggesting that the perceived pain intensity varied among children. Eland also presented a revised series of cartoons to another group of hospitalized children, who again did not rank-order the pictures similarly. However, each child's ranking was consistent during repeated testing, indicating that children did order the pictures subjectively, according to their own pain experience.

Although projective methods for assessing pain seem particularly suited for use with small children and for use in cross-cultural developmental studies, few methods have been rigorously evaluated. In fact, much of the research on projective methods for assessing pediatric pain has failed to demonstrate how qualitative differences in children's responses constitute quantitative differences in their pain attitudes, experiences, or expressions. At the present time, projective methods may be most valuable as part of an individual pain assessment to provide information about children's general understanding of pain and their methods for coping with pain. More research is necessary to determine how children's responses may vary according to their age, sex, and pain history, as in Jeans and Gordon's (1981) analysis of children's drawings, so that coding schemes can be developed to allow more meaningful comparisons among children and to facilitate an evaluation of the efficacy of different therapeutic modalities.

Direct Measures

Direct psychological measures of children's pain include verbal self-reports, structured interviews, questionnaires, visual analog scales, and various interval scales (e.g., poker chips representing pieces of hurt, faces varying in emotional expression, or pain thermometers graded in intensity). The common purpose for these measures is to obtain objective information about children's subjective pain experience. Children can directly describe many aspects of their pain experience and their coping abilities in their own words. They also can use quantifiable scales to depict the magnitude of their pain sensations. Direct pain measures potentially provide the most comprehensive information about children's perceptions. However, the reliability, validity, and determination of scale type (nominal, ordinal, interval, or ratio) for children's pain measures have not always been determined. The assumption that the ruler-like divisions on a pain measure represent equivalent differences in subjective pain perception has not always been examined for children. The type of scale produced by a pain measure is an essential consideration when evaluating children's pain and determining analgesic efficacy.

Self-Reports

Since pain is a multidimensional experience, methods for pain assessment in children should be multidimensional, providing information not only about the sensory dimensions of their pain (the quality, severity, location, and duration), but also about relevant situational and emotional factors. Children's verbal descriptions of their pain episodes, their feelings, their expectations, and their perceived control provide necessary information to identify the environmental and internal factors that may exacerbate their pain. This information is critical for the design of an optimal pain management program for a child. As described in Chapter 1, children do not necessarily perceive the same pain from the same pain-inducing stimulus. It is necessary to observe and to listen to children in order to understand which factors are influencing their pain perceptions.

Clearly, children's verbal descriptions of their pain may be biased. Hospitalized children may report that they have strong pain, in order to obtain analgesics more promptly from medical staff; conversely, they may deny that they have pain, in order to delay painful analgesic administrations. However, usually children's response biases may be modified so that they can respond accurately and openly about their pain. When relevant situational and emotional factors are evaluated, in addition to the frequency or strength of their pain complaints, it is often possible to identify why children's pain reports are biased. For example, hospitalized children may perceive that their pain medication does not arrive promptly when they need it. Their subsequent fear of increased pain may lead them to request medication more frequently or to complain more vociferously about the strength of their pain. Information about dosing intervals and children's voiced pain complaints can be obtained from reviewing medical charts. Information about children's motivations and fears can be obtained in brief interviews with children and their families. Since children perceive much of their medical treatment as unpredictable and beyond their control, their expectations for obtaining appropriate pain relief may be extremely low. When unpredictability, lack of control, and lowered expectations for pain relief are affecting children's pain or pain reports, a concrete charting system can be designed to enable them to follow the time course for their medication. The simple system, which they can help to draw with their parents, provides them with a sense of increased control and higher expectations for pain relief. The initiation of charts on which children and parents can easily follow the course of analgesic administration and invasive medical treatments can often minimize their response bias in reporting pain.

Children who minimize their pain reports because they fear more painful analgesic administrations often respond to a brief educational program in which they learn about the various factors that can increase or decrease their pain. They then rate their pain and consequent physical limitations at various intervals throughout the day. The objective of this program is to help children identify any natural variations in their pain, such as after participation in child life activities, during meals, during play with other children, and after analgesic administration. (This program is described in more detail in Chapters 6 and 7.) At the same time, children can learn simple strategies to use during injections and can gain some control about the choice of the type of administration or the site for an injection. This educational approach can minimize children's response biases in verbally reporting pain by providing them with a framework for understanding and coping with their treatments. The fear of pain is often greater than the actual pain produced by an injection, particularly when children assist their nurses in preparing the injection site and use simple techniques to help reduce the pain produced during the injection. When children realize from their own experience that they have much less pain after a brief injection when injections are a predictable part of their treatment and when they can reduce the pain induced by the injection, the children generally will not bias their pain reports.

Response biases, either exaggerating or minimizing pain, are also a potential problem for children with recurrent or chronic pain. However, if a comprehensive pain assessment is conducted for such children in which the situational, familial, and emotional factors that contribute to the children's pain and their pain behaviors are evaluated, it is possible to determine the extent to which children's fears about further medical treatment or their motivations to avoid school or familial responsibilities may bias their verbal pain reports. The key to determining the reliability and validity of children's pain information is to evaluate the context in which children perceive their pain. An understanding of their frame of reference for reporting pain, and of the factors that may influence their pain and their pain behaviors, enables health professionals to accurately interpret children's descriptions of their pain.

Interviews

Children's interviews have traditionally had a minor role in pain assessment, largely because of assumptions that children cannot provide reliable and valid information about their medical problems. Yet the interview is ideally suited to the assessment of children's understanding of their pain, as well as the factors that influence it. Information about the perceived cause, the treatments required, the prognosis for a medical condition, the reactions of family members or friends, and children's own expectations and attitudes toward the treatment can be obtained in a brief structured format. A "structured format" is a set of standard questions addressed to all children in a similar manner. A structured format ensures that all children will be interviewed in a consistent manner to obtain similar information about their pain problem and the manner in which the pain affects their lives and families. A "semistructured format" enables the interviewer to obtain the same information in a consistent manner from all children, but also in a flexible manner, so that any individually relevant aspects of a pain problem may be discussed in depth with each child.

Several structured interviews with age-appropriate pain questionnaires have been designed to assess children's knowledge about pain. Schultz (1971) interviewed 74 children aged 10 and 11 about the feelings that they associated with pain and the meanings that they attached to pain. The predominant meanings for children were fear of bodily harm, death, and anxiety. Tesler, Ward, Savedra, Wegner, and Gibbons (1983) later extended this research to investigate the types of coping strategies children used when they experienced pain. Their Pediatric Pain Questionnaire included eight questions about children's actual pain experiences, the words they used to describe pain, the colors associated with pain, the emotions they experienced with pain, their worst pain experiences, the ways they coped with pain, the positive aspects of pain, and the location of their current pain. The final form of the questionnaire was administered to 12 hospitalized children aged 9–12. Children were clearly able to identify, remember, and describe a wide range of painful events.

Although children can communicate directly about their pain in interviews, a question arises as to the best format for a structured interview or pain questionnaires. After completing semistructured interviews with 994 children aged 5–12 concerning their concepts, knowledge, and understanding of pain, their pain language, and their coping strategies, Ross and Ross (1984a, 1984c) described the three components critical for an accurate interview. These components are the type of question used, the psychological climate in the interview situation, and the child's perceptions of his/her role and capabilities. A comprehensive interview should consist of both a "generate" and a "supplied" format. The generate format requires children to generate or provide information (e.g., "What do you do to lessen your headache?"). This format is appropriate when children's opinions, attitudes, beliefs, and expectations are sought. The supplied format requires children to choose among certain supplied responses (e.g., "Which words best describe your headache pain?"). This format is appropriate when factual information about pain characteristics or children's life events is sought. As described by Ross and Ross (1984a, 1984c), the generate approach is far superior to the supplied format in terms of the quality and extent of information that can be obtained. The major drawback for the generate format in research studies of pediatric pain is that a great many children must be interviewed in order to know how to classify or code their responses. The supplied format is much more convenient for data collection, yet this format limits the type of information that the interviewer will receive. Examples of supplied and generate questions included on a questionnaire for chronic and recurrent pain (the Children's Comprehensive Pain Questionnaire, or CCPQ) are shown in Figure 2.4.

Gaffney (1984) used a generate format when she interviewed 600 children (30 boys and 30 girls at each age from 5 to 14 years old) about their understanding of pain. Her 10 questions were constructed to elicit children's natural definitions for

Do you usually have any warning that you are going to get a headache?
   Yes ___ No ___ Sometimes ___
Verbatim response: _____
When you have a headache, what else is happening to your body? (Note: After child
answers, specifically ask about nausea, dizziness, weakness, aura.)

_____

_____
_____

Where is your pain located? Tell me and then show me on your body.

_____

(Check areas)	Head:	Frontal	Abdominal:	Upper	Limb:	Arm
		Parietal		Lower		Leg
		Temporal		Left		Left
		Occipital		Right		Right
		Eyes				
		Other				

What words describe your pain? _____

(Prompt, after response:)
Sharp ___ Aching ___ Stinging ___ Hammering ___ Dull ___
Throbbing ___ Burning ___ Pounding ___ Cutting ___
When you have a headache, is your pain

steady (the same)?	usually,	always,	sometimes,	never
up and down?	usually,	always,	sometimes,	never
increasing (getting bigger)?	usually,	always,	sometimes,	never

When you have a headache, is there a time in the day or night when the pain is worse?
(Inquire, after response, about waking up, morning, afternoon, bedtime, and meals.) ___

_____
_____
_____

FIGURE 2.4. Supplied and generate questions from the Children's Comprehensive Pain Questionnaire (CCPQ), used to assess recurrent and chronic pain in children from 5 to 17 years old. (For a version of the full questionnaire, see the Appendix to this book.)

pain and their beliefs about the causes, cures, and subjective experience of pain. A classification system was developed by analyzing the content and themes expressed in children's verbatim answers (Gaffney & Dunn, 1986). Children's understanding of pain followed a developmental pattern, consistent with Piagetian theory (see Chapter 1 for further discussion).

   Two structured interviews and pain questionnaire formats that have been developed recently are the Varni–Thompson Pediatric Pain Questionnaire (VTPPQ) and the CCPQ, mentioned above. The VTPPQ is completed independently by the child, parent, and physician. It includes visual analog scales, color-coded rating scales, and verbal descriptors to provide information about the sensory, affective, and evaluative dimensions of children's chronic pain (Varni, Thompson, & Hanson, 1987). The scale has been initially evaluated for 25 children

(4-19 years old) with juvenile rheumatoid arthritis. The VTPPQ also provides information about the child's and family's pain history, symptomatology, pain relief interventions, and socioenvironmental situations that may influence pain.

The CCPQ consists of generate and supplied format questions, as well as quantitative visual analog and affective facial scales to assess multiple dimensions of children's recurrent or chronic pain. The CCPQ provides quantitative information about the sensory dimensions of children's pain (i.e., intensity, quality, duration, frequency, and location), emotional factors, and situational factors (the children's expectations for obtaining future pain relief, their ability to control the pain independently and with pharmacological intervention, and the relevance of the pain to their lives). Qualitative information is obtained about children's perceptions of the positive and negative consequences of their pain; their reliance on themselves, parents, or medication during painful episodes; their identification of probable causative factors; the nature and diversity of their pain-coping strategies; the children's pain history and pain behaviors; the parents' criteria for evaluating the presence and intensity of their children's pain; the number and efficacy of pain reduction methods used; the parents' own pain history; and the parents' and siblings' responses to the children during painful episodes. The CCPQ has been used with 300 children (aged 5-16) who experienced recurrent headaches, abdominal pains, limb pains, and various other chronic pains. Initial validity and reliability studies indicate that the questionnaire and the structured interviews provide an accurate, thorough, and objective assessment for many dimensions of children's pain. A version of the CCPQ is given in the Appendix to this volume.

When one is interviewing children about their acute, recurrent, or chronic pain experiences, it is quite misleading to use only a supplied format. Although there are features common to a particular type of pain (e.g., arthritic pain), there are other features that are unique for each child. A supplied format will not provide information about the unique aspects of children's pain. Health professionals may sometimes question children to confirm a medical diagnosis after they have already interviewed parents about the pain complaints. They use a supplied format to inquire about the presence or absence of various symptoms, and may not provide children with an opportunity to elaborate about their painful condition. Since pain is not simply an accompanying symptom of disease that disappears as the disease is treated, valuable information that may be used to understand and control children's pain is never obtained. The interview must be conducted in a comfortable atmosphere for children—an atmosphere in which they feel that their information is valuable for the interviewer's eventual understanding of the cause of their pain and for the selection of an appropriate treatment. As an example, our pain assessments for children with recurrent headaches begin with a brief and age-appropriate description of the pain research program, the major dramatic changes in our understanding about the plasticity and complexity of pain mechanisms (see Chapter 3), and information that research on children's headaches from the children's own perspective is relatively new. In fact, the pain management program in our clinic is the direct result of combining what we know about nociceptive systems with what we have learned during the past few years from the children and families themselves. During the individual interviews, children are first asked to explain the purpose of the assessment, in order to ensure that they have an accurate and realistic perception of the procedures. They are reminded that their answers will be confidential and will not be repeated to their parents. In order to maintain a comfortable and relaxed interview, we space questions so that difficult or emotionally arousing items are interspersed with easier items. Children should not feel attacked by a barrage of questions about a chronic or recurrent pain. These questions are necessary, but other topics may and often should be introduced informally to provide children with a brief rest if they become tired or discouraged.

Structured or semistructured interviews should be incorporated into all clinical pain assessments. The principal questions necessary to assess situational, familial, and emotional factors relevant to children's pain, as well as the sensory dimensions of their pain, can be included in a general format that is applicable for all types of children's pain. Additional questions or items can then be added to provide information that is unique to a particular type of pain.

Two basic semistructured interviews and pain questionnaires have evolved from the assessment and management of children referred for various pain complaints to our pain clinic. Children referred for management of acute pain evoked by medical procedures are interviewed in a format different from that used with children referred for management of recurrent or chronic pain. Yet the main objectives of both types of interviews are similar—that is, to collect information about children's previous pain experiences, their understanding of their medical condition and necessary treatments or their pain syndrome, and their coping abilities; and to identify the situational, familial, and emotional factors that affect their pain. In addition, children complete standardized inventories to evaluate their attitudes about pain in comparison with those of other children of the same age, sex, and health status. An outline of these assessment procedures is shown in Table 2.2.

TABLE 2.2.   Principal Features of the Pain Interview

Presenting pain problem	*Situational factors*
History	Child's learned pain behaviors
Intensity	Clinical environment
Frequency	Child's understanding of pain
Location	Child's expectations
Duration	Child's perceived control
Therapeutic interventions	Relevance of disease or pain-inducing stimuli
Pharmacological	*Contributing environmental factors*
Nonpharmacological	School
Role of parents and siblings	Peers
	Physical activities

The interviews are described in more detail in Chapters 7, 8, and 9, since they provide the framework for the management of acute, recurrent, and chronic pain, respectively. Information obtained from interviews and the use of standardized questionnaires can provide a comprehensive pain assessment for use in designing a treatment program. A sample pain report is included here for a child who was referred for the management of recurrent headaches.

PAIN ASSESSMENT REPORT

A. B. is a 13-year-old girl who was referred to the Paediatric Pain Programme by Dr. X. to participate in a study of recurrent headache pain syndrome. A. B. and Mrs. B. were seen on 24 February 1987 for a pain assessment.

A. B. was nervous and fidgety throughout the assessment. She was limited in her understanding of what happens to her during headache pain experiences. She became very frustrated with questions that she perceived as difficult. She has been experiencing one severe headache every 3 months and one to two mild headaches weekly for the past 11 years. The severe headaches last a minimum of 5 days. In the past year, her headache pain duration has increased to a maximum of 14 days. A. B. is able to differentiate between the two headache types. Her common headaches are dull, aching, and occur all over her head, while her less frequent headaches are sharp, throbbing, accompanied by dizziness, incoordination, nausea, vomiting, photophobia, and sonophobia. A. B. has taken a variety of medications, such as Inderal and Fiorinal, with minimum pain relief. She feels that she has no control over her pain. She is completely incapacitated during severe pain episodes. During mild episodes, she is able to continue with her usual activities. A. B. reports that her headaches usually start in the morning; the pain increases until noon. She is unsure of what may trigger her headaches, although she suggested that certain foods or weather conditions may precipitate them. She is now avoiding many foods that she associates with headache occurrence. She also identified parties, dances, concerts, school, and other events that are noisy as headache triggers. She also experiences frequent stomach pain.

A. B.'s scores on the Anxiety Inventory indicate that she is more anxious than most girls her age. Her scores on other standardized measures indicate that depression, preoccupation with sickness, anxiety, and social problems may be contributing to her pain experiences. Her scores on the Family Assessment Measure indicate that inadequate communication and emotional expression are problems within her family.

Mrs. B. had difficulty completing assessment measures. She was reluctant to complete measures regarding family functioning. She reports that A. B. has been experiencing frequent abdominal cramps. She also experienced frequent back pain at age 8, which she no longer experiences. Mrs. B. identified weather conditions (especially hot temperatures), noise, siblings, anger, fear, parties, dances, movies, physical activity, fatigue, mental concentration, tests, and the school bus as headache triggers. A. B. tries to avoid foods and situations that are known triggers. Overall, Mrs. B. identifies stress related to high social and academic goals and expectations as a primary factor precipitating her daughter's headaches. A. B. works hard at maintaining peer relationships and her academic standing. In doing so, she often becomes worried and excessively concerned about her performance. Mrs. B. describes

A. as having low self-esteem, in that she is very worried about the opinion of other children at school. She describes other family members as being unable to admit mistakes or to accept another's point of view.

These characteristics do not allow for an adaptive discussion or resolution of stressful problems. The family moved to Canada 3 years ago. They have found it difficult to adjust to the different climate and culture. A. B. has experienced some peer and school problems since she first arrived. Mr. and Mrs. B. are attempting to ignore pain complaints and praise normal functioning. A. is no longer allowed to stay at home with a headache or call home from school for permission to return home. This has increased her ability to cope adaptively with her headache pain.

Recommendations and Conclusions

A. B. has been experiencing headache pain since she was 2 years old (duration of 11 years). She differentiates between two headache types. Her usual headache is a mild, dull, and aching pain. The less frequent headaches are severe, sharp, and throbbing. These headaches are accompanied by nausea, vomiting, dizziness, incoordination, photophobia, and sonophobia. These descriptions are characteristic of both tension and migraine headaches. There are several situational, familial, and emotional factors contributing to A.'s headache pain experiences. She has probably developed a number of learned or conditioned environmental stimuli as headache triggers, particularly foods and weather conditions. (In their search to understand headache pain occurrences, children often associate a neutral stimulus with headache occurrence, so that the neutral stimulus can eventually trigger a headache because of the children's anxiety about that stimulus. Parents' responses may reinforce headache occurrence, in that they reduce their expectations for the children and their responsibilities during headaches. The headaches then allow the children to avoid unpleasant situations for long periods of time.) There is stress related to the B. family's move to Canada. The entire family has had difficulty adjusting to the new culture and climate. A. has experienced peer and school problems. Emotional factors, such as low self-esteem, depression, and preoccupation with sickness, as well as her inability to identify, discuss, and resolve stressful problems, also contribute to her recurrent pain experiences. A.'s stomach pain may also represent a recurrent pain syndrome.

Consequently, it is recommended that A. participate in a headache pain management program to modify the factors that are contributing to her headaches and to teach her some nonpharmacological methods of pain control. If it becomes evident that familial and emotional factors represent long-standing problems, she will be referred to the appropriate counseling agency. It is important that the underlying factors that precipitate her headaches be addressed. If they are not, she will continue to experience headaches and may develop new somatic complaints.

Structured pediatric interviews are limited to the extent that children must be able to comprehend specific questions and communicate verbally with the interviewer. However, they should not be restricted to specific answers or response categories. Although a limited choice of possible answers is convenient for research data analysis, it limits the quality of information that the interviewer receives from a child or parent. The interviewer must be trained to pursue hesitant or superficial responses, in order to elicit the most accurate and thorough information about a child's pain experience. Interviewers cannot simply check off appropriate responses on a structured interview and obtain a true picture of children's pain. They must listen, guide, think, and elicit as much information as possible. Although the design and standardization of brief, structured interviews may be geared toward an objective assessment of the symptoms, emotional reactions, and behaviors associated with children's pain problems, such interviews must be administered by trained and conscientious individuals.

Pain Rating Scales

Children's self-reports and interviews provide a basic framework for conducting clinical pain assessments prior to designing appropriate treatment programs, as well as for conducting research studies about developmental aspects of children's pain perceptions. However, some basic quantifiable scales must also be used to measure the level of children's pain directly, in order to evaluate the efficacy of different therapeutic treatments. Quantitative pain scales for children include category scales, graded thermometers, facial scales, and visual analog scales. Children select a level on the scale that describes their pain. The numerical values associated with the different levels on these scales are usually selected by adults. Rating scales vary according to the type (words, poker chips, faces, numbers) and the number of levels that are included. Rating scales that include a discrete number of levels (e.g., no pain, slight pain, mild pain, moderate pain, strong pain) are described as "category scales." The common problem in interpreting children's pain from their responses on rating scales is that the pain scores derived from children's responses are often based on numbers that were arbitrarily assigned by the investigator (e.g., no pain equals 1; mild pain equals 2; moderate pain equals 3) and may not reflect true differences in children's pain levels. The perceptual change between scores of 1 and 2 (no pain and mild pain) may not be the same as the change between scores of 2 and 3 (mild pain and moderate pain). Yet the numbers are often interpreted as if they represent absolute and accurate amounts of children's pain. Similarly, a pain level scored as 4 may not represent four times the strength of a pain scored as 1; again, however, pain scores are usually treated as though they represent numbers on an interval or ratio scale.

As described previously, measurement is the assigning of numbers by rules to represent properties of objects or events. The numbers, as symbols of these properties, can be manipulated in accordance with the rules of mathematics. When the properties of the number system reflect the properties of a perception, such as pain intensity, new information about the manner in which pain is perceived as strong or weak may result from the mathematic manipulations. Often, the properties of a number system only partially reflect the properties of events, so that the permissible mathematical operations are limited. There are four types of measurement scales that describe the different relationships between the properties of an event or perception and the number system; the type of scale must be identified so that the mathematical properties for the pain scale are known. The four scale types are "nominal," "ordinal," "interval," and "ratio."

The different numbers on a nominal scale represent only different categories or identities, such as the numbers designating players on a sports team. The numbers on an ordinal scale represent a set position or order among numbers, such as the rank-ordering of children according to their height. The numbers on an interval scale denote that there are equal intervals between numerical values; the difference between two consecutive numbers (e.g., 1 and 2) is equivalent to the difference between any other two consecutive numbers. The Fahrenheit scale for temperature is an interval scale. In an interval scale, both the size of the differences between numbers and their ordinal relation are relevant. A ratio scale, which has all the properties of nominal, ordinal, and interval scales, also has a natural origin that represents a true zero amount. The ratios of the scale values, rather than only their absolute values, are important. A fivefold increase is equivalent to the 1:5 ratio between 1 and 5, 2 and 10, 5 and 25, and so on. Ratio scales are highly desirable, because they have all three basic properties of the number system and therefore can provide the most comprehensive representation of the properties of objects or events (for review, see Gescheider, 1976).

Since each scale type has a certain number of permissible mathematical calculations, it is essential to know the specific scale type prior to interpreting children's pain on a rating scale. Serious errors may arise from inappropriate statistical analysis when the scale type is not known. Incorrect conclusions about children's pain perception or the efficacy of a treatment program may develop when the actual scale of measurement is not as precise as has been assumed. Although investigators aim to develop procedures to rate pain sensations that yield interval or ratio scales, it is not unusual to read a report on children's pain in which pain scores on an ordinal scale have been statistically analyzed and interpreted as scores on an interval or ratio scale. Caution must be used in developing children's pain scales to ensure that the type of scale is determined and that the clinical interpretations are valid.

Rating scales in which words are used to denote different levels of pain have been validated for adults (Gracely, 1980; Gracely, McGrath, & Dubner, 1978; Melzack, 1983), but generally have not been validated for children. Although a four- or five-level verbal scale is convenient to use for assessing children's pain, caution must be used in assigning numerical values to the words and in interpreting children's pain from their choices. As described earlier, the language children use to describe pain depends on their age, cognitive level, and previous pain experience. This information must be considered in evaluating children's responses on verbal rating scales.

Hester (1979) developed a poker chip measure to assess pain in children evoked by their immunizations. Children chose the number of chips (none to four) to correspond to the "pieces of hurt" that they experienced from the injection.

Children from 4 to 7 years of age were able to use the poker chips. Their responses correlated positively with the behavioral distress that they demonstrated during their injections. Although the number of poker chips selected by the children provided a quantitative index of their pain, it is not known whether the four numerical values represent true and meaningful differences that parallel four different levels of children's pain perception.

Rating scales in which a series of faces vary in the amount of distress that they depict have also generally not been validated as pain measures. The faces are usually assigned numerical values that reflect their order within the series from an adult's perspective. The numbers do not necessarily correspond to the perceived level of pain or fear depicted from children's perspective. Figure 2.5 illustrates a series of faces we have used to measure the affective dimension of pain in children. The numerical values shown below each face were determined from the children's own perspective, rather than our perspective (P. A. McGrath, deVeber, & Hearn, 1985). Children did not perceive the faces as varying equally in affective magnitude. If numerical values had been arbitrarily assigned from an adult perspective, they would have been very misleading as a measure of children's pain affect. Instead, the affective values were obtained by asking 200 children (from 3 to 17 years old) to directly scale the feelings depicted by the faces. Children over 5 years of age rated the faces consistently, regardless of their age, sex, or health status. Their own perceptions of affective magnitude determined the number values assigned to each face. These faces were then used by children to measure the affect associated

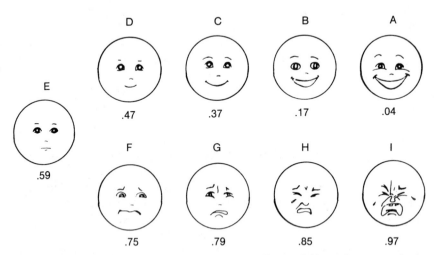

FIGURE 2.5. Affective facial scale used to measure pain affect in children. The numerical values shown below these faces represent the magnitude of pain affect depicted by the face from children's own perspective. The scale ranges from 0 to 1, where 0 equals "happiest feeling possible" and 1 equals "saddest feeling possible." Children from 5 to 17 years of age used standard psychophysical methods to rate the feelings associated with these faces to construct a scale of pain affect.

with different pain experiences. This facial affective scale has subsequently been integrated as one of the measures used for all children referred to our clinic for the management of acute, recurrent, and chronic pain.

Another facial scale has been developed as a pain measure for young children. The Oucher Scale consists of six photographs of a child's face in different expressions of pain, positioned at 20-unit intervals (0, 20, 40, 60, 80, 100) along a 0–100 vertical numerical rating scale (Beyer, 1984). Initial research showed that children ranked the pictures in the sequence as arranged by the investigators and that the numerical scale is a valid tool for assessing postsurgical pain (Aradine, Beyer, & Tompkins, 1988; Beyer & Aradine, 1986, 1988). However, the faces clearly depict the affective or suffering dimension of pain, whereas the numerical scale presumably depicts the strength of pain. The scale may be confounded by using the faces as markers along the numerical scale. As yet, there is not sufficient evidence to demonstrate that the six faces represent six levels of pain from children's perspective to correlate with the numbers selected from the adult perspective.

Similar measurement problems may exist for some of the pain thermometers available to assess children's pain. These consist of vertical or horizontal scales graduated from 0 to 10 or from 0 to 100, as shown in Figure 2.3. Zero is usually designated as "no hurt," and the other endpoint is designated as "most hurt possible." Children point to the level that indicates their pain. Often there are numerical values indicated on the thermometer. A question arises, though, as to the extent to which children's abilities to use numbers or to recall numbers may influence their responses on thermometer scales. Although they are promising tools, many facial pain scales and pain thermometers do not yet constitute precise measures of pediatric pain. There is insufficient information available about children's ability to use these measures regardless of their age, sex, and previous pain experience, and there is generally little information available on the type of numerical scale produced from the children's own perspective.

Cross-modality matching procedures, in which children adjust the strength of one perception (e.g., the brightness of a light) to match the perceived strength of another dimension (e.g., their pain), have been used by children as young as age 4 to assess their sensations (Bond & Stevens, 1969; Teghtsoonian 1980). Cross-modality matching procedures may be ideally suited for use by children as pain measures, since they do not require children to understand numbers or to understand certain pain words. Visual analog scales (VASs), a form of cross-modality matching in which the length of a line is adjusted to match the strength of a perception, have been demonstrated to be reliable and valid measures of pain in adults. In fact, VAS-derived numerical pain estimates have the properties of a ratio scale rather than an interval scale (Price, McGrath, Rafii, & Buckingham, 1983). Although VASs have been used in pediatric studies for assessing pain, little information on the reliability and validity of these measures was available for children of different ages or different pain conditions until recently.

A series of studies has examined children's ability to use VASs to measure different dimensions of their acute, recurrent, and chronic pain (McGrath, 1987a,

1987b; McGrath & deVeber, 1986a, 1986b; McGrath, deVeber, & Hearn, 1983). Children from 3 to 16 years of age used VASs and affective facial scales to rate the intensity and unpleasantness of several types of pain—acute pain evoked by medical procedures or evoked naturally in their daily activities, recurrent pain episodes, postsurgical pain, phantom limb pain, and chronic pain. Generally, children above 5 years of age were able to use VASs in a reliable and valid manner to describe their perceptions, regardless of their sex, age, or health status. VASs are practical and versatile methods for assessing childhood pain because they can be used to measure different dimensions of pain and different types of pain, and can be used in a variety of medical and dental situations. VASs have been integrated with behavioral and physiological indicators of postsurgical pain in children. Abu-Saad (1984a, 1984b) demonstrated that children were able to use such scales to indicate the severity of their pain, and advocates the use of VASs as a valuable method for multidimensional assessment of pediatric pain.

Determining the Reliability and Validity of a Pain Measure for Children

In order to determine the reliability and validity of a pain measure in adults, experimental pain is often induced in healthy volunteers. Discrete and quantifiable levels of noxious stimulation (electrical, chemical, or mechanical) are applied to evaluate how well the adults' scores on the pain measure reflect the controlled changes in the intensity of the noxious stimulus. Investigations of pain induced by electrical tooth pulp stimulation, thermal stimulation, and chemical stimulation have demonstrated that there is a direct and predictable relationship between pain strength and stimulus intensity when all other intervening variables are controlled. The nature of this relationship provides a framework for the evaluation of the precision of a pain measure. As an example, Figure 2.6 illustrates the relationship obtained when pain strength is plotted as a function of five levels of experimental tooth pulp stimulation.

Method validity can be determined by comparing the relationship between perceived pain and stimulus intensity that is obtained by using a potential pain measure to the relationship that has been established empirically. Interventions that will decrease pain (both pharmacological and nonpharmacological) can be administered to patients to determine whether the pain measure indicates a reduction in pain sensitivity that corresponds to the extent and duration of the intervention (as shown by the open circles in Figure 2.6). The reliability of the pain measure can be determined by comparing pain responses to several levels of noxious stimulation, among different individuals, and between different testing times. Method bias can be determined by comparing pain responses when there are different administrators or sets of instructions. Patient bias can be determined by using various randomization sequences or "catch trials" (trials in which no stimulus is delivered).

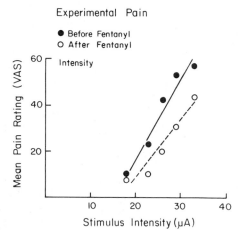

FIGURE 2.6.   The average pain strength produced by five levels of electrical stimulation applied to the upper teeth of healthy adult volunteers is plotted as a function of stimulus intensity before and after the intravenous administration of a short-acting narcotic, fentanyl.

Much research on pain in adults has included thresholds as measures of pain sensitivity. Thresholds provide indirect assessments of pain by determining the minimal amount of noxious stimulation that must be applied until an individual detects the stimulus (the "detection threshold") or notices a painful sensation (the "pain threshold"). "Tolerance threshold" is the maximum amount of stimulation that an individual can tolerate. Pain is expressed in units of the stimulus that produces pain (e.g., degrees Centigrade for noxious thermal stimulation or microamperes for tooth pulp stimulation). Direct assessments of pain, by contrast, provide estimates of how pain sensations vary in strength, quality, or aversiveness throughout the range from pain to tolerance. Pain is then expressed in units of subjective magnitude rather than in units of stimulus magnitude. Direct scaling techniques can provide a more flexible method for pain measurement because they are not defined by a particular type of noxious stimulation, as threshold measures are. Pain responses from direct scaling measures can provide quantitative estimates of perception for a variety of different pain experiences, and therefore can facilitate comparisons among different types of pain and across different individuals.

Although both direct and indirect pain measures are dependent on individuals for standardization, in that either their threshold or their estimates of subjective magnitude provide the basis for the "pain scale," both measures are useful for evaluating clinical pain. The intrinsically personal nature of subjective measures of pain has often caused clinicians to doubt the accuracy of a patient's pain report; however, the same suspicions could be expressed about the measurement of any perceptual experience, such as brightness or loudness. Yet clinicians use both direct and indirect scaling techniques to reliably assess patients' auditory and visual perceptions.

Because ethical concerns limit the use of experimental pain for validating children's pain measures, a different approach may be used. First, children may use the proposed pain measure to scale another perceptual experience (e.g., size, brightness, or heaviness) related to an objectively measurable stimulus. Figure 2.7a illustrates the relationship obtained in one study when children used VASs to rate the perceived size of five circles varying in diameter. The resulting psychophysical relationship obtained between perceived size and actual physical size could be compared across children of different ages, sexes, and health conditions to evaluate whether the children used the measures consistently. If so, then the measures could be used to assess the children's pain.

Figure 2.7b shows children's VAS-derived pain levels reported for five pain situations selected from the Children's Pain Inventory (CPI). This inventory is designed to provide hypothetical pain situations varying in intensity, instead of the graded levels of experimental pain that are usually administered in validity studies with adults. The CPI includes 30 situations, 25 that represent usually painful experiences and 5 that represent usually nonpainful experiences. Both familiar recreational and medical situations are included to provide situations that represent different levels of noxious stimulation, different amounts of child control, and different meanings for children, so that a variety of combinations of pain intensity and pain affect are depicted. Familiar medical situations for oncology, arthritis, and headache patients are also included, so that children's pain responses for the hypothetical situations can be compared later with their pain ratings during the actual situations. Children make VAS responses to rate the pain intensity and select a face from the set of nine faces to rate the pain affect associated with each situation. (Both the intensity and affect forms of the CPI are given in the Appendix to this volume.) The children whose VAS responses are shown in Figure 2.7b were able to use both VASs and affective facial scales to rate the strength and affect associated with the situations. These measures were then used by the children to rate their acute pain evoked by medical procedures in the clinic, as well as acute, recurrent, and chronic pain that occurred naturally in their lives.

Figure 2.8 illustrates a sample of the VASs and affective scales from a child's pain diary. This child was diagnosed with recurrent headaches. He monitored his pains for 1 month after assessment prior to intervention. The nine faces were randomly numbered and printed on a cover sheet. The type of pain, date, intensity (VAS), and affective magnitude (facial scale) were recorded for each pain. Pain intensity is scored by measuring the length of the line from the left endpoint to the child's mark; pain affect is determined by substituting the numerical values depicted in Figure 2.5 for the face the child selected.

A goal of research on pain measurement is to ensure that the numerical response values correspond accurately with perceptual changes. Consequently, it is often important to perform some simple calibration studies so that the relationship between pain measures and noxious stimulation can be defined. These calibration studies can be done prior to answering a major clinical research question or at the same time as the clinical study. As an example, all children who are referred to our

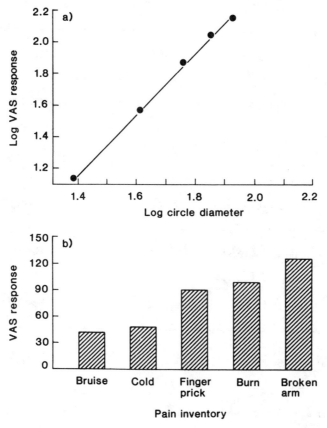

FIGURE 2.7. (a) The logarithmic mean VAS value depicting children's perceptions of the size of five circles is plotted as a function of the circle diameter. Each circle is based on the average of two responses from 175 children. (b) The histograms represent the mean VAS values for perceived pain strength associated with five experiences selected from the Children's Pain Inventory (CPI).

clinic for pain management complete a brief scaling task as part of their pain assessment interview. They use VASs to rate the sizes of seven circles varying in diameter. Each circle is presented twice in random order. A mean VAS-derived value (0–160 mm) is computed for each circle, and the mathematical function that describes the relationship between perceived circle size and actual circle size is determined for each child. The slope, y-intercept, and R^2 coefficient of determination (goodness of fit) of the function are compared with normative data from other children in the same age group, to ensure that the child is able to use VASs to make proportional judgments about his/her perceptions. The calibration task is easy to administer, and the numerical calculations can be performed quickly with a calculator (the seven circles, the VASs, and a scoring sheet are provided in the

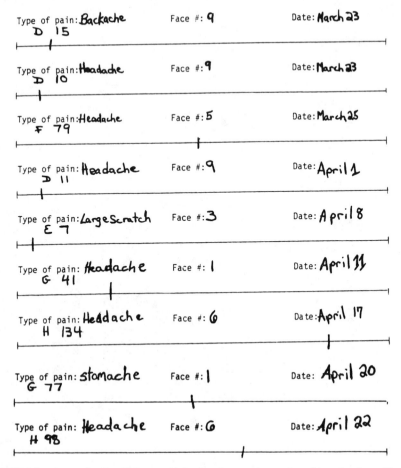

FIGURE 2.8. A sample of a 13.6-year-old boy's pain experiences from his pain diary. He was diagnosed with recurrent headache syndrome. He completed a diary for 1 month in which he used the VAS to rate the strength of any pains he experienced and the affective facial scale to rate the pain affect. Pain strength is determined by measuring the line from the left margin to his mark; pain affect is determined by substituting the affective value for the face he chose to match how he felt "deep down inside, not necessarily the face that other people saw." The faces were shown on a card in random order with number codes. The actual face values (A–I, shown in Figure 2.5) and VAS values are shown on the left below the type of pain.

Appendix). This task enables us to evaluate objectively how well or how poorly children will use the pain-scaling procedures.

In the study whose results are depicted in part in Figures 2.7 and 2.8, the relatively simple two-stage validation procedures enabled us to determine that children's VAS responses were consistent over time and that the responses accurately reflected children's perceptual changes. Children under 5 years of age were generally not able to complete the study, either because they could not comprehend the methods or because they were unwilling to participate in the entire study. Children who were unable to use the measures frequently responded by choosing only the VAS endpoints, apparently making a qualitative distinction as to large or small and then choosing the appropriate extreme value. All other children easily completed the scaling procedures.

Although there were no significant differences in pain intensity or pain affect on children's CPIs according to their sex, there were significant differences in pain profiles according to children's age and health status. Children seemed to respond differently, depending on their previous pain experience, so that younger children with less pain experience rated certain pain situations as more painful than children who had experienced a wider variety or intensity of pains (because of chronological age or health status).

The demonstration that VASs and affective facial scales were reliable and valid measures of the strength and unpleasantness associated with pain has led us to include both of these direct scaling procedures in a comprehensive pain assessment for children with acute, chronic, or recurrent pain. As an example, all oncology patients use VASs and affective scales to rate pain produced during their necessary medical procedures. These include physical exams, intravenous chemotherapy, intramuscular or intravenous injections, finger pricks, blood-sampling techniques, lumbar punctures, bone marrow aspirations, and portacatheter injections or cleaning. The direct scaling of their pain enables us to evaluate the efficacy of our pain management program more precisely. The mean pain intensity and pain affect associated with various medical treatments for child oncology patients are shown in Table 2.3. Although the ratings are generally related to the type of procedure, such as low to moderate pain ratings for weak to moderate noxious stimuli, specific pain ratings depend clearly on the child's age and sex, and on the situation in which he/she experiences a noxious stimulus. As emphasized in Chapter 1, emotional and contextual factors can significantly enhance or reduce the painfulness of a constant noxious stimulus. Consequently, children who may be referred initially because of extreme fear of pain related to procedures, or because of difficulties in coping with an initial diagnosis of cancer or a relapse, may report excessively high levels of pain associated with relatively mild noxious stimuli. As children learn appropriate coping strategies for reducing the pain and as the context is modified to improve their control and alter their expectations, the pain decreases for the same procedure.

Although the various pain management programs are outlined in later chapters according to the type of pain for which they are intended (acute, chronic, or recurrent), it is clear that relatively simple direct scaling techniques, such as VASs and affective facial scales, may be incorporated into a structured interview for clinical pain assessment and then used in the clinic to provide a precise evaluation of treatment efficacy. Table 2.3 illustrates that pain affect for children is not simply and directly proportional to the type or intensity of noxious stimulation. Children's pain experiences are determined by a noxious stimulus in relationship to their expectations, their fears, their perceived control, and the significance or relevance

TABLE 2.3. Mean Pain Intensity and Pain Affect Associated With Medical
Treatments for Oncology Patients

Procedure	Pain intensity	Pain affect
Checkup (n = 46)	2.3	.27
Finger prick (n = 46)	6.3	.40
Intramuscular injection (n = 55)	64.4	.85
Lumbar puncture		
Without pain management (n = 17)	51.3	.79
After pain management (n = 7)	15.9	.22
With sedation (n = 16)	80.2	.83

Note. Pain intensity was rated on a VAS with endpoints of 0 and 160 mm. Pain affect was rated on an affective facial scale with endpoints of 0 and 1 (1 = "saddest feeling possible").

of the pain-producing stimulus to their lives. Thus, statistical differences in mean pain affect values among various medical procedures may not have real clinical significance unless an effort is made to accumulate objective information about the situational factors that will affect children's pain perceptions.

Summary and Recommendations for an Integrated Approach to Pain Measurement

Although behavioral, physiological, projective, and direct report methods are available for assessing children's pain, several issues must be considered prior to the selection of a particular pain measure. First, does the measure fulfill the four criteria of reliability, validity, minimal inherent bias, and versatility? If insufficient information has been published about a potential pain measure, these criteria could be evaluated in basic psychophysical studies prior to the clinician's use of the pain measure. Children could use the proposed measure to rate their percep-tions of discrete levels of a non-noxious stimulus (e.g., the brightness of a light or the loudness of a tone). In this manner, it would be possible to assess the reliability and validity of the measure for children's perceptual judgments as a function of their sex, age, and health status. Once children's abilities to use the measure have been demonstrated, clinical evaluations could continue by requesting children to use the measure to assess the pain evoked by different medical or dental proce-dures, to determine whether the new measure reflects the intensity and unpleasant-ness of their experiences. Test–retest reliability could be determined, and children's responses on the measure under a variety of different pain management ap-proaches could be compared. The integration of basic psychophysical research with clinical evaluation will provide valuable information about the reliability, validity, and practical feasibility of any pediatric pain measure, and the type of numerical scale it produces.

Second, the choice of physiological, behavioral, or psychological pain mea-sures is restricted by children's age and cognitive level. Clearly, infants will not be able to use direct scaling techniques to describe their pain. Physiological or behavioral measures must be used to assess pain when children are unable to communicate or are too young to comprehend the use of direct scaling techniques. Although behavioral and physiological responses that are specific indices of in-fants' pain have not yet been identified, their general body movements, facial expressions, and cry patterns can provide reliable, valid, and quantitative informa-tion about their overt distress. The criteria for pain-related behaviors and the time periods for observing children must be standardized to minimize differences in children's distress scores resulting from differences among raters. Physiological monitors must be calibrated and standardized to minimize differences resulting from differences in recording techniques. Infants' facial expressions may have the most potential as practical and convenient measures of infant distress, since they can be used in many clinical situations in which the infants' behaviors may be restricted by medical equipment. As yet, the analysis of facial expression, body behaviors, and cry patterns requires trained observers. In the future, abbreviated clinical scales could be developed to facilitate on-site evaluations of infants' overt distress. Although infants' overt distress reflects their pain, fear, and general physio-logical arousal, it should provide a means of evaluating the efficacy of pharmaco-logical and nonpharmacological approaches to controlling their pain. The optimal evaluation of their distress may require the use of concurrent measures in which observational and physiological methods are integrated.

Similarly, for children aged 1–4, it will not be possible to use direct scaling techniques consistently to assess their pain. Instead, behavioral and physiological measures must be used to infer their pain from their overt distress. Behavioral, physiological, and psychological techniques should be integrated as children become older. Correlating the information from the three categories of measures should provide more comprehensive information on children's pain experiences and pain behaviors. Caution must be used both in the initial selection of anxiety and pain-related behaviors and in the subsequent observation and scoring of behaviors. Children's behaviors undoubtedly vary according to the number of people present at the time of observation and whether they are peers, parents, child life workers, or medical staff. Children respond to stress and pain with different behaviors, depending on their age, sex, cognitive level, and familial pattern. Behavioral scales should incorporate this individuality in pain expression by including information as to the nature of each child's specific behaviors and the normality of the observed clinical behaviors for each child.

The major problem in using a behavioral pain scale is that children's behav-iors are not simply and directly proportional to the strength or unpleasantness of their pain experience. Their behaviors are complex expressions of their pain and emotions that are influenced by several situational and familial factors. It is misleading to interpret a high or a low pain level solely on the basis of children's distress behaviors. Children's distress behaviors may reflect their anxiety, their lack of concrete age-appropriate information about an invasive medical treatment, and their lack of simple pain-coping tools. However, it is also misleading to ignore children's pain behaviors when evaluating their pain experience. A consideration of the nature and frequency of children's distress behaviors, as well as of their parents' responses to those behaviors, is essential for a comprehensive evaluation of children's pain.

Direct scaling techniques that can be incorporated into a semistructured interview format are the best source for obtaining objective information about children's pain experiences. VASs may be adapted to assess multiple dimensions of children's pain experiences. They provide a convenient and practical method for assessing pain in children above 5 years of age. Children's subjective ratings of pain strength and unpleasantness must be evaluated in relation to their age, sex cognitive level, and previous pain experience. Children's VAS-derived pain scores will not provide clinically meaningful information unless concrete information about their frame of reference, against which they evaluate the strength and unpleasantness of each new pain, has been obtained. This information may be collected on brief standardized inventories as part of a comprehensive plan assessment.

The third issue that must be considered in the selection of pain measures is that an adequate description of pain (particularly chronic pain, in which the source of noxious stimulation may not be precisely identified) requires information on many dimensions of the sensation, such as quality, location, duration, and frequency—not only pain intensity. The design of a comprehensive pain management program requires information on the emotional, motivational, and situational factors that can modify the perception of pain. Consequently, a systematic multidimensional approach is necessary for the evaluation and management of acute, recurrent, and chronic pain in children.

The fourth issue that must be addressed in selecting a pain measure for children is the nature of the pain that is to be assessed. Acute pain evoked by invasive medical procedures is a relatively simple type of pain to measure, because it is amenable to observational, physiological, and direct scaling techniques. However, for chronic or recurrent pain, it is not possible to consistently observe children's behavior or record their physiological responses throughout the day, when their chronic pain may fluctuate. It is necessary, then, to incorporate measures that evaluate salient features of such children's pain experience on a continuing and long-term basis. As a consequence, a combination of direct scaling approaches with behavioral scales that record general behaviors (e.g., school attendance, physical activity, and medication requirements) is preferable to the type of behavioral distress scales that have been developed for clinical situations. It is important to begin to consider the characteristics of pain, as well as the characteristics of children, in selecting adequate pain measures.

Of the many methods available for assessing pediatric pain, VASs and category scales may offer the most versatility for evaluating pain developmentally and for assessing pain at different time intervals for acute, chronic, and recurrent pain.

Direct scaling techniques that incorporate interviews, VASs, and category scales to identify qualitative distinctions in children's pain experience are probably the most useful tools for conducting comprehensive initial pain assessments. These methods have also been used to evaluate the efficacy of different pain management programs for chronic pediatric pain (McGrath, 1987b; McGrath & Hinton, 1987). We feel that VASs are important tools that should be incorporated in any battery of pain measures for children above 5 years of age, in consideration of their ease of administration, their flexibility for tapping multiple dimensions of children's pain experience, and the ease of conducting calibration studies to ensure that children comprehend the use of the scales. A multidimensional approach to pain management may be augmented by the use of physiological and behavioral scales, as well as psychological scales, depending on the particular interest of the clinician or investigator. For infants and young children who are unable to directly report their subjective experience of pain, efforts should be made to integrate behavioral and physiological measures, with proper attention to the time sampled, a quantification of the stimulus eliciting pain, and (when possible) an estimate of the number of previous exposures to this stimulus the infant has received. Although the measurement of pain in infants and children is more difficult than the measurement of pain in adults because of the complexity of the developing child, there are several practical methods that may be adapted for clinical use in measuring any type of pain that children experience.

3

The Plasticity and Complexity of the Nociceptive System

General approaches, specific techniques, and new ideas for how to control pain in children are inextricably woven into the fabric of our existing knowledge about how children perceive pain. Information about the underlying physiological mechanisms that transform a noxious stimulus into the perception of a particular pain, with unique attributes of quality, location, duration, intensity, and aversiveness, provides the essential framework for developing and refining pharmacological and nonpharmacological methods of pain control for children. During the past 15–20 years, an exciting array of information about the nature of nociceptive processing has accrued from anatomical, physiological, neurochemical, medical, and psychological research on pain. We now know that the nociceptive system is a much more flexible and complex sensory system than was previously believed. The system that mediates our pain perceptions is a marvel of subtlety and complexity. It is not a fixed and rigid system that transfers a certain amount of pain from a constant stimulus; instead, the nociceptive system is plastic, in that it has the capacity to respond differently to the same noxious stimulus. Thus, an injection will not necessarily produce the same amount of pain for all children. The nociceptive system will respond differently, depending on the context in which children receive the injections. When children use a simple coping strategy (e.g., squeezing a hand in proportion to the pain that they feel), or when they are actively involved in preparing an injection site (e.g., choosing the site, cleaning the site with an alcohol swab), they will generally experience less pain. This chapter describes some of the features of nociceptive processing that are responsible for this plasticity. (For additional detailed reviews of nociceptive processing, see Basbaum, 1980; Dubner, 1980; Dubner & Bennett, 1983; Dubner, Gebhart, & Bond, 1988;

Fields & Basbaum, 1978; Kerr, 1980; Kruger & Liebeskind, 1984; Melzack & Dennis, 1978; Ng & Bonica, 1980; Price, 1988; Wall, 1988; Wall & Melzack, 1984; Willis, 1985.)

The quality and intensity of all pain sensations are not simply related to the nature and extent of the tissue damage evoked by a noxious stimulus; the neuronal activity evoked by the stimulus is also modified by internal pain-suppressing systems. An appreciation for the plasticity and complexity of nociceptive processing provides the basis for a careful and conscientious evaluation of the different interventions available for reducing pain in infants and children. In fact, an understanding of the general features of nociception, endogenous pain-inhibitory systems, and the variety of environmental and internal factors that can modify pain is necessary not only for the selection of the most appropriate therapeutic modality, but also for the optimal application of that modality. Inaccurate expectations about the probable mode of action or presumed efficacy of a treatment by health professionals, children, or parents may alter the treatment's analgesic potency, whether it is a pharmacological or a nonpharmacological intervention. The rationale for the choice of a particular treatment for children, in consideration of the condition or injury evoking their pain and the relevant situational and emotional factors that may affect their pain, creates the critical background necessary to maximize the analgesic potency of any treatment. Consequently, both children and their parents require some understanding of the mode of action and presumed efficacy of a treatment.

Generally, children above 5 years of age are able to understand simple mechanisms of pain and pain control, particularly nonpharmacological methods of pain control. Some children as young as 3 are able to grasp the concept that their brains can ignore pain under certain conditions. From infancy throughout early childhood, children seek parental reassurance when they are distressed emotionally or hurt physically. They learn that their parents' reassurance can reduce their distress, anxiety, pain, and suffering. Information about the variety of factors that can activate internal pain-suppressing systems provides a reasonable explanation for why their pain may be reduced when they receive parental reassurance through a hug or kiss. Children can easily learn other nonpharmacological methods for reducing their pain if they receive an age-appropriate rationale with concrete practical examples.

However, parents may have difficulty in believing that deceptively simple, noninvasive coping strategies, such as distraction, visual imagery, and self-hypnosis, can truly block their children's pain. Their biases about nonpharmacological interventions may inadvertently lower the efficacy of a therapeutic approach. It is essential to teach parents that children's pain is not determined solely by the intensity of a noxious stimulus, but that many situational and contextual factors can modify their pain. A brief description of current research, which includes pictures or figures depicting the different nociceptive responses or pain intensities evoked by the same noxious stimulus when it is presented in two different contexts, can provide convincing evidence to parents that many factors are important for pain control. When children and parents understand that a variety of factors affect pain, families become a meaningful part of any pain therapy rather than an unintentional impediment. Knowledge of the mechanisms underlying children's pain perception is an essential prerequisite for selecting an appropriate intervention and for providing optimal pain relief with that intervention.

Although a comprehensive description of each component of nociceptive processing is beyond the scope of this book, the main features of the nociceptive system, including endogenous pain-inhibitory systems and the variety of internal and external factors that may activate them, are briefly reviewed in this chapter. The emphasis is on the plasticity and complexity of the nociceptive system—that is, on how the same noxious stimulus can produce qualitatively and quantitatively different pains. The structures that detect tissue injury and initiate the pain signals, and the pathways that convey these signals, are described, with a focus on how these signals may be modified at many levels within the nociceptive system. Because our current knowledge about pain and nociceptive mechanisms in children represents the culmination of centuries of studies on the nature of sensation and perception, the chapter begins with a brief historical perspective.

A Historical Perspective

The origins of our contemporary understanding of nociception may be traced throughout recorded history in the search for the physical, emotional, or spiritual mechanisms responsible for human pain. Questions about pain and suffering have been raised by all cultures. Why is there pain without an obvious physical injury? What are the mechanisms for pain with and without injury? Where is pain experienced—the heart, the soul, or the brain? Is pain an emotion, a sense, or a special combination of senses? How can pain be reduced? The nature of these questions shows that ancient people, like contemporary researchers, were intrigued by the multidimensionality of pain and were perplexed by the seemingly inexplicable varieties of pathological pain conditions. Although the plasticity and complexity of pain have generally been implicitly recognized, it is only comparatively recently that theories of nociception have been able to account explicitly for a variety of pain phenomena. People's explanations for pain have been guided by, and occasionally restricted by, the prevailing scientific and medical ideas of their time. The evolution in theoretical explanations for pain provides the perspective needed for our current understanding of nociceptive mechanisms in children and for our current approaches to pediatric pain management.

Although all cultures have been able to explain pain produced by physical injury, pain experienced without a discernible injury has been regarded as mysterious. When physical causes for pain were not evident, ancient people attributed the pain to spiritual causes, such as the intrusion of foreign objects or evil spirits into the body, or to the abnormal loss of vital substances from the body (Keele, 1957). Often, the evil spirits were viewed as a punishment, so that the appropriate treatment consisted of supplicating the responsible gods. In *The Wisdom of India*, both spiritual and physical pain are described as evils (Yutang, 1942). Keele (1957) cites several examples of these attributions throughout history, including the Biblical character Job's description of his pain as the "arrows of the Almighty . . . within me" (Job 6:4), and the Egyptians' beliefs that evil spirits could invade the body through the left nostril or left ear. Treatment for pain often involved extricating the evil spirits and restoring the balance of body fluids. The attribution of pain to evil spirits inflicted as punishments by offended gods is a common theme in many cultures. In fact, the derivation of the word "pain" has been described variously as from the Greek word *poine*, meaning "penalty" or "punishment"; from a Sanskrit root *pu*, meaning "sacrifice"; and from the Latin word *pena*, meaning "punishment" (Bonica, 1953; Dallenbach, 1939; Keele, 1957; Tainter, 1948). These derivations clearly indicate the ancient cross-cultural belief that pain is a consequence of a wrongdoing by the sufferer.

The *Canon of Medicine* of Avicenna (see Gruner, 1930), written in the 10th century A.D., describes pain as one of the unnatural states to which the animal body is liable. Avicenna cited 15 types of pain and the various agents and methods to alleviate pain. These included agents that produced relaxation (e.g., dill, linseed); agents that were hot and combined with a glutinous substance (e.g., the gum of prunes); oils in laxatives; opium and root bark of mandrake; poultices (the most efficient poultices were made with flour of orobs boiled in vinegar); cupping; walking; listening to agreeable music (e.g., a mother's lullaby to her child in pain); and being occupied with something very engrossing. The multidimensional nature of pain and the complexity of pain relief from diverse pharmacological and nonpharmacological methods have been noted throughout recorded history.

In addition, both the unique emotional aspect and the sensory aspect of pain have been recognized throughout history. However, cultures differed as to which aspect was regarded as the more important characteristic of pain. Cultures that regarded the emotional or suffering aspect as more important tended to regard pain in terms of the emotional or spiritual, locating pain experience in the heart or blood vessels. The Egyptians, Indians, Chinese, and Greeks emphasized the heart rather than the brain as the center of sensation. Cultures that regarded the sensory aspects as more important defined pain in terms of the physical stimuli or body senses and located pain within the body. Both views are evident in the writings of the great Greek philosophers. Alamaeon, Pythagoras's disciple, conducted intensive investigations on the senses and proposed that the brain rather than the heart was the center for sensation and reason (Bonica, 1980; Keele, 1957). Aristotle, however, proposed that pain occurred when an excess of vital heat produced an increase in the sensitivity to touch; the sensitivity arose from the flesh and was conveyed by the blood to the heart, where pain was experienced (Aristotle, ca. 330 B.C./1902). Like many of his contemporaries, Aristotle emphasized the aversive component of the pain experience, describing pain as "a quayle"—a quality of the soul opposite to pleasure. His explanation for pain comprises the "emotional theory" of pain: The aversive or unpleasant component is common to all pain experiences, and therefore is the main feature that defines pain. Aristotle's influence on philosophical and scientific thought delayed the recognition of pain as a separate sensation.

After Aristotle's death, the observations of Herophilus and Erasistratus in Egypt on anatomy and physiology led to their proposals that different sets of nerves were responsible for sensation and movement and that the brain was the center of sensation (Keele, 1957). Galen discovered and further developed the work of Herophilus and Erasistratus on the central nervous system. His explanations of the physiology of pain were a notable exception to the prevailing ideas of the Greco-Roman period (Procacci, 1980). Galen believed that the brain was the center of sensation, that organs and tissues were innervated by nerves differentiated for specific functions, and that the smallest nerves were the ones important for pain. Despite Galen's extensive research on sensory and peripheral nerves and the spinal cord, his work was obscured for over a thousand years while Aristotle's views gained momentum.

Since the early philosophical inquiries about how our knowledge of the world is derived from our sensory experiences in the world, advances in the understanding of pain perception and nociceptive mechanisms naturally paralleled advances in medicine and science. Theories to account for pain reflected existing knowledge in science—specifically, anatomy, physiology, and medicine. In the 1600s, general acceptance of the emotional theory of pain lessened as more information about the nature of sensory and motor systems accrued. Descartes, who regarded the brain as the center of sensation and motor function, described pain as a sensation in his book *L'Homme (Treatise on Man)*, published in 1664. Pain was conducted by "delicate threads" in nerves that connected different body tissues to the brain. Burning, for example, caused minute particles of fire to pull upon the delicate cord of the nerve to produce a pain in the brain, just like pulling at the end of a rope to strike a bell (Descartes, 1664/1972). His views of pain precede the "specificity theory," in which pain is defined as a distinct sensation similar to hearing, vision, taste, smell, and touch, and mediated by nerves exclusively designed for nociceptive processing.

Scientific knowledge about the brain and the peripheral and central nervous systems increased dramatically during the 17th and 18th centuries. Erasmus Darwin, grandfather of Charles Darwin, conducted extensive studies on the sensory systems and recognized that the nerves that responded to touch were different from those that responded to painful heat (Darwin, 1794; Dallenbach, 1939). However, he regarded pain as a general sensation resulting from excessive stimulation of any sensory system. Overstimulation by light, sound pressure, distention, heat, or cold could cause pain. His observations and deductions foreshadowed the "intensity theory" of pain, in which pain is regarded as the result of excess activity in regular nerve fibers and not simply the result of activity in specific pain fibers.

The observation that the spinal nerves mediating sensations were independent and distinct from the nerves mediating motor activities (Bell & Bell, 1827; Magendie, 1822a, 1822b), and the discovery that there were certain spots in the skin that, regardless of how they were stimulated, always produced specific sensations of warmth, cold, pressure, or pain (Blix, 1884; Goldscheider, 1884), gave renewed impetus to research on the pain system as a distinct sensation. About this time, Muller (1842) proposed the "doctrine of specific nerve energies," in which he stated that the brain received information about external objects and internal body structures because of the nature of the specific nerves that were activated. Each of the five senses conducted a particular form of energy specific to that sensation. Muller theorized that the nerves of feeling provided several sensations: tickle, shudder, itch, pleasure, pain, fatigue, suffocation, warmth, cold, touch, and movement. He did not believe that each of these feeling nerves had a separate nerve system, but rather that they transmitted different sensations because of differences in the state of the organism at the time of arousal. Muller's doctrine emphasized that human perceptions were determined by the properties of sensory nerves or by their connections and terminations in the brain.

The growing acceptance that the various sensations could be attributed to identifiable physiological mechanisms significantly altered the nature and direction of pain research. Investigations focused on identification of the receptors, nerves, pathways, and brain sites that were responsible for pain perception. Theorists attempted to incorporate each new scientific finding into their explanations for pain sensation. In addition, information from clinical observations of unusual pain states (described in Chapter 1), such as causalgia, tabes dorsalis, and phantom limb pain, provided more information about pain mechanisms. Pain associated with these disorders had been inexplicable according to the predominant emotional, specificity, or intensity theories of pain.

The specificity theory—that pain is a specific sensation with its own sensory mechanisms—was explicitly formulated by Schiff (1858; cited by Boring, 1942) after he demonstrated that pain and touch were mediated by independent sensory systems. The intensity theory—that pain is not a specific sensation, but results from intense stimulation of any sensory organ—was first suggested by Erasmus Darwin (1794) and explicitly formulated by Urb (1874; cited by Boring, 1942). In 1884, Goldscheider modified this theory by postulating that the intensity of the noxious stimulus, the subsequent activation of nerves peripherally, and the summation of neural excitation centrally were the critical determinants of pain. He proposed that pain was mediated by tactile nerves that produced excitations in the grey matter of the spinal cord; the summation of these excitations then produced pain. By the end of the 19th century, there were four conflicting theories on the nature of pain: emotional or affective, specificity, intensity, and "patterning" theories. Although there was empirical evidence in support of each theory, a progressive accumulation of anatomical, physiological, and clinical data showed each by itself to be inadequate. In particular, the inability of the specificity theory to account for why pain persisted after patients had their "pain nerves" cut and why severe pain was produced by nonnoxious stimuli in other patients, led to renewed interest in patterning and central summation theories. As an example, Livingston (1943/ 1976) described how the view that pain was a primary sensation evoked when an intense stimulus activated a specific sensory ending and the activity was conducted along fixed pathways did not account for observations of referred pain, neuralgia pain, or phantom limb pain. His elegant, precise, and personal observations about patients and their apparently inexplicable pain conditions provide a practical and fascinating insight into the complexity of the pain problems faced by clinicians and the inadequacy of the then-current pain theories for understanding pain patients.

Goldscheider (1884), who studied cutaneous pain sensation, proposed that excessive skin stimulation activated all types of receptors and produced convergence and summation of activity in the brain stem and spinal cord. Pain resulted when excitation exeeded a critical level, either because there was increased activation of a variety of receptors that may normally have responded to nonnoxious stimuli or because pathological conditions enhanced the summation of nonnoxious stimuli. Noordenbos (1959) added the concept of sensory interaction to a patterning theory. He proposed that rapidly conducting large-fiber pathways could inhibit or suppress activity in the slower-conducting fiber pathways conveying noxious information. An increase in the understanding of the plasticity and complexity of nociceptive processing may be traced to research generated by this "gate control" theory.

The essential questions about our common pain experiences remain the same as those posed by the early philosophers: "Why do we feel pain when there is no apparent physical damage causing it?" and, conversely, "Why, when there is physical damage, do we not always feel pain?" However, we are much closer to answering these questions today. Pain is not the inevitable result of physical damage, and the intensity of pain is not simply proportional to the severity or type of an injury. Although the relationship between injury and pain is generally true, such as for the acute pain produced by an injection, there are many exceptions to this relatively simplistic relationship. The mechanisms responsible for the modifiability of pain perception are described in the following sections.

Nociceptive Mechanisms

"Nociception" or "nociceptive processing" refers to the detection of a noxious stimulus and the transduction and transmission of information about the presence and the quality of that stimulus from the site of stimulation to the brain. "Nociception" is not synonymous with "pain." Pain is a psychological experience, the human perception; nociception is the activity in the nervous system that may lead to pain. "Neurons" are the basic elements of nociceptive processing. These are nerve cells, composed of a cell body and two types of extending processes, "dendrites" and "axons" (Figure 3.1A). Dendrites are multiple short branches that detect information about tissue damage; the axon is a single long process that relays the information about tissue damage throughout the nervous system. Some

A.

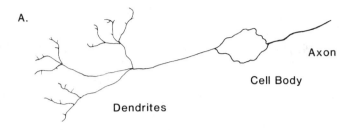

Axon

Cell Body

Dendrites

B.

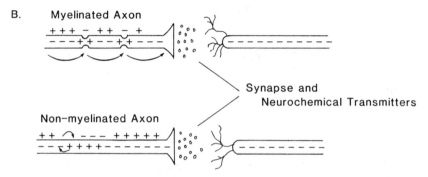

Myelinated Axon

Synapse and
Neurochemical Transmitters

Non-myelinated Axon

FIGURE 3.1. (A) A neuron with axon and dendritic processes is illustrated. (B) Propagation of electrical impulses is depicted along a myelinated and a nonmyelinated axon.

axons are "myelinated"—that is, their neural membranes are electrically insulated by myelin sheaths.

Nociceptive information is conducted by electrical impulses that are generated in a neuron and then transmitted along the length of the axon. The inside of an axon is negatively charged ($\sim$ 70 mV) in comparison with the region outside the neuron, because of an imbalance in the concentrations of positive and negative ions. A noxious stimulus excites a neuron by producing a localized change in the "permeability" of the membrane—that is, the ability of the membrane to allow positive and negative ions to pass through the membrane. Neural excitation can alter the balance of positive and negative ions at the site of stimulation. Membranes differ in permeability and in their "excitatory thresholds," the minimal amount of stimulation required to activate them. When stimulation is sufficiently strong to excite the neuron, there is a sudden inflow of positive ions that positively charges the inside of the axon at the site of stimulation (depicted in Figure 3.1B). This electrical charge propagates along the length of the axon in nonmyelinated axons or jumps from node to node (nonmyelinated regions) in myelinated axons. The conduction of electrical impulses along an axon is referred to as "depolarization."

Nerve fibers or axons are classified into three major groups according to the diameter of the axons and their conduction velocities. These are A, B, and C fibers with alpha, beta, gamma, and delta subcategories. The A group includes all the myelinated large-diameter axons of somatic nerves, with fast conduction rates from 2.5 to 120 m per second. The B and C groups consist of smaller-diameter fibers with slower conduction velocities. The B group includes all the myelinated axons of autonomic nerves; the C group includes all nonmyelinated fibers. Approximately 10–25% of the A-delta fibers conduct impulses evoked by noxious stimuli; other types of A and B fibers do not conduct nociceptive information. Many fibers in the C group respond to noxious stimulation, whereas others respond to innocuous stimuli.

Electrical activity is transferred from one nerve to another by "neurochemical transmitters," substances that are released at the end of a nerve (the "terminal") by depolarization. Neurochemical transmitters diffuse throughout the region between two (or more) nerve endings, called a "synapse." Several neurotransmitter substances have been identified, such as acetylcholine, norepinephrine, dopamine, serotonin, and substance P. The effects of neurotransmitters at a synapse may be excitatory or inhibitory, depending on the nature of the substance released and the type of neurons at the synapse. In excitatory synapses, the electrical activity from one nerve generates similar electrical activity in the second nerve by causing its depolarization. In inhibitory synapses, the electrical activity from one nerve hyperpolarizes the second nerve (the inside of the nerve becomes more negative), so that the second nerve is more resistant to stimulation. The relatively simple mechanism of excitatory and inhibitory synapses provides the first manner in which the transmission of nociceptive impulses to the brain may be blocked. Complex systems of excitatory and inhibitory mechanisms are possible at very early levels in the processing of a noxious stimulus.

The perception of pain usually begins with the application of a noxious stimulus. The stimulus generates neuronal impulses that are conducted along the peripheral nerves, designated as "primary" or "first-order" neurons. These neurons synapse in the dorsal horn of the spinal cord onto "second-order" neurons, whose cell bodies are located within the dorsal horn. Axons of the second-order neurons then synapse onto "interneurons," neurons that synapse with other neurons in the spinal cord, or onto "projection neurons," neurons that project along several pathways to the thalamus and cortex. Neural projections also descend from the brain and synapse onto neurons in the spinal cord, where they can modulate the activity evoked by primary nerves.

Nociceptive Receptors and Fibers

"Nociceptors," the receptors that respond to tissue injury, are the dendritic processes of primary neurons. Nociceptors consist of freely branching nerve endings that are located in skin, blood vessels, subcutaneous tissue, muscle, fascia, periosteum, viscera, and joints. The axons of nociceptors are designated as "primary nociceptive afferents." Nociceptive afferents are not uniformly sensitive to noxious stimuli. They vary in their characteristic responses to mechanical, thermal, and chemical stimulation and in their conduction velocities (Beitel & Dubner, 1976; Perl, 1968, 1980; Price & Dubner, 1977). Anatomical and physiological studies have shown that A-delta and C primary afferents are critically involved in relaying nociceptive information (Collins, Nulsen, & Randt, 1960; Dyck, Lambert, & Nichols, 1971; Dyck, Lambert, & O'Brien, 1976; Gasser, 1943; Hallin & Torebjork, 1976; Price, 1988; Zotterman, 1933).

A-delta primary afferents are a functionally mixed group of fibers because they include fibers that respond to innocuous mechanical stimulation (low-threshold mechanoreceptive afferents); fibers that respond to cooling the skin (thermoreceptive afferents); and also afferent fibers that respond almost exclusively to intense thermal and/or mechanical stimuli (nociceptive afferents). The two major categories of A-delta fibers that respond exclusively to noxious stimuli are high-threshold mechanoreceptive afferents, which respond maximallly to noxious mechanical stimuli, and A-delta heat-nociceptive afferents, which are maximally sensitive over the range of skin temperatures to which humans report pain. Unmyelinated C primary afferents are also a functionally mixed group because they include fibers that respond to mechanical, thermal, and noxious stimuli. However, C fibers respond almost exclusively to levels of stimulation that are noxious, whether mechanical or thermal stimuli. C polymodal nociceptive afferents respond to noxious thermal, mechanical, and irritant chemical stimuli. Although their thresholds to mechanical and thermal stimuli are at levels that do not produce pain in humans, they are maximally sensitive to stimuli in the noxious range.

The responses of A-delta heat nociceptors and C polymodal nociceptors to heat pulse stimuli at 37–51°C are shown in Figures 3.2A and 3.2B. As shown, the neuronal responses in these afferents increase when temperatures are increased. However, the pattern of the increase is different for the A-delta heat and C polymodal nociceptors; A-delta heat-nociceptive afferents show a more abrupt and steep response increase at 45°C, approximately pain threshold. The C fibers show a gradual montonic increase as temperature increases throughout the noxious heat range.

Activity in the A-delta and C fibers produces two qualitatively distinctive pains in humans. Most people have experienced these "first" and "second" pain sensations after stubbing a toe or dropping a heavy object on their feet. An immediate stinging, sharp, and well-localized pain sensation (related to activation of A-delta fibers) is followed about 1–2 seconds later by a burning, diffuse, and poorly localized pain sensation (related to activation of C fibers) that lasts longer than the stinging pain and also outlasts the original noxious stimulus.

Although there are primary afferents specialized for the conduction of nociceptive information, activity in primary nociceptive afferents alone does not predict the level of pain evoked by a noxious stimulus. As an example, the application of brief noxious heat pulses to the hand will evoke "first" and "second" pain in

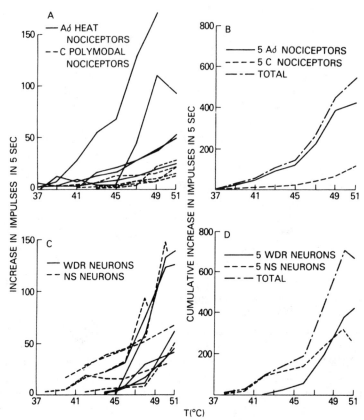

FIGURE 3.2. (A) Responses of five A-delta heat and five C polymodal nociceptive afferents to increases in receptive field temperature (Hu & Dubner, unpublished observations). The magnitude of the response, expressed as the increase in impulses in the 5-second period after the onset of the stimulus, is plotted against the final temperature of individual trials. (B) Cumulative temperature responses of the five A-delta heat nociceptive afferents, five C polymodal nociceptive afferents, and both groups combined. (C) Responses of five wide-dynamic-range (WDR) and five nociceptive-specific neurons (NS) to receptive field skin temperature increases applied as described above. Both groups respond with the highest frequencies to skin temperatures in the noxious range (45–51°C). (D) Cumulative temperature responses of the five WDR, five NS neurons, and both groups combined. From "Neurons That Subserve the Sensory-Discriminative Aspects of Pain" by D. D. Price and R. Dubner, 1977, *Pain*, 3, p. 313. Copyright 1977 by Elsevier Science Publishers. Reprinted by permission.

humans. When pulses are administered repeatedly at 3-second intervals, the strength of the "second" pain sensation increases with repeated stimulation, even though the pulses are the same intensity (Price, Hu, Dubner, & Gracely, 1977). However, the activity in polymodal primary nociceptive afferents that is evoked by the constant noxious stimulus decreases with repeated stimulation. Central summation mechanisms, and not activity in nociceptive afferents, must be responsible for the increased pain.

Dorsal Horn Circuitry

Extensive research has been conducted on the anatomical organization and connections of primary nociceptive afferents within the spinal cord. The dorsal horn has been shown to be an important site for the modulation of sensory information (Basbaum & Fields, 1984; Besson, 1980; Casey, 1980; Cervero, Iggo, & Ogawa, 1976; Dubner, Hoffman, & Hayes, 1981; Dubner et al., 1984; Fields, Dubner, & Cervero, 1985; Fitzgerald, 1981, 1982; Iggo, 1980; Kumazawa & Perl, 1978; Melzack & Wall, 1982; Perl, 1985). The dorsal horn is divided into layers of "laminae" on the basis of the different types and densities of cell bodies within the region (see Figure 3.3). Large- and small-diameter primary afferent fibers are distributed randomly throughout peripheral nerves, but they differentially innervate the dorsal horn laminae. The differential termination of primary nociceptive and non-nociceptive afferents within the dorsal horn constitutes the basic map or circuitry for the modulation of nociceptive input. Laminae are distinguished by their anatomical and physiological properties: their afferent terminations, the response properties of second-order neurons and their synaptic connections, and the presence of descending axonal projections from the brain. The laminae do not have rigid boundaries, so that the dendrites of a cell body within one lamina may extend into neighboring laminae. The outermost lamina, the marginal zone or lamina I, receives input from small-diameter primary afferents, including the primary nociceptive afferents (Gobel, 1979; Light & Perl, 1979a, 1979b). Lamina I consists mainly of Golgi type I neurons or projection neurons whose axons ascend to the brain stem (Gobel, 1979).

Lamina II consists of an outer layer containing small, closely packed neurons with a large number of dendritic processes and an inner layer with a less dense texture and fewer dendritic terminals (Gobel, 1979). Nociceptive and non-nociceptive small-diameter afferents project to the outer and inner layers of lamina II, respectively. Lamina II contains predominantly two types of interneurons, "stalked cells" and "islet cells" (Bennett, Abdelmoumene, Hayashi, & Dubner, 1980; Gobel, 1979; Gobel et al., 1980; Ramón y Cajal, 1928/1982). As shown in Figure 3.3, the cell bodies of stalked cells are located in the dorsal half of lamina II, near the I–II border. The axons of stalked cells generally extend dorsally into lamina I, whereas the dendrites extend ventrally across lamina II with some extension into laminae III and IV. Because the dendrites of stalked cells penetrate to the inner and outer layers of lamina II, they receive both nociceptive and non-nociceptive input. The

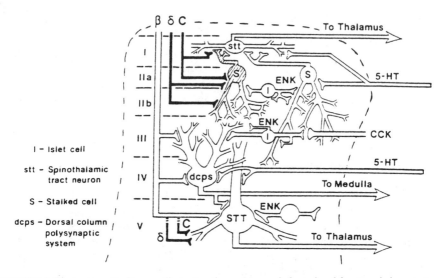

FIGURE 3.3. A schematic diagram illustrating the major morphological and functional characteristics of neurons and neural interconnections within dorsal horn layers (or laminae) I through V. Sensory projection neurons are indicated in layers I, IV, and V. These include NS and WDR spinothalamic tract neurons, as well as dorsal column postsynaptic (dcps) neurons. Layer I neurons receive mainly excitatory and perhaps some inhibitory connections from stalked cells in layer II. Stalked cells are either NS (left neuron in layer IIa) or WDR (right neuron in layer IIa), depending on the ventral extent of their dendrites. Those extending into only layer II are NS, whereas those extending more ventrally (wherein mechanoreceptive afferents synapse) are WDR. NS stalked cells receive their input from synapses on their spines in layers IIa and IIb. WDR stalked cells receive nociceptive afferent input in layers IIa and IIb, as well as in layers III and IV. Layer V projection neurons may receive connections from layer IV neurons, as well as direct primary afferent input. Several types of inhibitory interneurons are shown; some of these are enkephalinergic or dynorphinergic. The layer II NS islet cell receives exclusive input from nociceptive afferents, and it inhibits the output of stalked cells via various types of inhibitory synaptic connections. The more ventral islet cells receive input from sensitive mechanoreceptive afferents. Other types of low-threshold mechanoreceptive inhibitory neurons exist in the dorsal horn. From *Psychological and Neural Mechanisms of Pain* (p. 131) by D. D. Price, 1988, New York: Raven Press. Copyright 1988 by Raven Press. Reprinted by permission.

islet cell is a small interneuron with longitudinal dendrite projections within the lamina where the cell body is located. Small-diameter myelinated low-threshold mechanoreceptive afferents terminate in the inner portion of laminae II and III.

Lamina III consists primarily of islet cells, a few inverted stalked cells, and an interneuron with axonal projections to the inner zone of lamina II (Gobel, 1979). Lamina III cells may be particularly concerned with low-threshold afferents that terminate in the region (Bennet et al., 1981). Lamina IV neurons receive input from large-diameter myelinated afferents. They are most effectively activated by light mechanical stimuli (Price & Mayer, 1974; Wall, 1984a, 1984b). Lamina V neurons receive input from both large- and small-diameter afferents and respond to both innocuous and noxious stimuli. The axons of many of these cells project to the brain. These neurons are excited by both mechanical and thermal stimuli and can be excited into a state of continous discharge or "windup" by repetitive stimulation of C fiber afferents (Mayer, Price, & Becker, 1975; Price & Dubner, 1977). The neurons also display considerable cutaneous, muscular, and visceral convergence.

To summarize, the laminar organization is characterized by specialized dorsal horn cells that receive differential or convergent input from large- and small-diameter primary afferents and from interneurons with longitudinal or dorsal-ventral projections. The dorsal horn organization provides a framework for a multiplicity of excitatory and inhibitory synaptic connections that may modulate nociceptive transmission from primary nociceptive afferents to second-order projection neurons. A central neuron with an input from a primary nociceptive afferent may also receive excitatory or inhibitory input from other nociceptive and non-nociceptive afferents, either directly by convergent input or indirectly by synaptic connections with excitatory or inhibitory interneurons. (See Bennett et al., 1980; Fields & Basbaum, 1984; Price, 1984a, 1988; and Wall, 1967, 1978, 1980, for more detailed reviews of the possible excitatory and inhibitory mechanisms.) Figure 3.3 illustrates one model of the modulating influences within the dorsal horn (Price, 1988).

Two types of nociceptive neurons have been identified in the spinal cord: "nociceptive-specific" (NS) and "wide-dynamic-range" (WDR) neurons (Price & Dubner, 1977; Hayes, Price, & Dubner, 1979). NS neurons respond exclusively or nearly exclusively to intense mechanical or thermal stimuli and receive convergent input from both A-delta and C nociceptive afferents. NS spinothalamic tract neurons are located primarily in lamina I, but are located to a lesser extent in laminae IV and V. These neurons receive exclusive excitatory input from impulses in small-diameter fibers, including high-threshold A-delta mechanosensitive afferents and C polymodal nociceptive afferents. Two general types of NS neurons have been identified: high-threshold NS neurons, which respond to only definitely noxious mechanical stimuli; and moderate- to high-threshold NS neurons, which respond to firm, nonpainful pressure of the skin but respond with a higher-frequency impulse discharge to noxious stimuli (Kumazawa & Perl, 1978; Price, Dubner, & Hu, 1976; Price, Hayes, Ruda, & Dubner, 1978). The latter type of cell may signal information about a strong but not painful stimulus, as well as about a noxious stimulus (Price, 1984a, 1988). As shown in Figures 3.2C and 3.2D, the responses of NS neurons to graded noxious skin temperatures (44–51°C) increase monotonically; this is consistent with psychophysical research showing that pain strength increases montonically over the same temperature range (Hardy, Wolff, & Goodell, 1952; Price, Barrell, & Gracely 1980). There is evidence that NS neurons are inhibited by stimulation of large fibers in the dorsal column (Foreman, Beall, Applebaum, Coulter, & Willis, 1976) or transcutaneous electrical nerve stimulation (TENS; Cervero et al., 1976), two methods that produce analgesia.

WDR neurons respond to low-threshold stimulation, but respond maximally to noxious mechanical or thermal stimuli (Figures 3.2C and 3.2D). They exist in high concentrations in lamina V and to a lesser extent in laminae I, II, IV, and VI (Price et al., 1976; Price et al., 1978; Price, Hayashi, Dubner, & Ruda, 1979). They receive convergent input from A-beta, A-delta, and C afferents. The sensitivity of WDR neurons to innocuous as well as noxious stimuli suggests that they relay information about the quality of the sensation, as well as about pain strength. Many WDR neurons in laminae I and V are spinothalamic tract neurons, which convey messages directly to the thalamus. The "receptive fields" (the body regions in which neurons respond to stimulation) for WDR neurons are organized into concentric zones. In the central zone, the neurons respond differently as the stimulus intensity increases from gentle touch to firm pressure to noxious pinch. Neuronal impulses increase progressively as the stimulus intensity increases. These central zones are surrounded by less sensitive zones, in which only firm pressure and noxious stimuli will elicit an impulse discharge. Finally, these zones are surrounded by another, even less sensitive zone, in which only noxious stimulation will evoke an impulse discharge. The receptive field zones can expand or contract. Recordings from WDR neurons in alert monkeys showed that the size of the receptive field expanded when a monkey performed a thermal discrimination task and contracted when it was performing a visual discrimination task (Hayes, Dubner, & Hoffman, 1981; Hoffman, Dubner, Hayes, & Medlin, 1981). It is almost incredible that the size of the receptive fields of WDR neurons can increase or decrease depending on an animals' attention. This observation provides an exciting clue for explaining how pain may be blocked in humans by cognitive-behavioral methods.

WDR neurons respond to noxious mechanical or noxious thermal stimulation with a higher frequency of impulse discharge than that evoked by any form of innocuous stimuli. There are several parallels between the physiological characteristics of WDR neurons and the psychological characteristics of human pain experience (Price, 1984b, 1988). Responses of WDR neurons to graded levels of noxious thermal stimuli increase monotonically over a 45–51°C range. The rate of increase in impulse discharge in these neurons is the same as the rate of increase in pain sensations when humans experience the same noxious heat pulses. Also, like humans' ratings of pain, the responses of WDR neurons to noxious thermal pulses can be influenced by the psychological set of the organism. The responses of these neurons to temperatures from 45° to 49°C are higher when the monkey is performing a thermal discrimination task, when thermal stimuli are quite relevant to a successful performance, than when performing a visual discrimination task, when thermal stimuli are not relevant.

In summary, neuronal impulses from thermoreceptive, nociceptive, and mechanoreceptive afferents excite various types of second-order neurons in the dorsal horn. Impulses from primary nociceptive afferents are not passively reproduced onto the second-order pathways for subsequent projection to the brain, but are actively transformed by a complex network of excitatory and inhibitory control mechanisms.

Ascending Pathways to the Brain

Nociceptive information is conducted in ascending pathways from the spinal cord and trigeminal nuclei to the brain stem and thalamus. Several different pathways convey nociceptive information, such as the spinothalamic, spinoreticular, spinomesencephalic, spinocervical, and second-order dorsal column tracks (Bowsher, 1957; Dennis & Melzack, 1977; Melzack & Wall, 1982; Willis, 1985; Willis & Coggeshall, 1978). Evidence indicates that the relative importance of these nociceptive pathways varies among species. Similarly, the exact origin and destination of the various pathways are also species-dependent (Willis, 1984). The spinothalamic tract has been regarded as the most important pathway for conducting nociceptive information in humans (White & Sweet, 1955; Willis, 1984). Clinical and behavioral studies have shown that lesions interrupting the spinothalamic tract in the anterolateral quadrant of the spinal cord produce a loss of pain sensation below the level of the lesion on the contralateral side of the body in humans (Foerster & Gagel, 1931; White & Sweet, 1955). Although the precise locations of the cells of origin for the spinothalamic tract in the human spinal cord are not known with certainty, anatomical evidence indicates that there are numerous spinothalamic tract cells in laminae I and V, regions that contain both NS and WDR neurons (Willis, 1984, 1985). Although pathways ascending in the anterolateral quadrant are crucial for signaling pain in humans, other pathways also play a role, since pain may return months to years after an initially successful cordotomy (a surgical procedure in which the quadrant is lesioned) (Foerster & Gagel, 1931; White & Sweet, 1955, 1969). The return of pain in these cases is probably not due to regeneration of the anterolateral quadrant pathways, since another cordotomy does not necessarily restore analgesia. The pain probably is signaled by pathways other than those contained in the lesioned anterolateral quadrant. Pathways in the dorsal part of the spinal cord that may play a part in nociception include the spinocervical tract and the second-order dorsal column tract. Recordings from neurons in these tracts show that at least some cells are nociceptive (Angaut-Petit, 1975; Brown & Fyffe, 1981).

Many dorsal horn neurons are projection neurons whose axons ascend to the brain. The neospinothalamic tract is composed of long fibers that project directly to the ventrolateral and posterior thalamus, where they synapse onto neurons that project to the primary somatosensory cortex. Impulses are conducted rapidly along this pathway to facilitate perception of the location, intensity, and duration of the noxious stimulus. The paleospinothalamic tract is composed of long and short fibers that project to the reticular formation, the medulla, the midbrain, the periaqueductal grey (PAG), the hypothalamus, and the medial thalamus, and that synapse with neurons projecting to the limbic forebrain structures and to many other parts of the brain. Impulses conducted along the paleospinothalamic tract stimulate suprasegmental reflex responses that modulate ventilation, endocrine function, and circulation.

Some NS, WDR, and non-noxious responding neurons in the superficial and deep layers of the spinal cord dorsal horn are spinothalamic tract neurons that project primarily to the contralateral thalamus. The spinothalamic tract terminates in the ventral posterior lateral nucleus and the central lateral nucleus (Bowsher, 1957; Mehler, 1962; Willis, 1984). For many years, investigators were unable to identify neurons responding to noxious stimulation in the primary somatosensory cortex. However, recent work has demonstrated the location of these neurons in the primary somatosensory cortex (Guilbaud, Peschanski, & Besson, 1984; Kenshalo, Giesler, Leonard, & Willis, 1980; Kenshalo & Isensee, 1980; Lamour, Willer, & Guilbaud, 1982). The thalamus is much more than a simple relay station for the transfer of information between ascending pathways and the cerebral cortex. Electron-microscopic examination of the thalamus has shown a complex array of synaptic interactions among cells that project to the cortex; interneurons; axons from ascending tracts; and axons from the cerebral cortex, thalamic reticular nucleus, and other regions of the brain. Anatomical evidence of multiple synaptic connections has been supplemented by physiological descriptions of the varied excitatory influences among different types of neurons. The circuitry of the thalamus facilitates a wide variety of synaptic interactions betwen ascending projections from the spinal cord and brain stem and neurons of the cerebral cortex.

Despite much progress in mapping ascending pathways, many questions remain unanswered about the supraspinal mechanisms in nociception. The characteristics of neuronal responses and the mapped anatomical relationships suggest that distinct nuclei may be differentially involved in the sensory-discriminative, motor, motivational, or affective functions of nociceptive processing, corresponding to the different aspects of pain perception (for review, see Guilbaud et al., 1984; Price, 1988; Willis, 1985).

Endogenous Pain-Suppressing Mechanisms

Research on pain modulation by activation of endogenous pain-inhibitory systems represents an exciting area that has rapidly developed during the last two decades (Akil & Watson, 1980; Basbaum & Fields, 1978; Cannon, Liebeskind, & Frenk, 1978; Fields, 1985; Fields & Basbaum, 1978, 1984; Hammond, 1985; Kosterlitz & McKnight, 1980; Mayer & Price, 1976; Terenius, 1978, 1984, 1985; Yaksh & Rudy, 1976). Since Melzack and Wall (1965) first proposed the existence of a descending pain-modulating system as part of their gate control theory of pain, much evidence has accumulated from anatomical, physiological, and behavioral studies to support their hypothesis of a central system that modulates neuronal responses to noxious stimuli. The dual discoveries of opiate receptors and endogenous opioids (endorphins) in the same regions of the brain from which stimulation-produced analgesia (SPA, in which electrical stimulation produces profound loss of pain sensation) could be elicited, and the reversal or antagonism of SPA by the relatively specific opiate antagonist naloxone, established the concept of an endogenous opioid-mediated analgesia system. Endogenous opioid peptides are distributed at both spinal and supraspinal levels, at sites coincident with the mapping of opiate receptors and enkephalin-containing neurons.

During the 1970s, several laboratories reported the discovery of opiate receptors in the mammalian brain (Akil, Watson, Berger, & Barchas, 1978; Atweh & Kuhar, 1977; Pert & Snyder, 1973; Simon, Hiller, & Edelman, 1973; Snyder, 1977; Terenius, 1978). In 1975, Hughes et al. isolated the first two endogenous opioid peptides, leu- and met-enkephalin. These peptides have pharmacological properties similar to those of morphine. Since their discovery, several other peptides with properties similar to analgesics have been identified in the brain and pituitary (Cox, Goldstein, & Li, 1976; Goldstein, Tachibana, Lowney, Hunkapiller, & Hood, 1979; Weber, Roth, & Barchas, 1981). The class of opiate-like peptides has been referred to by the generic term "endorphins." The analgesic effects of these peptides may be prevented by the administration of the opiate antagonist naloxone. The functions of endogenous opioids for pain control have usually been studied by blocking the opioid receptor with naloxone and then examining the subsequent effects on pain perception.

SPA is a highly specific and powerful suppression of pain-related behavior by electrical stimulation of certain discrete brain sites (Mayer & Liebeskind, 1974; Reynolds, 1969). During SPA, animals are alert and respond to most environmental stimuli, except for noxious stimuli. Electrical stimulation in analogous brain sites in patients with chronic pain produces a similar loss of pain without any other sensory loss. Research on SPA in animals and humans has demonstrated the importance of endogenous opioids in the control of pain (Adams, 1976; Cleeland, Shacham, Dahl, & Orrison, 1984; Hammond, 1985; Hammond & Yaksh, 1981; Kofinas, Kofinas, & Tavakoli, 1985; Sjolund & Bjorklund, 1982; Sjolund & Eriksson, 1980). The cerebrospinal fluid obtained from stimulated human patients was assayed to determine the presence of endogenous opioids. There was a significant rise in opioid peptides during electrical stimulation (Akil et al., 1978). Although studies of SPA are critical, in that they demonstrate the role of endogenous opioids in pain regulation, they also indicate the complexity of pain modulation. Naloxone reversibility of SPA is dependent on the specific parameters of stimulation, including the site, frequency, and duration of stimulation.

During SPA, nociceptive cells in the spinal cord dorsal horn are selectively inhibited by stimulation at analgesia-producing brain stem sites (Guilbaud, Besson, Oliveras, & Liebeskind, 1973). Figure 3.4 illustrates the major strucures that have been implicated in generating analgesia (Fields & Basbaum, 1984). Originally, Basbaum and Fields (1984) proposed the PAG as the origin of an endorphin-mediated analgesia system. However, considerable anatomical data have been obtained about possible inputs to the PAG. Some of these inputs may be critical for initiating the descending pain-inhibitory systems. The PAG is still considered a critical component of this system, along with the rostral ventromedial medulla (RVM) and the superficial layers of the dorsal horn, as shown in Figure 3.4. The

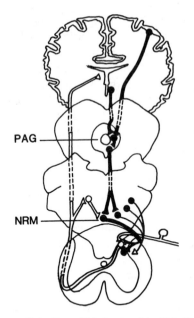

FIGURE 3.4. A diagram illustrating the critical structures that contribute to the control of pain transmission neurons. The periaqueductal grey (PAG), at the midbrain level, is an important site for brain stimulation-produced analgesia and for analgesia produced by microinjection of opiate analgesics. The nucleus raphe magnus (NRM), at the medullary level, is the site for serotonin-containing cells. Cells in the NRM and the adjacent nucleus reticularis magnocellularis receive excitatory effects and neuronal input from PAG. They project afferent axons to the spinal cord via the dorsolateral funiculus to terminate among NS sensory projection neurons in layers I and V and the spinal cord dorsal horn (area with synaptic connections shown in lower right portion of figure). Collaterals from this area project to structures involved in descending inhibition, as well as pain-processing brain structures (shown by the open pathways on the left side of the figure). At the spinal level, descending pathways inhibit nociceptive projection neurons through direct connections, as well as through interneurons in the superficial layers of the dorsal horn. In addition to this brain stem spinal cord network, connections from neocortex and hypothalamus to the PAG have recently been documented. Adapted from "Endogenous Pain Control Mechanisms" by H. L. Fields and A. I. Basbaum, 1984, in P. D. Wall and R. Melzack (Eds.), *Textbook of Pain* (p. 143). Edinburgh: Churchill Livingstone. Copyright 1984 by Longman Group Limited. Adapted by permission.

PAG receives afferents from the frontal cortex and hypothalamus and projects to neurons in the RVM; RVM neurons, in turn, project to and control pain transmission neurons in the superficial dorsal horn. Both PAG and RVM contain opioid peptides and produce analgesia when stimulated. Thus, pain modulation is subserved by a spatially extensive system that is distributed along the entire system, including neocortical limbic brain stem and spinal components (Basbaum & Fields, 1978, 1984; Fields & Basbaum, 1984). Endogenous opioid peptides are widely distributed and overlap extensively with spinal and midbrain regions important for nociceptive processing. Lesions or local anesthetic injections onto the RVM will abolish the analgesia produced by stimulation of PAG (Behbehani & Fields, 1979), supporting the hypothesis that the pain-modulating action of the PAG is relayed through the RVM. Stimulation of the RVM selectively inhibits dorsal horn neurons that respond maximally to noxious stimulation. This inhibition is blocked by lesions of the dorsolateral funiculus (Fields, Basbaum, Clanton, & Anderson, 1977; Willis, Haber, & Martin, 1977).

An endogenous endorphin-mediated analgesia system may be activated by various methods, such as prolonged noxious stimulation or by exposing animals to a variety of stressful stimuli. A naloxone-reversible analgesic effect can also be demonstrated with classical conditioning paradigms. In these situations, an innocuous stimulus (e.g., a tone) is paired with a stressful analgesia-inducing stimulus (e.g., prolonged foot shock) until the relatively neutral stimulus begins to elicit analgesia by itself.

Animal behavior studies indicate that stress, fear, pain intensity, and pain duration are all important factors for activating endogenous endorphin-mediated analgesic systems. As an example, Watkins and Mayer (1982) proposed that activation of an endorphin-mediated analgesia system is associated with learned helplessness. When animals are unable to avoid a stimulus that is painful, they develop analgesia. These investigators suggest that an animal's ability to control a noxious stimulus is a major factor that determines whether an endorphin-mediated analgesic system is activated. They conducted an experiment in which they delivered identical electrical stimuli to paired groups of rats. Only one of the rats in the group could terminate the shock by actively turning a wheel. Although all rats in the group received exactly the same shock, only rats that could not control the shocks developed significant naloxone-reversible analgesia. Thus, the fear or stress produced by lack of control may be an important factor for activating this system. There is also evidence that pain-modulating pathways without endorphins exist; however, their underlying pharmacology is not yet known.

Acute and Chronic Pain

The nociceptive mechanisms responsible for pain perception are complex interactive systems. The sensory nerves that detect and transmit information about tissue damage, and the descending pain-inhibitory systems that modify their activity, are important features of nociceptive processing. However, these mechanisms have been studied predominantly in response to acute pain produced by the application of a relatively short-duration noxious stimulus. Although mechanisms that are activated by a prolonged noxious stimulus are much less clearly understood, it is clear that chronic pain is not simply a prolongation of the same mechanisms induced by acute pain; rather, chronic pain activates different mechanisms (Wall, 1984a, 1984c).

When a nerve is damaged by a noxious stimulus, there are many immediate and long-term effects. For example, after an axon is cut, there is an immediate discharge followed by a period of relative insensitivity, described by Wall (1984a, 1984c) as "the calm before the storm." The cut ends then begin to seal and develop sprouts. The sprouts are spontaneously active, mechanically sensitive, and sensitive to adrenalin. Sprouts may establish contacts with other sprouts, thereby facilitating impulses from one axon to another. This mechanism may allow neuronal impulses from the region of damage to be transferred onto other nerve fibers (Seltzer & Devore, 1979). In addition to these changes at the site of injury, subsequent central changes may be traced. These occur in the axon proximal to the cut and in the spinal cord; they are alterations in the responsivity of neurons and in the inhibitory mechanisms in the spinal cord. Damage to the peripheral nervous system can lead to a variety of pathological pain states as a result of changes induced in the central nervous system.

In spite of new information on central processing and endogenous pain-inhibitory mechanisms, many clinical pain phenomena are still not satisfactorily explained. The explanations presumably depend on continued research about the relationships betwen the peripheral and central nervous systems and the mechanisms for conducting acute and prolonged pain. Special emphasis must be placed on investigation of pathological pain—pain produced in a non-normal fashion, in a way other than the application of an intense tissue-damaging stimulus. It is essential to begin to understand more precisely the immediate and long-term consequences of peripheral injury, both at the site of injury and in the central nervous system.

Critical Features of the Nociceptive System

The special features of the nociceptive system are not simply the different components of the sensory system—that is, the specific nociceptors, primary nociceptive afferents, nociceptive pathways, ascending from the spinal cord to the thalamus and cortex, and descending pain-inhibitory systems. Instead, the critical features of nociceptive processing are the facilitative mechanisms that modulate the impulses conveyed by nociceptive fibers. The central convergence of input from nociceptive and non-nociceptive peripheral fibers onto second-order neurons, the central mechanisms of excitation and inhibition, and the activation of endogenous pain-suppressing systems represent the special features that characterize nociception as a plastic and complex sensory system. Central neurons receive excitatory and inhibitory input from other nociceptive and non-nociceptive afferents and from neurons descending from the brain.

Certain types of skin sensations show evidence of temporal summation and prolonged discharge. Since responses of primary afferent neurons do not temporally summate or long outlast the duration of stimulation, such phenomena must occur centrally. Several studies have demonstrated that the spinal cord dorsal horn is the site of origin of temporal summation and afterresponses, and that such phenomena show striking parallels to the perceived intensity and qualities of pain experienced in humans (Price et al., 1978).

Noxious somatic stimuli sometimes evoke sensations that last longer than the stimulus application. These afterdischarges, lasting several hundred milliseconds, can be evoked in spinothalamic tract neurons by single electric shocks to A-delta and C fiber afferents or by brief noxious heat stimuli. Some non-noxious stimuli also evoke prolonged afterresponses in spinothalamic neurons and after sensations. As an example, if a very gentle and tactile stimulus (e.g, a fingernail) is applied along the line between your upper lip and the skin above the lip, a tingling sensation is experienced that persists after the finger is withdrawn. These sensations will stop abruptly when you rub the stimulated region. It has been shown that a similar stimulus applied to a monkey's foot will evoke 20- to 60-second after-discharges in WDR spinothalamic neurons. These afterdischarges can be abruptly ended by rubbing the stimulated region. WDR neurons are the only type of dorsal horn neurons that exhibit tactile evoked afterresponses. The relationship between the WDR neurons and tactile evoked responses may partially account for certain pathological pain syndromes, in which very gentle stimulation provokes intense paroxysmal pain.

Response characteristics of WDR and NS spinothalamic neurons also reflect a variety of inhibitory mechanisms related to nociception (Price, 1984a, 1988). The most familiar type of inhibition is initiated by stimulation of low-threshold mecha-noreceptive afferents. Most low-threshold mechanoreceptive afferents have rapid conduction velocities and large-diameter axons. Repetitive stimulation of these afferents, by electrical stimulation of the dorsal columns or by low-intensity electrical stimulation of peripheral cutaneous nerves, can inhibit the responsivity of the second-order neurons that receive input from high-threshold primary affer-ents. The inhibition of WDR and NS neurons by dorsal column and peripheral nerve stimulation led to the development of analgesia produced in humans by dorsal column stimulation or by TENS (described in detail in Chapter 5). WDR neurons can also be inhibited by intense stimulation of body zones that are quite remote from the neuron's receptive field (LeBars, Dickenson, & Besson, 1979). Both spontaneous impulse discharge and the nociceptive responses of monkey WDR neurons can be inhibited by intense mechanical stimulation of the contralateral foot or hand, or many zones within the trigeminal region. A similar phenomenon has been shown for humans, when intense pressure is applied to the contralateral hand and "second" pain evoked by electrical stimulation of C afferents in the hand is almost completely suppressed (Melzack & Wall, 1965).

Both opiate- and non-opiate-related systems descend to dorsal horn laminae I, II, and to some extent V. Inhibition of nociceptive responses of WDR and NS neurons are probably mediated partly by serotonergic and noradrenergic mecha-nisms, as well as by enkephalinergic interneuronal mechanisms within the dorsal horn itself (Basbaum & Fields, 1984; Fields & Basbaum, 1984; Glazer & Basbaum, 1981; Ruda, 1982). These descending controls may be triggered by intense somato-sensory input or by psychological factors that occur during stress. Current investi-gations are revealing the complex interactions within the dorsal horn related to the variety of descending inhibitory controls.

In summary, a stimulus that produces tissue damage initiates a sequence of neural events that can lead to the perception of pain. However, the perception of pain is not simply and directly related to the quality or extent of tissue damage. The neural excitation initiated peripherally by a noxious stimulus may be influ-enced at many sites within the central nervous system. A barrage of impulses are conducted along both nociceptive and non-nociceptive primary afferents to syn-apse onto second-order neurons in the spinal dorsal horn. Peripheral afferents collect specific information from sites in the periphery and deliver impulses to the six laminae of the dorsal horn, which are major sites for the modulation of nociceptive input. Activity in primary afferents can inhibit the transmission of nociceptive information to second-order projection neurons. Central neurons that respond to nociceptive afferents may be modulated by peripheral afferents other than those that excited them, and also by systems descending from the brain stem. The dorsal horn gating mechanisms are extremely complex networks of excitatory and inhibitory interactions. Fibers of projection neurons ascend from the spinal cord along several pathways to the thalamus and cortex. The ascending nociceptive tracts provide information about the sensory-discriminative aspects of pain, arouse the motivational–affective aspects of pain, activate descending analgesia systems, and initiate autonomic and motor responses. The perception of pain depends upon the complex interactions between nociceptive and non-nociceptive impulses in ascending pathways, in relation to the activation of descending pain-inhibitory systems.

The critical features of nociception—specificity, convergence, inhibition, summation, and descending control—have important implications for the management of pediatric pain. However, the clinical application of this knowledge has unfortunately lagged behind the scientific advances in our understanding of the plasticity of nociception. It is necessary to begin to adapt the principles of pain management gained from adult and animal studies to children who experience acute, chronic, or recurrent pain problems.

4

Pharmacological Interventions for Alleviating Children's Pain

A surplus of over-the-counter and prescription drugs is available for alleviating pain and suffering. Pharmacological interventions for pain relief comprise a major competitive industry, as is readily evidenced by the diverse array of advertisements in medical journals, in magazines, in newspapers, and on television. These advertisements present colorful and provocative claims as to the analgesic power of a variety of products. Drugs for controlling pain in children may be promoted with special claims about the drug's potency, lack of side effects, and pleasing taste.

Despite the availability of many drugs for pain control, the prescription and administration of analgesics to infants, children, and adolescents constitute a controversial issue. Clinical reports indicate that children do not always receive the analgesics required to alleviate their pain. This issue, the appropriate selection and administration of analgesic medication for children, provides the foundation for this chapter. The major categories of analgesic drugs, their probable modes of action, and their current prescription and administration in pediatrics are reviewed. Emphasis is placed on a description of the principles of analgesic selection and administration for optimal pain management, rather than on a delineation of the specific analgesic and risk properties of individual drugs.

Do Children Receive Adequate Types and Doses of Pain Medication?

Much attention has been focused recently on whether infants, children, and adolescents receive appropriate and adequate medication to alleviate their acute, recurrent, or chronic pain. Several articles have been published that highlight the special problem of undermedication for children and that raise serious questions as to the scope of the problem. Investigators have reported major discrepancies between adults and children in the prescription or subsequent administration of analgesics (Anand & Aynsley-Green, 1988; Anand & Hickey, 1987; Beyer, DeGood, Ashley, & Russell, 1983; Eland, 1974; Schechter, Allen, & Hanson, 1986; Swafford & Allan, 1968). Retrospective chart reviews, in which the prescription and administration of drugs (type of drug, dosage, administration route, and efficacy, as assessed by voiced pain complaints) are examined, were performed in these studies for adults and children who had similar medical problems and presumably similar pain experiences. Swafford and Allan (1968), in a survey of children admitted to an intensive care unit during a 4-month period, reported that only 14% of the children (26 of 180) received any narcotics for pain relief. Only 3% of the child patients who had general surgery received analgesics, presumably because "pediatric patients seldom need relief of pain after general surgery. They tolerate discomfort well" (Swafford & Allan, 1968, p. 133).

In a later study, Eland (1974) examined differences between 18 adults and 25 children in the type and administration of analgesics. Although the children had medical conditions similar to those of the adults, the adults received 372 narcotic and 299 non-narcotic analgesic doses during their hospitalization, whereas the children received only 24 analgesic doses. In fact, 13 children received no analgesics, despite diagnoses that included traumatic amputation of the foot, excision of neck mass, and heminephrectomy. It is possible that adults and children were not matched equally with respect to their medical diagnoses and surgical traumas, so that adults may have experienced stronger pain; nevertheless, the difference in medication doses is still surprising. This tendency to undermedicate children is still evident in recent studies (Beyer et al., 1983; Schechter et al., 1986).

In 1977, Eland and Anderson summarized some of the common explanations offered by medical staff for why children do not receive potent narcotic analgesics:

- Children's nervous systems are immature, so that they are unable to experience the same pain intensity as adults.
- Children possess an enhanced ability to recover from illness or trauma, so that they do not require the same medication as adults.
- The risks of addiction or respiratory depression are high when children receive narcotic analgesics.
- Children are unable to communicate their pain to medical staff.
- Nurses are distressed by administering painful injections to relieve children's pain.

These justifications or myths may be attributed to a lack of general understanding about the basic principles of nociceptive mechanisms; to a lack of specific knowledge about children's ability to perceive pain; to an absence of trustworthy methods for measuring pediatric pain; and to communication difficulties among medical staff, nursing staff, patients, and the families of patients about children's pain experiences and behaviors. More recently, nurses and medical staff have provided similar reasons as to why children may be undermedicated. A study on the incidence of postoperative pain in children indicated that there was an implicit practice of administering the minimal analgesic doses at the maximal time intervals between doses because of fear of addiction (Mather & Mackie, 1983). Common themes reflecting misunderstanding of how children feel pain and the manner in which they express pain emerge in several studies of why medical and nursing staff are reluctant to prescribe and administer analgesics to children.

Mather and Mackie (1983) surveyed the incidence of pain in 170 children (69 girls, 101 boys) recovering from surgery. Analgesic medication was not ordered for 16% of patients, and the narcotic analgesic medication that was ordered was not administered to another 29%. This study was unique in that it consisted of prospective interviews with children and pain assessments during their surgical recovery, rather than only retrospective chart reviews. Each patient was visited two to four times during each of 3 postoperative days. Interviews and assessments were conducted by the same registered nurse, who had specialized in pediatric nursing. A 4-point pain severity scale (no pain, mild pain, moderate pain, severe pain) was used to assess each child's pain experiences. In addition to the pain responses, the investigators collected data on each child's age and sex; type of surgery; preoperative medication ordered (dose, frequency, and route of administration); postsurgical analgesics ordered (dose, frequency, and route of administration); postsurgical analgesics given (number of doses, total dose); side effects of medication; and a global estimate of analgesic efficacy. At least 90% of the patients were premedicated prior to surgery, predominantly with a commercially available mixture of papaverine and hyoscine. Postoperative medications were ordered for 84% of the patients. The most common prescription included a narcotic and a non-narcotic analgesic, rather than narcotic medication alone. Meperidine and acetaminophen were the most frequently ordered narcotic and non-narcotic medications, respectively. The primary drugs (the more potent analgesic drugs, including narcotics) that were ordered were not administered to approximately 40% of children. Although non-narcotic analgesics, principally acetaminophen, were substituted generally for narcotic analgesics, analgesics were not administered for some children.

Overall, only 25% of patients were pain-free on the day of surgery, regardless of the medication that they received, and approximately 40% of the patients experienced moderate or severe pain. There was no apparent relationship between the type of surgery and the prescription of analgesic medication. The incidence of moderate or severe pain reported by children during the postoperative period was high, regardless of their analgesic treatment. In addition, the prescribing patterns of the medical staff who managed these patients were not consistent. The interpretation of the analgesic medication orders by nursing staff, which often led to substitutions of non-narcotic analgesics for more potent narcotic analgesics, also contributed to poor analgesia for children.

Several issues critical to the management of children's pain are evident in this study. Who should assume principal responsibility for the choice and administration of medications? In many cases, adequate medications were not ordered. Since the majority of orders were written for narcotic primary and non-narcotic secondary medication, the attending nurses decided which medications were actually administered, based on the children's needs. In addition, most orders were written p.r.n. (*pro re nata*, as necessary or according to circumstances), which requires further judgment as to the time intervals between drug administration. Although p.r.n. should provide the optimum treatment in theory, since medication administration is scheduled by patient need, there are difficulties with this administration route. Patients are usually required to experience and report pain before pain medication is administered. There was also a large variability among dosage regimens in the study, both in the size of doses and in the minimal time interval specified between doses. As an example, some high-clearance drugs, with typical plasma lives of 3-4 hours, require dosing intervals of 3-4 hours for effective pain relief. Some children had lengthy intervals between doses; as a result, the doses were insufficient to provide analgesia. Furthermore, individual variability should be recognized and doses administered accordingly. Nearly 50% of the prescriptions written for meperidine were for doses of less than 1 mg/kg, with the stated pediatric dose in the formulary of one of the hospitals as 1-2 mg/kg. Many of the doses ordered were inadequate, regardless of the frequency with which doses were actually administered. Mather and Mackie (1983) emphasize that the primary potent drug that was ordered was not administered in 46% of all cases. In many of these cases, another less potent drug was substituted.

Beyer et al. (1983) compared the postoperative prescriptions and administrations of analgesics after cardiac surgery for 50 children with those for 50 adults. Children were prescribed significantly fewer narcotics. They received only 30% of all the analgesics that were administered, whereas adults received 70%. Schechter et al. (1986) conducted a chart review to investigate the use of analgesics with 90 children and 90 adults who were selected randomly from hospital charts. They then matched children with adults according to their sex and four diagnostic categories: hernias, appendectomies, burns, and fractured femurs. Adults received an average of 2.2 doses of narcotics per day, whereas children received only 1.1 doses. Significant differences in dosing practices were also noted between the diagnostic categories. For example, there was a greater discrepancy in narcotic administration between children and adults for medical diagnoses that required longer hospital stays. Adults received more narcotics. There were also significant differences in dosing among different hospitals, with an urban hospital administering more doses per day than a rural hospital. Narcotics were ordered less often for infants and young children than for older children; when they were ordered, however, the frequency of administration was similar for all children.

The true extent to which infants and children are undermedicated—whether because of a failure to recognize their pain or because of a general reluctance to assume responsibility for the selection and administration of appropriate analgesics—is not known. Although clinical studies indicate that undermedication for children can be a serious problem, more research is necessary to determine its prevalence. As described in Chapter 3, our understanding of pain, pain control, and the responsible nociceptive mechanisms has changed dramatically during the past 20 years. However, there is an unfortunate lag between the scientific accumulation of knowledge about the plasticity and complexity of the nociceptive system and the application of that knowledge to the management of pain in pediatrics. Reliance on an outdated concept of pain as a rigid, inflexible system dictates a relatively inflexible approach to pain management that may account in part for the reliance on minimal analgesic medications for children. Education about nociceptive mechanisms, including endogenous pain-inhibitory systems and the factors that activate them, must be provided more consistently to health professionals so that children's pain can be assessed and managed in accordance with what is truly known and not merely assumed about their perceptions. At present, there is little objective, prospective information available about the prevalence of different types of pain in children or about the efficacy of the different analgesic medications used to manage children's pain.

Analgesic Medications

The term "analgesic" describes a category of drugs that act to reduce pain selectively, without producing a loss of consciousness. (By contrast, general anesthetics produce both pain reduction and loss of consciousness.) Of all analgesic prescriptions, 99% derive from only two families of compounds: the aspirin type and the opium type. There are several names for similar pain drugs, because similar mixtures may be advertised and sold either by their chemical composition or by their product trade names. In general, pain relief is produced by drugs that act centrally to inhibit the transmission of nociceptive signals to the brain or by drugs that act peripherally to inhibit the metabolism of pain-producing substances in body tissues. Narcotics relieve pain by their actions on the central nervous system, whereas aspirin and similar drugs relieve pain by their actions on the peripheral nervous system. Analgesics vary in pain-reducing potency, in the extent to which they produce undesirable side effects, and in their probable mode of action. Selection of an appropriate analgesic for children requires consideration of the nature of the pain and the potency, side effects, and physiological properties of the available analgesics. (For reviews, see Beers & Bassett, 1979; Dundee & Loan, 1983; Gladtke, 1983; Houde, 1979; Huskisson, 1984; Jaffe & Martin, 1980; Littlejohns & Vere, 1981; Mitchell, Lovejoy, Slone, & Shapiro, 1982; Twycross, 1984.)

Non-Narcotic Analgesics

The non-narcotic analgesics include antipyretic drugs to lower body temperature and anti-inflammatory drugs to reduce swelling. These are the drugs of choice for controlling low-intensity pain, fever, and inflammation. The most commonly prescribed antipyretic analgesics for children are aspirin compounds and aceta-minophen. Antipyretic drugs have a long history of therapeutic use, with a high level of effectiveness, a low level of toxicity, and limited abuse potential.

Aspirin

In 1763, the Reverend Edward Stone wrote to the Royal Society in London that the extract of willow bark reduced fever and alleviated suffering from rheumatism. Leroux identified the active ingredient in the willow extract in 1827. He named it "salicin" for the scientific name of the tree from which it was isolated, *Salix alba*. The subsequent synthesis of acetylsalicylic acid replaced the analgesic use of salicylates derived from naturally occurring sources. Dreser introduced acetylsali-cylic acid into the medical formulary in 1899, and it was later marketed by Bayer as "aspirin." Although aspirin has been widely used for its analgesic, antipyretic, and anti-inflammatory effects since 1899, its probable mechanism of action has been described only recently. Aspirin and other nonsteroidal anti-inflammatory drugs reduce pain in part by selectively inhibiting prostaglandin synthesis at the site of injury (Smith & Willis, 1971; Vane, 1971). However, the exact mechanism by which prostaglandins contribute to inflammation and pain is not yet known. Prostaglandins E_1 and E_2 are often released at the site of an injury. They may sensitize nociceptors to histamine and bradykinin, chemical substances released by inflammation that produce pain. Thus, the inhibition of local prostaglandin production should desensitize nerves and reduce pain.

Aspirin is the drug of choice for the relief of mild to moderate pain. It is most effective for controlling low- to moderate-intensity pain associated with inflamma-tion. After oral administration, aspirin is absorbed rapidly from the gastrointestinal tract, with peak blood levels occurring in approximately 2 hours. Once absorbed, the aspirin is metabolized to salicylic acid in various tissues. Asprin is a very safe drug for children, but it does have several side effects. The most frequently reported of these are gastrointestinal upset and bleeding. Aspirin-induced gastrointestinal injury results from a local irritation of the mucosal lining that allows diffusions of acid into the mucosa, with subsequent tissue damage. Aspirin is contraindicated for patients with gastrointestinal ulcers. Since aspirin inhibits prostaglandin syn-thesis, it can adversely affect platelet function (Roth & Majerus, 1975). Aspirin is also contraindicated for children with liver disease, hemophilia, Vitamin K defi-ciency, or platelet coagulation deficiencies, because it interferes with platelet aggregation. Furthermore, caution is recommended in the administration of as-pirin to children with influenza, because of a possible connection between the use of aspirin and the development of Reye's syndrome (American Academy of Pediat-rics, Committee on Infectious Diseases, 1982; National Surveillance for Reye Syndrome, 1982). Although there has been no unequivocal evidence of causation, epidemiological surveys of children with Reye's syndrome implicate aspirin as a factor.

Aspirin should be administered with milk or food to minimize gasterointestinal upset. When children drink a large amount of water with aspirin, the tablet dissolves more rapidly, so that there is less local gastrointestinal irritation. Aspirin has been mixed with many compounds to buffer its gastrointestinal effects, but generally these compounds are less effective buffers than food, milk, or antacids. Acetylsalicylic acid preparations are available for children in tablets, gums, and suppositories. The specific doses required for optimal analgesia vary with the form of the drug due to differences in absorption, as listed in hospital formularies and in *The Pediatric Drug Handbook* (Benitz & Tatro, 1981).

Acetaminophen

Acetaminophen, also known as paracetamol (e.g., Tylenol, Panadol, and other brands), was introduced by Von Mering as an analgesic and antipyretic in 1893. It is the major metabolite of phenacetin and acetanilid. Phenacetin was introduced into medicine as an analgesic in 1887; however, it was removed from the market because it had serious toxicity. Acetaminophen has antipyretic and analgesic properties equivalent to those of aspirin, but lacks aspirin's anti-inflammatory properties. It also does not have aspirin's gastrointestinal and hematological side effects or the possible connection with Reye's syndrome. Acetaminophen is probably the most commonly prescribed analgesic for mild to moderate pains. Its antipyretic properties make it a popular choice for the treatment of colds and influenza. Acetaminophen is an effective alternative to aspirin in patients who are aspirin-sensitive or who have bleeding problems. However, since acetaminophen does not have anti-inflammatory properties, it is not as effective as aspirin for children who have pain of an inflammatory origin. Acetaminophen's mechanism of action is still unclear. Although it is a weak inhibitor of prostaglandin synthesis, it appears to be more active in the central nervous system than in the periphery, unlike aspirin.

Acetaminophen is rapidly and completely absorbed from the stomach and upper small bowel, with peak levels occurring in 30–60 minutes after oral administration. Its plasma half-life is approximately 2 hours. The usual dose for children is similar to that for aspirin. Acetaminophen is available in elixirs, tablets, drops, and suppositories. Rectal absorption is more erratic than oral absorption. Acetaminophen is a good alternative analgesic for children who should avoid aspirin, since it provides comparable analgesic efficacy with significantly fewer side effects.

Combination Drugs

A variety of combination analgesics have been developed in order to combine the analgesic effects of aspirin or acetaminophen with compounds to reduce possible side effects or to elevate mood. These include primarily caffeine and buffers against gastrointestinal irritation. Combination drugs may also mix antihistamines or antispasmodics with aspirin or acetaminophen. As yet, though, no over-the-counter combination drugs have been demonstrated as more effective for the reduction of mild to moderate pain in children than aspirin or acetaminophen.

Nonsteroidal Anti-Inflammatory Drugs

Nonsteroidal anti-inflammatory drugs (NSAIDs) are similar in potency to aspirin. They are used primarily to treat inflammatory disorders and acute pain of mild to moderate intensity. The most commonly used drugs have been ibuprofen (Motrin), naproxen (Naprosyn), tolmetin (Tolectin), and indomethacin (Indocin). The NSAIDs inhibit prostaglandin synthesis. Their anti-inflammatory and analgesic effects occur peripherally, whereas their antipyretic effects occur centrally.

The NSAIDs are well absorbed from the stomach and upper portion of the small intestine after oral administration. However, some of these drugs can produce several gastrointestinal, hepatic, renal, and hematological side effects. More research must be conducted to evaluate which NSAIDs offer more analgesia than aspirin in light of their known side effects. For example, ibuprofen has been studied extensively for the control of postoperative dental pain in adults. The 400-mg dose was more effective than placebo, aspirin, acetaminophen, and combination analgesics containing codeine (Dionne, Campbell, Cooper, Hall, & Buckingham, 1983). Another NSAID, zomepirac (Zomax), was used as a potent analgesic for a brief time. It was removed from the market voluntarily by the manufacturer after five deaths occurred from anaphylactoid reactions associated with its administration (Householder, 1985). As yet, many NSAIDs have not been approved as analgesics for children.

Narcotic Analgesics

Morphine

"Narcotic analgesics" and "opioid analgesics" are two terms for a class of drugs with similar pain-reducing properties. The term "narcotic" derives from the Greek word for stupor, *narcosis*, because these analgesics produce a drowsy stupor along with pain relief.

Opium, a drug extracted from the dried juice of the unripe capsule of the opium poppy, has been used as an analgesic, antitussive, and antidiarrheal for many centuries. The first medical document, the Ebers Papyrus of 1550 B.C., recommends opium for crying children, presumably for its sedative and analgesic properties. The Greeks dedicated opium to the gods of night, death, sleep (Hypnos), and dreams (Morpheus). Hippocrates prescribed it as a hypnotic. However, in the Roman era, Galen used opium specifically to reduce pain. Morphine was isolated from opium in 1806 by Serturner and named after Morpheus. Morphine is the most commonly prescribed analgesic drug for the relief of severe pain. It is the standard by which the analgesic properties of all opioid drugs are determined.

The specific mechanisms by which opioid drugs produce analgesia are not completely understood. High-affinity, sterospecific binding sites for opioids have been identified in the mammalian brain (Pert & Snyder, 1973), and several subtypes of opiate receptors have been described, such as mu, delta, kappa, sigma, and epsilon (Hughes et al., 1975). The opioid receptor sites are located in specific areas of the midbrain, medulla, and spinal cord. Opioids inhibit the release of nociceptive neurotransmitters. Opioids may also activate pain-inhibitory pathways in the brainstem that exert descending pain control. Opioids affect both the intensity and unpleasantness of pain. Patients may report that they still feel a sensation after morphine administration, but often that they no longer perceive it as a painful sensation. Morphine reduces anxiety and induces euphoric feelings.

Data on morphine kinetics in children have only recently become available. Dahlstrom, Bolme, Feychting, Noack, and Paalzow (1979) reported that infants, young children, and older children metabolized morphine in essentially the same way. There was no difference in sensitivity to morphine between children of different ages. The morphine level in blood peaked at 30 minutes after intramuscular (i.m.) or subcutaneous (s.c.) administration and almost immediately after intravenous (i.v.) administration. Although the half-life of morphine is assumed to be approximately 2 hours, significant variation in the mean duration of action of morphine (from 2.5 to 4.5 hours) has been shown, depending on children's age and dosage (Kaiko, 1980).

Morphine is well absorbed after parenteral administration, but poorly absorbed after oral administration. ("Parenteral" refers to administration routes other than oral, such as s.c., i.m., i.v., or rectal.) Therefore, the oral dose of morphine is higher than the equivalent parenteral dose. Although morphine is usually administered s.c. or i.m., both a continuous i.v. infusion of morphine for children in pain with terminal malignancy and a continuous s.c. infusion with a syringe pump may be used (Miser, Davis, Hughes, Mulne, & Miser, 1983; Miser, Miser, & Clark, 1980). Morphine is prescribed in high doses at flexible dosing regimens for the treatment of chronic pain in adults with malignant disease. The extent to which children with malignant disease require maximal doses at frequent time intervals has not yet been documented. deVeber (1986) cited case histories of children with chronic pain from cancer who required much higher doses of morphine to obtain adequate pain relief than that usually recommended.

Morphine produces a selective analgesia, in that it does not alter other sensory systems. However, it has several adverse effects, such as lightheadedness, dizziness, sedation, nausea, vomiting, and sweating. A dose-related respiratory depression accompanies morphine administration, because of a decrease in responsiveness to carbon dioxide pressure (PCO_2) in the brain stem respiratory center. Maximal respiratory depression occurs approximately 7 minutes after i.v. administration, 30 minutes after i.m. administration, and 90 minutes after s.c. administration. Morphine stimulates the chemoreceptor trigger zone that leads to nausea and vomiting. There may be a vestibular component to this phenomenon, because more ambulatory than recumbent patients become nauseous. Morphine decreases motility in the stomach and duodenum, significantly slowing the passage of gastric contents into the small bowel. It decreases peristaltic contraction in the large and small bowel, constricts the ileocecal valve, and increases the tone of the anal sphincter so that the passage of gastric contents is severely slowed, producing constipation. Morphine also, of course, has the potential for drug abuse because it can produce mental and physical dependency.

Codeine

Codeine, a naturally occurring opium alkaloid, is structurally related to morphine. Codeine is the basic weak narcotic analgesic used to control moderate pain associated with various causes. Codeine is also used as an antitussive to relieve exhausting, nonproductive coughs that do not respond to non-narcotic antitussives. Codeine is approximately one-twelfth as potent as morphine parenterally, but between one-third and one-fourth as potent orally. Codeine is well absorbed orally, with peak levels about 1–1½ hours after ingestion. Since it is resistant to degradation after oral administration, codeine's oral efficacy is approximately two-thirds that of its parenteral activity, so that it has the highest parenteral-to-oral ratio of any opiate. The most common side effects for codeine are nausea, constipation, dizziness, and sedation. The addictive potential for codeine is fairly low, however, and tolerance is very slow to develop.

Codeine is available in pure preparations or in combination drugs with aspirin or acetaminophen. Although the comparative efficacy of these drugs has not been described precisely for children, the combination drugs may provide more analgesia than codeine, aspirin, or acetaminophen alone. Codeine is not as effective as aspirin for reducing pain due to inflammation, since narcotics do not have anti-inflammatory properties.

Synthetic and Semisynthetic Narcotics

Several synthetic and semisynthetic derivatives of codeine or morphine have been in clinical use since the early 1900s. These drugs are obtained by a relatively simple structural modification of the morphine or codeine molecule (semisynthetic) or by production of a compound with a structural resemblance to the molecule (synthetic). The drugs are classified according to their structural similarity to morphine or codeine; their analgesic potency relative to morphine or codeine; their agonist (facilitating) or antagonist (blocking) relationship to morphine; their abuse potential; and their adverse side effects. Meperidine (Demerol), hydromorphone (Dilaudid), fentanyl citrate (Sublimaze), oxycodone (Percocet,

Percodan), and pentazocine (Talwin) are among the most commonly prescribed synthetic and semisynthetic opiate drugs.

These various analgesic drugs were derived from the opioid agonists to produce the quality of analgesia produced by morphine without the problem of loss of consciousness, tolerance, and addiction associated with morphine administration. Although an ideal narcotic analgesic drug, with maximal pain-reducing potency and no side effects, has not yet been developed, these derivatives provide valuable alternative analgesics that vary in potency, duration of action, and side effects. Drugs may be selected according to the specific needs of the patient and according to the nature of the pain. As an example, fentanyl (Sublimaze), a synthetic drug that resembles morphine, produces profound analgesia for a much shorter period (15–30 minutes) than morphine. Consequenty, this drug is useful for relatively short-duration invasive medical investigations in children, such as cardiac catheterizations.

Diamorphine hydrochloride (heroin) is a semisynthetic derivative of morphine that produces analgesia more quickly than morphine, but that lasts for a shorter time period. Heroin produces more respiratory depression than morphine. Other side effects include vomiting, constipation, and sedation. Heroin is illegal in the United States and Canada, but it is permitted in Great Britain for strictly controlled use with adult patients who have severe pain because of malignant disease. Although there are few controlled studies evaluating the analgesic efficacy of heroin in comparison with morphine, these studies have not shown any difference in their efficacy (Levine, Sackett, & Bush, 1986). The scientific evidence suggests that morphine and heroin produce similar analgesia and have similar adverse effects. Many individuals have advocated the use of heroin for terminal patients with severe pain.

The use of heroin represents an emotionally charged issue because of the common fear that patients' pain cannot be controlled adequately with only morphine. However, there has been insufficient research to substantiate this fear. The mechanisms of heroin-induced analgesia are similar to those of morphine; heroin is converted within the body into morphine and presumably affects comparable supraspinal sites. Although more research should be conducted to unequivocally resolve the question of whether heroin can provide better analgesia for adults with chronic pain than morphine, the issue is not yet relevant to pediatrics (and, in any case, is irrelevant in the United States and Canada). Insufficient data are available about the prevalence and control of chronic pain associated with malignant disease in children and the possible need for other narcotic analgesics. Until such data are available to show that the available narcotic analgesics, properly prescribed and administered, are not adequate for children, it is premature to consider the use of heroin for pediatric pain control.

Methadone (Dolophine) is not closely related to morphine, but produces similar analgesic and respiratory effects. Methadone analgesia has a longer duration than morphine analgesia. Unlike morphine, methadone has good oral absorption, with a parenteral-to-oral ratio of 1:2. It is the most effective orally administered potent narcotic. Orally administered methadone is recommended for the control of moderate to severe pain. Methadone produces less nausea and vomiting than morphine. Although physical dependence can occur, methadone is used to treat narcotic addiction. It enables individuals to function without euphoric and sedative side effects and prevents physiological withdrawal. Preliminary studies comparing the analgesic efficacy of methadone and morphine in children indicate that methadone provides prolonged analgesia, despite individual variability in duration due in part to the size of the loading dose (Berde, Holzman, Sethna, Dickerson, & Brustowicz, 1988; Berde, Sethna, Holzman, Reidy, & Gondek, 1987).

Oral Narcotic Mixtures

Oral narcotics have been mixed with other drugs to provide medication that enhances analgesia while minimizing aversive side effects. The "Brompton cocktail," probably the best-known of these mixtures, was developed at Brompton Hospital in England. The cocktail initially contained morphine, cocaine, gin, and honey to provide an effective narcotic–stimulant combination. The name is now used to describe several different analgesic mixtures that usually combine morphine, cocaine, and alcohol. The particular ingredients in the various cocktails are often selected according to the specific needs of the patient, rather than according to the nature or intensity of the pain. The cocktail has been used primarily to lessen pain caused by cancer (Melzack, Ofiesh, & Mount, 1976). Some mixtures include phenothiazines to potentiate the analgesic affects of morphine and to relieve anxiety. Although several cocktails are used for children, children may find the taste of some of the inactive ingredients, particularly alcohol, aversive (Twycross, 1979). It should be possible to adjust the ingredients so that the aversiveness of the solution is not a major problem. Methadone, with better oral absorption than morphine, should provide a better oral narcotic mixture.

Since children tend to prefer to swallow pain medications, oral narcotic mixtures can provide a practical administration route for a combination of drugs selected according to the needs of the children. Oral narcotic mixtures can be quite useful for relieving pain and anxiety in children scheduled for invasive medical procedures in ambulatory clinics.

Adjunctive Drugs

Adjunctive Drugs in Combination Analgesics

"Adjunctive drugs" are drugs that do not have specific analgesic properties, but that have a role in the treatment of pain. These drugs may help relieve children's pain by elevating their moods, reducing their anxiety levels, minimizing the adverse side effects of the primary analgesic ingredients, or potentiating the analgesia. Combination analgesics, which usually mix aspirin or acetaminophen with an opioid such as codeine, are often designed to provide maximal pain relief by activating both central and peripheral mechanisms to increase analgesia; these mixtures may include various adjunctive drugs as well.

Caffeine, a central nervous system stimulant, is contained in some oral analgesic combinations. Caffeine was used more commonly before 1977, when a Food and Drug Administration advisory review panel concluded that the contribution of caffeine to analgesia had not been adequately demonstrated. In 1984, Laska and colleagues reviewed many unpublished studies in which caffeine was used in combination analgesics. He concluded that in doses greater than 65 mg, caffeine provided modest analgesia as well as mood elevation. Barbiturates and other sedatives have also been added to analgesic combinations, such as Fiorinal (which includes aspirin, caffeine, and butalbital), in order to relieve anxiety and tension so as to decrease pain.

An accurate evaluation of the efficacy of adjunctive drugs or fixed-dose combination analgesics has been complicated by many methodological problems. Also, studies have often been conducted on drug formulations that have since been altered. For example, early investigations of the analgesic efficacy of aspirin and oxycodone (Percodan) were actually conducted with a drug combination that contained caffeine and phenacetin as well. A dental model, in which the postsurgical pain produced after the extraction of impacted third molars is monitored, has been used extensively to investigate varying combinations of analgesic drugs in adults (for review, see Dionne, 1986). In general, the analgesic efficacy of combination drugs is dependent on dose, the proportion of narcotic to non-narcotic ingredients, and the source of pain.

Psychotropic Drugs

Psychotropic drugs influence a patient's emotional state by their actions in the brain. (For reviews, see Combrinck-Graham, Gursky, & Saccar, 1980; Monks & Merskey, 1984.) Tranquilizers, antidepressants, and psychostimulants are the primary categories of psychotropic drugs that have been used to alleviate pain. Since the perception of pain involves sensory, motivational, and affective components, it is possible to modulate this perception by altering the motivational and affective components as well as the sensory components. There is also evidence that some psychotropic drugs have analgesic properties independent of their psychological effects. As yet, no studies have been conducted to evaluate the analgesic properties of psychotropic drugs in children.

Tranquilizers. The major tranquilizers, neuroleptics, are used to treat a wide range of mental disorders. The drugs more commonly used in pain relief include the phenothiazines and butyrophenones. The phenothiazines are typically administered to reduce the anxiety that occasionally accompanies pain, particularly cancer pain. In addition, they have antiemetic properties that control the vomiting associated with narcotic administration. Chlorpromazine (Largactil) is used to calm emotions by depressing emotional centers in the brain, lowering the responsiveness of the reticular formation, and potentiating the effects of narcotic analgesics. The administration of phenothiazines for pain control is still somewhat controversial because of adverse side effects and because some may increase pain. Butyrophenones are often used in combination with narcotic analgesics to induce analgesia and emotional tranquility and to reduce vomiting.

The minor tranquilizers, or anxiolytics, have also been used to control pain. These drugs reduce anxiety and tension without severely affecting consciousness. The anxiolytics used for pain control are the benzodiazepines and the propanedioles. Small doses of benzodiazepines such as diazepam (Valium) produce a sense of calmness and an increased ability to cope with stress. These drugs are often used to sedate children before surgery or during invasive medical procedures. The propanedioles produce intense drowsiness and are generally used for adults for the management of pain due to muscle spasm, in which anxiety and tension exacerbate the pain. Although anxiety can increase pain, and this may lead to the assumption that anxiolytic drugs should reduce pain, antianxiety drugs independently administered are not potent analgesics.

Antidepressants. Antidepressants, the category of drugs used to relieve all forms of depression, are also used for pain relief. Tricyclic compounds and the monoamine oxidase inhibitors are effective in alleviating reactive depressions in patients with chronic pain. Patients obtain pain relief concomitant with a reduction in their depression. Clinical studies have shown that many patients who receive tricyclic medications alone report significantly less pain, despite the fact that only a small percentage of these patients show symptoms of depression. The onset of analgesia for chronic pain conditions after tricyclic administration is more rapid (3–7 days) than the usual onset of an antidepressant effect in clinically depressed patients (14–21 days).

There is sufficient evidence in humans that tricyclic antidepressants are beneficial for relieving many chronic pain conditions, such as headaches, arthritis, low back pain, and some neuropathies. Animal experiments indicate that tricyclic antidepressants modulate nociceptive information-processing in the central system. Interactive studies, in which opiates and antidepressant treatments have been used, indicate that the antidepressants can enhance morphine analgesia. The action of tricyclic antidepressants is mediated partly by inhibition of serotonin reuptake. As described in Chapter 3, the serotonin neurons of the spinal cord and the nucleus raphe magnus of the brain stem are closely related to pain-processing structures. Amitriptyline may increase morphine analgesia by blocking serotonin uptake in the terminals of monoaminergic neurons, with the result that the higher levels of serotonin potentiate the effectiveness of the serotonin-dependent descending analgesia system (Botney & Fields, 1983). Therefore, the tricyclics may have a direct effect on the central nervous system that allows morphine to be more effective. They also have a sedating effect, so that pain patients, who usually have disturbed sleep cycles, can sleep more naturally.

Our clinical observations have shown that tricyclics in combination with a cognitive-behavioral program can effectively reduce the frequency and intensity of recurrent headaches in adolescents, when depression is a primary factor responsible for the development or maintenance of the recurrent pain episodes. The possible side effects associated with administration of tricyclic antidepressants are dry mouth and drowsiness for the first 5 days, urinary retention, and constipation. Tricyclics should not be administered in conjunction with monoamine oxidase inhibitors, because their interaction can produce convulsions and occasionally coma.

Monoamine oxidase inhibitors are used for the treatment of depressive illness in adults and for the management of psychogenic pain in adults. They produce an increase in the concentration of monoamines such as norepinephrine and dopamine, and inhibit the enzymes of the monoamine oxidase group that increase brain amine concentrations. These drugs are generally not used with children.

Physical Drug Dependence

The fear of drug dependence is one of the common reasons why children may receive inadequate doses of narcotic analgesics for the control of severe pain. Yet there is little evidence that addiction is a valid concern in pediatrics (Porter & Jick, 1980). Although drug dependence is possible, there are no published reports describing physical or psychological dependence on narcotic analgesics in children. Drug "dependence" occurs when children become so accustomed to the effects (physiological or psychological) of a drug that they require the drug on a continuous or periodic basis. Children may develop "tolerance" to a drug, so that they require progressively higher doses of the drug to achieve the same physiological effect. Children with prolonged pain may require progressively higher doses of narcotics to achieve adequate analgesia. Yet drug tolerance should not be equated with drug addiction. Physical dependence develops when an individual's body requires the drug to function; there is a physical disturbance if the drug is withdrawn. Drugs that produce physical dependence include morphine, morphine-like substances, some of the tranquilizers, barbiturates, and alcohol.

Physical dependence is a common phenomenon, and mild withdrawal symptoms are evident in most patients who have taken narcotic analgesics for over 2 weeks and then stop taking them. Mild symptoms, such as restlessness, rhinorrhea, or sleeplessness, may develop approximately 8–12 hours after the last dose of a narcotic. Major withdrawal symptoms, such as irritability, tremor, nausea, diarrhea, or muscle pains, will develop 48–72 hours after the last dose. Although dependence can be easily controlled by gradually tapering medication and usually does not constitute a major problem for the clinician or patient, the term "dependence" has become more or less synonymous with the term "addiction" in common parlance, so that the fears associated with narcotic analgesia for children may be exaggerated.

Unlike dependence, which is common, addiction is an extremely rare phenomenon in patients entering the hospital for control of pain. Addiction represents a pattern of drug use in which an individual is wholly absorbed in the compulsive use and procurement of a drug, and has a tendency to relapse after withdrawal (Yaffe, 1980). Twycross (1978) described a low incidence of addiction even in adult patients with terminal malignancies who received narcotics for prolonged periods of time. Although the majority of patients with severe chronic pain due to malignant disease are adults, not children, and the majority of studies on the potential for dependence on narcotic analgesics have been conducted with adults, there is little empirical evidence to indicate that children should be denied narcotic analgesics for fear of dependence or addiction.

Guidelines for Analgesic Administration

As reviewed here, a variety of analgesics are available to control pain in infants and children. The primary concern in pediatric pain control is how to select and administer the most appropriate analgesic to reduce a child's pain. Several guidelines for analgesic administration in children are listed in Table 4.1. It is first necessary to evaluate the severity and etiology of the pain—that is, the peripheral or central origins of the pain and the probable role of inflammatory mechanisms. The drug's pharmacological properties, indications, side effect liability, adverse reactions, and dosage routes must then be considered. The rational prescription of analgesics for children requires matching the analgesic efficacy of an appropriate drug or combination of drugs with children's pain level, after careful consideration of the drug's side effects and the onset and duration of analgesic action. Antipyretic analgesics with anti-inflammatory properties are generally prescribed to control mild to moderate pains in children. More potent narcotic analgesics are required to relieve moderate to severe pains. The specific dosing regimens, analgesic

TABLE 4.1.   Guidelines for Analgesic Administration

- Determine children's pain level
  - Mild—Aspirin and acetaminophen
  - Moderate—Codeine
  - Strong—Morphine, methadone
- Evaluate physical source
  - Peripheral or central
  - Inflammatory processes
- Consider situational and emotional factors
- Select appropriate administration route, dosage, and dosing interval
- Consider need for adjunctive drugs
  - Tranquilizers
  - Antidepressants

potency, side effects, and contraindications are listed in hospital formularies and in *The Pediatric Drug Handbook* (Benitz & Tatro, 1981).

The mode of administration of an analgesic drug is probably a more important consideration for children than for adults. Children may become afraid of injections, so that they either do not request pain medication or deny pain when checked by medical staff. Optimal analgesic administration for children requires flexibility, when possible, in selecting routes according to children's needs. Analgesics may be administered orally in tablets, elixirs, or gums; by i.v., i.m., or s.c. injections; and by suppositories. The use of portacatheters has increased in pediatrics, particularly for children who require administration of multiple drugs at weekly intervals. A catheter is surgically implanted within a vein, with a small tube extending outside the child's skin. Drugs are injected directly into the external tube. (Children's anxiety and pain reactions to catheters and injections are described in Chapter 7 on the management of acute pain.) Intermittent s.c. and i.m. injections are problematic for children with bleeding diathesis. Continuous i.v. or s.c. infusions with constant-infusion pumps can provide excellent pain relief for these children. Continuous-infusion techniques are indicated for children with severe pain for whom oral and intermittent parenteral narcotics provide insufficient pain relief or for whom intractable vomiting prevents the use of oral analgesics. These techniques can provide uninterrupted and safe pain control (Bray, 1983; Bray, Beeton, Hinton, & Seviour, 1986; Cousins & Mather, 1984).

The spinal administration of opioid drugs and local anesthetics has been developed as an alternative method of pain control for adults with cancer pain (for reviews, see Bromage, 1984; Cousins & Mather, 1984; Moulin & Coyle, 1986; Yaksh, 1981). However, the injection of analgesics and anesthetics into the subarachnoid (intrathecal administration) and epidural space has only recently been conducted in children (Attia, Ecoffey, Sandouk, Gross, & Samii, 1986; Finholt, Stirt, & DiFazio, 1985; Glenski, Warner, Dawson, & Kaufman, 1984; Shapiro, Jedeikin, Shalev, & Hoffman, 1984). The principal criterion for the choice of intrathecal and epidural administration routes had been the presence of intractable pain despite adequate trials of conventional drugs administered via conventional routes. The demonstration that epidurally administered morphine provides safe, effective relief of children's postsurgical pain will undoubtedly lead to more clinical studies comparing the quality of analgesia, side effects, and recovery periods among varied administration routes for children.

Since the analgesic potency of drugs varies according to the administration route, the route for a desired analgesic must be selected primarily on the basis of which route will provide maximal pain relief within the necessary time frame. Although children generally prefer to swallow pain medications rather than receive injections, their choices are not based solely on a common fear of more painful injection routes. Usually children have not received any consistent instructions about their need to receive pain medication or about how to cope with injections, such as specific suggestions about how to reduce the painfulness.

Children often perceive injections as more threatening because they do not understand many aspects of their hospitalization and treatment. Most events, including the times and methods for receiving treatments, seem beyond their control. There may not be much consistency among personnel in conducting procedures, particularly invasive procedures that will hurt children. The preparation of a body site, the position in which a child is placed, and the manner in which a child may be distracted or encouraged to participate should be consistent, to enable the child to understand and comply with treatments. Behavioral management programs, in which even toddlers receive painful treatments in a structured and consistent manner in order to allow them some control and to provide them with accurate expectations about what will happen, will make medical procedures easier and less painful for all concerned.

The literature on pain control recommends clearly that pain medication should be prescribed in anticipation of pain and to prevent its recurrence, rather than to eliminate a strong pain after it has developed. This is particularly important for children, who may not understand that they can be pain-free despite a major injury. They may associate pain with their condition and with their general anxiety about hospitals or medical personnel, so that they do not realize that they can be comfortable even while their injury heals and while they are in the hospital. The constant experience of even mild pains may lead to behavioral and emotional problems that can intensify existing pain. When pain is immediately and effectively managed, children's anxiety is reduced because they realize that their suffering can be controlled.

Medication should be administered regularly and prophylactically in a time-contingent manner. When pain medication is prescribed on a p.r.n. basis, children experience pain before they are able to obtain pain relief. Since higher doses of narcotics are necessary to relieve existing pain than to prevent the recurrence of pain, such dosing schedules are not adequate. Pain problems may develop when children are hospitalized for a long period and receive analgesic medication according to a p.r.n. schedule. There may be variable or lengthy delays between the time when children request pain relief and when they receive it, particularly if there is a shift in nursing staff or if drugs are ordered during a busy period in the hospital pharmacy. Children may begin to request their medication at progressively shorter time intervals or may develop exaggerated pain behaviors in an effort to convince the medical staff that they truly need their medication. These problems generally do not occur when children receive analgesics on a time-contingent basis—that is, when the dosing interval has been determined according to the drug's duration of action and the child's need for pain relief.

Patient-controlled analgesia (PCA), in which patients press a button to administer incremental analgesic doses delivered to an i.v. catheter through a portable infusion system, has been used successfully by adults to control their pain, particularly postoperative pain. More recently, PCA has been used by children and adolescents (Brown & Broadman, 1987; Dodd, Wang, & Rauck, 1988; Means, Allen, Lookabill, & Krishna, 1988; Rodgers, Webb, Stergios, & Newman, 1988; Tyler,

1987). Children from 6 to 18 years old have used this technique to provide excellent pain relief with minimal side effects and adverse complications. Children could easily understand how to use the PCA button to titrate their analgesic requirements. In fact, studies have indicated that children preferred PCA and used less analgesia postoperatively on the PCA system than when drugs were administered by more conventional routes and schedules. PCA might be even more effective with children than adults, since control seems a more important component of pediatric pain management than of adult pain management. The knowledge that children are actively involved in controlling their own pain facilitates analgesic efficacy.

In addition to the proper drug choice, administration route, and dosing interval, it is necessary to remember that the children are the patients and that pain and pain control should be evaluated from the children's perspective. Parents may make decisions about how children should receive medication or how children should cope during treatments from their adult and personal perspective. As an example, some parents believe that children should not be informed in advance about painful injections. Also, they can inadvertently teach children to fear injections because they protect, soothe, and reassure the children during treatments, without allowing them also to learn to cope on their own and to make choices. Whereas some parents may prefer "not to look" during injections, their children may prefer to watch what happens. Their intent concentration during the procedure may lessen their pain. There are many simple tools (see Chapter 7) that children can use to reduce pain during analgesic administrations. They need to evaluate and choose which tool is best for them.

When children's pain is evaluated from their own perspective, they perceive that they have more control over their hospitalization, treatments, and pain, so that the aversiveness associated with their illness and treatment is diminished. They are able to cope more positively with their illness, pain, and painful analgesic administrations. Although young children may not be able to make valid decisions about their needs for analgesic medication, it is wrong to assume that *all* children are incapable of making *any* decisions about how to receive their medications and how to cope with their pain. Children should participate in various aspects of their medical treatment. When possible, they should be encouraged to choose an injection site, to learn some simple pain-coping strategies that can be transferred to all situations in which they receive invasive medical procedures, and to evaluate the efficacy of a sedative or analgesic. Children as young as 3 years old have been able to make decisions about whether they prefer to receive sedation, to use nonpharmacological methods such as relaxation or hypnosis, or to use a combination of drug and nondrug interventions prior to and during lumbar punctures or bone marrow aspirations. Although it requires more time to teach children in a concrete, age-appropriate manner about their treatment choices, the benefits are enormous. Children are generally less anxious and apprehensive about treatments, and they are even more responsive to the effects of sedative drugs. Not all children, even older children, will want to share decisions about their medical treatments or medications; however, most children are curious, interested, and motivated to participate actively in decisions with their parents and medical staff.

It is essential to remember that environmental, behavioral, cognitive, and pharmacological interventions for pain control should not be regarded as mutually exclusive. Instead, a particular treatment for pain control must depend on the nature and quality of pain, as well as on the needs of an individual child in a particular situation. When a pharmacological intervention is chosen as the principal mode of pain control, certain rules of administration should be followed. Appropriate drugs must be prescribed according to the extent of the child's suffering and must be administered in adequate doses. The selection of an appropriate analgesic should be based on the needs of each child and not solely on the source of the pain. Aspirin or acetaminophen are usually appropriate to control mild to moderate pain; aspirin or acetaminophen with codeine may provide pain control for slightly stronger pain. Parenteral morphine is effective for the control of severe pain. Oral methadone may be appropriate for some chronic or prolonged pain conditions.

As reviewed earlier, a variety of studies have shown that children may be undertreated, compared to adults who have the same pain-producing problem. Children may be prescribed weaker non-narcotic analgesics, whereas adults receive more potent narcotics. Also, children have often received fewer analgesics than the prescribed maximally allowable doses. The drug duration should be as long as possible to reduce the number of doses needed per day, especially for oral medication that is taken at home. Drugs should be selected to provide maximal analgesia for children. More attention should be placed on how to shift children after surgery from parenteral to oral analgesics to ensure consistent pain control throughout their hospitalization. Clinical studies indicate that children may experience abrupt changes in analgesic medication when they are transferred from intensive care units after surgery to hospital wards—often a dramatic change from i.v. morphine to oral acetaminophen.

Similar problems may develop for children with chronic pain. Rogers (1986a) describes an analgesic consultation for a 7-year-old girl with recurrent pelvic tumor. The patient experienced a cramping and occasionally stabbing pain in her abdomen. She was receiving 10 mg of i.v. morphine every 2 hours p.r.n. and had been on i.v. narcotics for 2 months. She was about to be discharged, but attempts to switch her medication to an oral analgesic (oxycodone plus acetaminophen—one Percocet tablet every 4 hours p.r.n.) had failed. Since a Percocet tablet contains approximately 5 mg of oxycodone, which is equivalent to about 1 mg of i.v. morphine, it is not surprising that the patient did not obtain adequate pain relief. Children do realize differences in analgesic efficacy (onset and duration of effect) between drugs. Oral analgesics have a slower onset of action than i.v. analgesics. Rogers's specific recommendation for this child was to use a combination of both drugs and administration routes, depending on the time course of action and the oral-to-parenteral ratios. Oral and i.v. analgesics were to be administered concurrently, while increasing the amount of one and concomitantly decreasing the amount of the other, until the desired degree of analgesia was obtained by the oral medication. Methadone was selected as the oral drug for this patient because it has good oral efficacy and a longer duration of action. The solution was to administer morphine (10 mg i.v.) plus methadone (5 mg orally) every 3 hours p.r.n. for the next 24 hours, then to decrease morphine by 2-mg decrements and, when necessary, to increase oral methadone by 5-mg increments. The morphine was discontinued in 5 days, and the patient's pain was controlled with 20 mg of oral methadone every 4 hours p.r.n. Rogers emphasizes that children, like adults, develop tolerance to narcotics and can require what one assumes are "adult" doses to obtain adequate pain relief.

Summary

Peripherally acting analgesics, including aspirin, acetaminophen, and NSAIDs, are generally prescribed to relieve mild pain in children. Centrally acting analgesics (opiate and opioid compounds) are most commonly prescribed to relieve moderate to severe pain. The choice of analgesic, administration route, and dosing interval requires consideration of the duration of action of the drug; the decision should be based not only on a strict adherence to its pharmacological properties, but also on a thorough pain assessment for each child. Exaggerated fears of addiction, lack of knowledge about the plasticity and complexity of nociceptive mechanisms, and general reluctance to trust children's abilities to describe their pain have led to many situations in which children have not received appropriate and adequate medications to control their pain. The exact prevalence of undermedication in infants and children is not known. However, clinical reports indicate that postsurgical pain management may be a common problem.

Pain management is a special discipline with direct relevance to pediatrics. Education programs must be provided to teach all health professionals that pain management in infants and children is not simply a corollary of disease management. Attitudes toward pain control for children are not always based on accurate information (Schechter & Allen, 1986). Most pediatric departments and children's hospitals do not subscribe to any of the three journals that are exclusively devoted to publications about pain and pain control. Many medical schools still promote the concept of a rigid nociceptive system, which dictates a relatively inflexible approach to pain control. More education is needed to dispel myths about children's nociceptive processing, their endogenous pain-inhibitory systems and the factors that can activate them, their abilities to use valid and reliable pain measures, and the efficacy of pharmacological interventions for controlling their pain. Much more research is necessary to evaluate the analgesic efficacy of the over-the-counter and prescription medications available for controlling pain in children, in accordance with the guidelines for the ethical conduct of drug studies in infants and children (American Academy of Pediatrics, Committee on Drugs, 1977; Cohen, 1980).

5

Nonpharmacological Methods for Alleviating Children's Pain

Laboratory and clinical research on nonpharmacological methods of pain control has increased rapidly during the past decade. The renewed interest in the use of physical, behavioral, and cognitive interventions to reduce pain is a natural consequence of increased knowledge about the complexity of nociceptive processing, the nature of endogenous pain-modulating systems, and the variety of factors that can modify human pain perception. The recognition that the pain system is plastic, in that the neuronal responses evoked by a constant noxious stimulus may be attenuated by modifying environmental or internal factors, has led to a wider appreciation of nonpharmacological approaches. Prior to the discovery of endogenous pain-modulating systems, the choice of a nonpharmacological intervention was frequently assumed as indicative of the psychological or functional nature of a pain complaint. However, today these methods are used to reduce several acute, recurrent, and chronic pain problems for both adults and children. Their widespread use suggests that nonpharmacological methods have acquired more credibility because of new knowledge about the descending pain-suppressing systems that are presumably responsible for their analgesic effects.

The emphasis of research investigations has evolved from basic questions about the efficacy of different nonpharmacological interventions for reducing pain to more complex questions about the nature of the analgesia produced. Recent studies have addressed such questions as whether hypnosis differentially affects the intensity and aversive dimensions of pain (Price & Barber, 1987) and whether hypnosis is equally effective for reducing different types of pain (Houle, McGrath, Moran, & Garrett, 1988). More attention in research is also being focused on identifying the components of a nonpharmacological intervention that are primarily responsible for the analgesia produced, and on selecting the most appropriate methods for each patient.

Nonpharmacological interventions are categorized as physical, behavioral, or cognitive, according to whether the interventions are focused primarily on modifying an individual's sensory systems, behaviors, or thoughts and coping abilities. Table 5.1 lists some of the nonpharmacological methods of pain control that have been used with children. Although each intervention is listed within a principal category, the three categories are not mutually exclusive. Instead, most nonpharmacological methods vary in the particular combination of physical, behavioral, and cognitive modulation that is involved. As an example, hypnosis may be considered primarily a cognitive intervention, because patients learn to reduce pain through their mental concentration; however, a hypnotic induction process often includes a physical component (progressive muscle relaxation) and a behavioral component (suggestions for performing physical movements or exercises that are usually incompatible with pain).

Some of the interventions listed in Table 5.1 are similar to those cited by Avicenna when he wrote the *Canon of Medicine* in the 10th century A.D. (Gruner, 1930). He included several nonpharmacological, as well as pharmacological (herbal), remedies for pain. He described physical stimulation by the application of heat and cold, various poultices, massage, and relaxing exercise—"walking about gently for a considerable time" to soften the tissues and relieve pain (Gruner, 1930, p. 529). In addition, he cited cognitive interventions such as listening to agreeable music and "being occupied with something very engrossing" to remove the severity of pain. Although these interventions are quite similar to the physical, behavioral, and cognitive techniques available many centuries later, much more is now known about how they modify pain.

This chapter describes the major nonpharmacological methods that have been used to alleviate pain in infants, children, and adolescents, and their probable modes of action. The selection and application of physical, behavioral, and/or cognitive interventions are reviewed according to both the nature of the pain and the specific needs of individual children and their families. The design and

TABLE 5.1.   Nonpharmacological Pain Interventions

Physical	Behavioral	Cognitive
Surgical techniques	Exercise	Distraction
Anesthetic blocks	Operant conditioning	Attention
Pressure, massage	Relaxation	Imagery
Hot and cold stimulation	Biofeedback	Thought-stopping
Electrical nerve stimulation	Modeling	Hypnosis
Acupuncture	Densensitization	Music therapy
	Art and play therapy	Psychotherapy

implementation of multistrategy pain management programs, which integrate several nonpharmacological methods for the control of common acute, recurrent, and chronic childhood pains, are described in later chapters.

Physical Interventions

Physical interventions for reducing pain consist of various techniques to inhibit the transmission of neuronal impulses generated by a noxious stimulus. Neuronal activity may be inhibited either by blocking the pathways that normally convey the nociceptive signals (e.g., by a surgical lesion of the primary or second-order afferents) or by activating internal pain-suppressing mechanisms (e.g, by an increased stimulation of non-nociceptive afferents). Surgical procedures and anesthetic nerve blocks interfere with normal nociceptive processing; electrical nerve stimulation, massage, application of heat and cold, and acupuncture activate internal pain-inhibitory systems.

Surgical Techniques and Anesthetic Blocks

Many neurosurgical procedures have been conducted to alleviate chronic pain in adults. However, since children do not experience chronic intractable pain to the same extent as adults, few if any of these major operations have been conducted in children. Consequently, only general information on the rationale for common surgical techniques and the current perspective on their use are presented in this section. Appropriate references are provided for more detailed information about surgical interventions used to control pain in adults.

The primary objective of all surgical procedures to relieve pain is to selectively lesion or cut the peripheral afferents or central ascending pathways that mediate a patient's pain experience. Usually patients have tried numerous pharmacological and nonpharmacological interventions without success, prior to consideration of a surgical procedure. Several surgical procedures have been performed to interrupt pathways at various levels of the nociceptive system to control pain—from a lesion in the most peripheral section of a nerve to lesions in successively higher levels of the nociceptive system, culminating in the destruction of a small area in the cortex. (Reviews of the more common techniques are provided by Bouckoms, 1984; Dubuisson, 1984; Lipton, 1984; Loeser, 1980; Miles, 1984; O'Brien, 1984; Spangfort, 1984; Sweet & Poletti, 1984; Tasker, 1984; Verrill, 1984; and Wood, 1984.)

Nerves may be destroyed by injecting toxic substances, such as alcohol or phenol; by burning with a high-frequency electrical current; or by cooling severely. The evolution of different surgical techniques for reducing pain is reviewed by Bonica (1953) and Melzack and Wall (1982). The latter authors emphasize that the surgical lesion of a nerve has multiple effects, in addition to the desired effect of blocking nociceptive transmission. Depending on the location in the peripheral or central nervous systems, lesions may permanently disrupt normal patterning of all sensory input, interrupt pathways that could be used to modify pain from endogenous mechanisms, change the temporal and spatial pattern of relationships among all ascending systems, and produce highly abnormal excitation in deafferented cells (central cells whose peripheral input has been cut). The enormous plasticity and complexity of the nociceptive system almost preclude the possibility of identifying and lesioning a single section of the system to abolish pain selectively and completely. In fact, many neurosurgical procedures have only temporarily reduced pain; the pain often returns at an even stronger level.

Nerve blocks or analgesic blocks, in which a local anesthetic is injected into or near nerves, have been used to reduce cancer pain in adults for over a century (for review, see Bonica, 1953, 1979b). Local anesthetics temporarily reduce the ability of nociceptive neurons to respond to tissue damage. The word "local" refers to the relatively concentrated area of action of the anesthetic solution. The concentration of analgesic solution may be adjusted so that it selectively affects small-diameter A-delta and C fibers. Local anesthetics may be applied topically to the skin surface, administered to infiltrate specific nerves, or used to temporarily block the site of an intended surgical lesion. Until recently, the primary use of local anesthetics in pediatrics has been for topical anesthesia or nerve infiltrations.

Topical anesthetics, which may be applied as creams, ointments, solutions, or sprays, slightly numb the surface for a brief period. They do not penetrate unbroken skin, but do penetrate mucous membranes and are used commonly in preparations for sore throats and, more recently, for venepunctures (Clarke & Radford, 1986). Local anesthetics, such as lidocaine (also known as lignocaine) and bupivacaine, are injected onto a nerve or infiltrated into a general area to produce insensitivity so that children do not experience pain. These anesthetics are used routinely to manage children's pain when they require invasive medical treatments, minor surgery, and restorative dental procedures (for review, see Mather & Cousins, 1986).

More interest in the use of peripheral and central blocks to reduce pain in infants and children during surgery has developed with the availability of longer-acting anesthetics, increased knowledge of pharmokinetics, and a more detailed understanding of the anatomy of various blocks in children (Bowler, Wildsmith, & Scott, 1986; Duncan, 1985). Research has been conducted to determine the safety of various anesthetics for children of different ages. For example, Eyres and colleagues demonstrated that the local anesthetics lignocaine (4 mg/kg by subcutaneous, caudal, and tracheal administration) and bupivacaine (2 and 3 mg/kg by caudal and lumbar epidural routes) were safe for children (Eyres, Bishop, Oppenheim, & Brown, 1983a, 1983b; Eyres, Hastings, Brown, & Oppenheim, 1986; Eyres, Kidd, Oppenheim, & Brown, 1978).

Caudal anesthesia has been used for several years for children requiring circumcisions, hypospadias repair, and hernia repair (Armitage, 1979; Bramwell, Bullen, & Radford 1982; Brown, 1985; Hassan, 1977; Jensen, 1981; Kay, 1974; Lourey & McDonald, 1973; Lunn, 1979; Mather & Cousins, 1986; Schulte-Steinberg, 1980; Schulte-Steinberg, & Rahlfs, 1978). Abajian et al. (1984) review their use of spinal analgesia during surgery in high-risk infants. They recommend that spinal analgesia be considered for infants with certain congenital anomalies, a history of prematurity, or a history of neonatal respiratory disease, all of whom are at risk for general anesthesia. Lunn (1979) compared the analgesic efficacy of caudal analgesia and intramuscular morphine for 40 boys after circumcision. The caudal analgesia was superior as assessed by a nurse rater blind to the drug administration, who evaluated children's distress behaviors postoperatively. Dorsal penile blocks reduced stress and pain in newborn infants during circumcisions (Kirya & Werthmann, 1978; Williamson & Williamson, 1983). The efficacy of dorsal epidural blocks for providing postoperative analgesia in four infants and three adolescents with respiratory distress was reported recently (Meignier, Souron, & LeNeel, 1983). The authors suggest that epidural analgesia is an alternative to postoperative controlled ventilation for children with respiratory distress. Blocks of the sciatic nerve (McNichol, 1985) and the tibial nerve (Kempthorne & Brown, 1984; Ratcliff & Kempthorne, 1983) have also been used to reduce pain in children. The former blocks have been used for orthopedic surgery in otherwise healthy children, whereas the latter have been used to relieve calf spasm in children with head injuries to allow the manipulation of their feet necessary for corrective plastering.

The application of regional anesthesia, in addition to topical and local anesthetic infiltrations, will probably increase in pediatrics as knowledge increases about the pharmokinetics of anesthetics in infants and children. The potential benefits of the wider use of nerve blocks to reduce pain in children during and after surgery are that they can provide localized analgesia without the risks of general anesthesia or the side effects of narcotic analgesia.

Physical Therapies

Physical therapies include a variety of techniques to relieve pain by stimulating different body regions with pressure, heat, cold or weak electrical currents. They represent familiar methods of pain relief that have been adopted naturally by people in all cultures throughout recorded history. Although the physiological mechanisms responsible for the pain reduction induced by various physical therapies are not yet completely understood, a number of studies have provided information about their probable modes of action.

Pressure, Massage, and Deep Rubbing

Children seem to massage or apply pressure naturally when they experience many types of pain, such as deep pain in their muscles, recurrent stomachaches or headaches, or acute pain after injections. Their massage helps to alleviate their distress and pain. Many methods of body massage are effective for lessening pain and promoting relaxation in adults, from light stimulation at the site of pain to deep stimulation at a body site distal from the painful region. However, there are no controlled studies to evaluate the efficacy of the varied techniques for alleviating pain in adults or in children. Pressure applied to a certain body region can induce analgesia in a distal painful region, such as when deep pressure is applied to a point located between the thumb and index finger (the *Ho-ku* point) to reduce dental pain. This form of pressure, "acupressure," is similar to acupuncture in that pain is suppressed by stimulation of low-theshold afferents. (Acupuncture is discussed in more detail later.)

Several health practitioners manipulate different body areas to stretch, align, and relax the various tissues and organs that presumably contribute to a patient's pain and discomfort. Chiropractors, osteopaths, physiotherapists, physiatrists, and orthopedists practice specialized forms of manipulation, which vary according to their particular disciplinary training, skills, and licensure. Although there has been no systematic study of the efficacy of these approaches for reducing children's pain, clinical reports have shown that children with chronic pain associated with disease (e.g., arthritis) or acute pain associated with injury benefit from therapy provided by physiotherapists, physiatrists, and orthopedists. The extent to which children are treated by chiropractors or osteopaths is unknown, but it is probably quite low. As an illustration, my colleagues and I recorded the number of health professionals and their disciplines that 200 children with recurrent pain syndromes had seen for diagnosis or treatment. Only 15 children had been treated by individuals other than medical doctors, and only 4 were treated by chiropractors.

The "laying on of hands" has been cited for centuries as a method for spiritual and physical healing. More recently, therapeutic touch, which combines emotional reassurance with gentle physical touching, has gained more popularity as an unconventional but effective method for reducing pain and discomfort. Several touch therapies have been developed, each with a distinct group of patient advocates. However, all lack true endorsement by the medical and scientific communities. A few physicians incorporate the use of touch in their medical practice to relax and reassure their patients, but the practice is not advocated generally.

There is no information available about the efficacy of therapeutic touch in pediatrics. Yet, because most children seek parental reassurance when they are hurt, and they receive strokes, hugs, and kisses that can alleviate their pain, children might benefit more than adults from the use of therapeutic touch. In fact, most children's hospitals are well aware of the need for children to be physically reassured during their hospitalization and medical treatment by nurses, physicians, and child life staff. Special concerns have been raised about the potential adverse effects of the lack of touching, holding, and physical comfort on the recovery of infants and children in intensive care units, where the environment often places enormous restrictions on child–staff interactions despite the advantages of the one-to-one nursing care provided in many centers. More recently, many children's hospitals have begun to advocate extensive visiting privileges for the parents of children in intensive care, except during their actual medical treatments. Parents provide a stabilizing influence for these children, who are in a strange and frightening environment of continuous daylight, noise, and high activity. In addition, parents may be crucial in assisting staff to discriminate between pain and anxiety for children who are unable to communicate verbally.

The effects of touch and massage are both physical and psychological. The skin and underlying tissue are stimulated, with firm pressure often applied at traditional acupuncture sites. The patient receives special personal contact and attention in a pleasant and relaxing context, in which the therapist communicates concern and empathy. Pain reduction is achieved from the combination of physical stimulation, relaxation, stress reduction, and psychological benefits. (Reviews of the role of manipulation, massage, and rehabilitative medicine in adult pain management are provided by Cyriax, 1984; Tappan, 1984; and Wells, 1984.)

Hot and Cold Stimulation

Varied and ingenious methods of alleviating pain by applying thermal stimulation—to raise or lower the body temperature, to heat or cool the skin surface, and to heat different tissues deep within the body—have been devised in many cultures. Poultices, such as the poultice made from the flour of orobs boiled in vinegar described by Avicenna in the 10th century A.D. (Gruner, 1930), are substances that are heated to a higher temperature and then applied to the skin to allow the heat to transfer to the skin surface to reduce pain. The 20th-century extension of this type of cutaneous thermal stimulation is the electric heating pad that is commonly used to relieve muscular aches and pains. Other superficial heating methods (those that produce the highest temperatures on the body surface, rather than in internal tissues) include hot packs, radiant therapy, and hydrotherapy.

Forms of heat used to treat deep pain are ultrasound and short-wave diathermy. In ultrasound, high-frequency waves of air pressure (sound waves at approximately 1 MHz, a frequency much higher than our auditory hearing range of 15,000–20,000 Hz) are focused onto the body. The sound waves are absorbed by solid tissues such as bone and are transformed into heat energy. Diathermy heats the body from the inside to the outside by electromagnetic radiation—the same energy that is the basis for visible light, radio waves, and microwaves. Although visible light does not pass through the body, as can be readily seen by the shadow cast when someone stands in front of a light, the radiation used in diathermy passes through the body and is absorbed by the deep tissues, where the electromagnetic energy is transformed into heat.

The application of cold to the skin in various forms, such as ice packs, ice water, ice massage, and superficial cooling agents (e.g., ethyl chloride spray) can also reduce pain. The most common techniqiue is to combine ice and water in a rubber pack and to apply the compress to the skin. In ice massage, a block of ice is rubbed over the skin to cool the skin and the underlying musculature. Evaporative agents cool the skin surface and produce a numbing sensation. Ethyl chloride spray is often used to lightly numb children's skin prior to invasive treatments.

The therapeutic application of heat and cold for children is more restricted than for adults. This is probably due primarily to differences between children and adults in the prevalence of the painful conditions that respond to these interventions, but it is also a result of the lag in the application of nonpharmacological methods to reduce children's pain. The selection of a particular thermal intervention is based on a consideration of the source of the disorder responsible for the pain and the presumed physiological mechanisms activated by the intervention (for reviews, see Lehmann & deLateur, 1982a, 1982b, 1984; Lehmann, Warren, & Scham, 1974). As an example, the pain and stiffness associated with rheumatoid arthritis are lessened by superficial heat, but intensified by cold. Deep heat produced in joints by ultrasound is not advocated for arthritis, because the heating of the synovium may exacerbate the condition.

The physiological mechanisms responsible for the pain relief produced by thermal stimulation are not yet completely understood. Different mechanisms are presumably involved in the varied modes of heat and cold application. Superficial heat produces vasodilation, with a subsequent increase in blood flow, whereas cold produces constriction and decreased blood flow. Activation of both types of thermal afferents may inhibit the responsivity of second-order nociceptive neurons, and therefore suppress pain through a spinal gating mechanism. Ice, which produces an aching pain, may reduce pain because of its action as a counterirritant by mechanisms similar to those of intense nerve stimulation and acupuncture (Melzack & Wall, 1982).

Electrical Nerve Stimulation

Various forms of electrical stimulation have been used as therapeutic interventions to reduce pain since the electrogenic torpedo fish was first used to treat arthritic pain and headaches at the time of Socrates (for review, see Kane & Taub, 1975). At present, electrical stimulation of peripheral and central nerves has been used to relieve many painful conditions in adults. Electrical stimulation has been applied to the surface of the skin; subcutaneously to peripheral nerves or to the region near them by surgically implanted electrodes; at the site of the sensory roots entering the spinal cord; and at different regions within the brain. In the most widely used form of cutaneous stimulation, known as "transcutaneous electrical nerve stimulation" (TENS), electrodes are placed on the surface of the skin and a mild electric current is administered. Electrical pulses applied to the surface of the skin directly activate peripheral non-nociceptive nerves.

The analgesic efficacy of many forms of electrical nerve stimulation was investigated in adults after Melzack and Wall (1965) proposed their "gate control" theory of pain; according to this theory, activity in large non-nociceptive primary afferents can inhibit the spinal effects of primary nociceptive afferents. Wall and Sweet (1967) investigated the effects of large-fiber stimulation and showed that electrical stimulation reduced chronic pain in patients and decreased sensitivity to experimental pain in volunteers. Since then, the clinical application of electrical stimulation for reducing pain has increased dramatically.

Many transcutaneous stimulators are available commercially. They generally consist of small battery-operated units, with electrodes attached to flexible wires. The intensity, frequency, width, and shape of electrical pulses may be varied for maximal efficacy. Patients adjust the intensity until they feel a tingling sensation. Pain is usually reduced during stimulation and for variable time periods after stimulation, depending on the type of pain and the intensity and frequency of stimulation. Studies have demonstrated that TENS effectively reduces pain associated with causalgia, postherpetic neuralgia, and rib fractures; chronic back pain; acute postsurgical pain; phantom limb pain; amputation pain; musculoskeletal pain; and joint pain from rheumatoid arthritis. A major advantage of TENS therapy as compared to narcotic intervention is that the TENS analgesia is continuous without respiratory depression or sedation.

The analgesia evoked by TENS has been attributed to a combination of three probable physiological mechanisms. First, TENS directly activates large, low-threshold peripheral afferents that can suppress the excitatory effects of the small, high-threshold primary nociceptive afferents on the second-order neurons in the dorsal horn. Second, TENS may activate an endogenous endorphin-mediated analgesia system, since the pain relief produced by low-frequency TENS was found to be inhibited by naloxone, a narcotic antagonist (Sjolund & Eriksson, 1979), and pain is not reduced by TENS for patients who have taken narcotics (Cooperman, Hall, Mikalacki, Hardy, & Sadar, 1977; Solomon, Viernstein, & Long, 1980). Third, TENS may decrease the abnormal excitability of damaged parts of peripheral nerves, because the stimulation causes nerve impulses to travel both centrally and also peripherally toward the damaged area on the nerve (Melzack & Wall, 1982). The use of electrical stimulation for reducing pain in adults is reviewed by several authors (Long & Hagfors, 1975; Melzack & Wall, 1982; Price, 1988; Woolf, 1984).

The analgesic efficacy of electrical stimulation applied to the sensory roots (Wall & Sweet, 1967) led to the development of several procedures for stimulating central pathways to reduce pain, described collectively as "dorsal column stimulation." Initially, electrodes were inserted directly onto the dorsal column, and the attached wires were led through a hole in the dura to an external radio stimulator. This surgical procedure has been generally replaced by a less invasive procedure, "percutaneous dorsal column stimulation," in which electrodes are inserted into epidural needles and positioned onto the top of the dura above the dorsal column. Several painful conditions in adults have been partially relieved by percutaneous dorsal column stimulation (for reviews, see Krainick & Thoden, 1984; Long,

Erickson, Campbell, & North, 1981; Melzack & Wall, 1982). Pain reduction is attributed to the same mechanisms presumed responsible for TENS analgesia.

During the last decade electrical stimulation at different brain sites has been used to reduce chronic and intractable pain associated with cancer, phantom limbs, and lumbar discs in adults. The primary stimulation sites are the periaqueductal region, the periventricular region, and the thalamic somatosensory relay nucleus. Pain reduction is variable, with some patients experiencing complete relief and others obtaining no relief, depending on the type of pain, the brain site, and the parameters of electrical stimulation. The physiological mechanism responsible for the analgesia produced by brain stimulation is presumably the endogenous endorphin-mediated analgesia system, responsible for stimulation-produced analgesia (SPA) in animals (for reviews, see Dieckmann & Witzmann, 1982; Gybels, 1979; Hosobuchi, 1980; Richardson & Akil, 1977a, 1977b; Turnbull, 1984).

Dorsal column and brain stimulation have not been used to date with children, primarily because few children experience chronic, intractable pain that is not amenable to conventional management; however, dorsal column stimulation may be useful for adolescents who suffer chronic pain associated with a well-defined organic etiology. The rationale for the selection of electrical stimulation as an intervention for adolescents should be similar to that used for adults, with the same stringent procedural guidelines. Although it is not surprising that major invasive techniques of electrical stimulation have not been used for reducing pain in infants and children, it is surprising that the less invasive TENS procedures have not been used more frequently. Despite the positive advantage of continuous analgesia without concomitant respiratory depression and sedation, TENS analgesia for children has been evaluated in only one clinical study cited by Schechter (1985). Epstein and Harris (1978) used TENS to reduce children's postsurgical pain. Sixty percent of the children required no additional pain relief treatment.

TENS is a physical intervention for reducing pain that may have special significance in pediatrics. The need to control pain after surgery in infants and children who have medical conditions complicating the usual risks of respiratory depression and sedation may be better achieved by TENS. Children whose neurological conditions must be continually monitored, infants recovering from cardiac surgery, or children with damaged lungs may all benefit from TENS alone or in combination with non-narcotic analgesics. In addition to postsurgical pain, TENS may reduce pain for children with chronic musculoskeletal pain and children who require repeated painful intramuscular injections. Although much clinical research is necessary to evaluate the efficacy of TENS for infants and children, the evidence from adult studies and the one pediatric study indicate that TENS should effectively reduce certain painful conditions in children. The availability of a noninvasive technique for alleviating pain should prevent many of the clinical abuses that develop when children suffer because of a reluctance to prescribe or administer narcotic analgesics.

Acupuncture

Traditional acupuncture is a complex process that is part of an ancient Chinese theory of medicine in which all diseases and pains are attributed to an imbalance in the vital life energy, called C'hi. A person's health depends on the balance of energy within the system, which flows along channels or meridians. Acupuncture restores the energy flow within the body to a proper state of balance. Extremely thin needles are inserted into some of the 365 classical acupuncture points located on the channels, and then are manipulated to restore the energy flow. The points are selected in traditional acupuncture not only according to the nature of the pain or disease, but also to the time of day, weather, and many other factors. (For reviews of the concepts and theory underlying the traditional practice of acupuncture, see Kaptchuk, 1983; Macdonald, 1984; O'Connor & Bensky, 1981; Takagi, 1982.)

Although acupuncture has been used for over 2,000 years in China, the serious study of acupuncture analgesia in Western society did not begin until the 1970s, when scientific exchange was initiated with the People's Republic of China. At that time, physicians, anesthetists, and scientists were able to observe a variety of surgical procedures in which acupuncture was used to prevent pain. Spoerel (1975) related his impressions of the diverse aspects of acupuncture after observing 106 operations. Many sites or loci for insertion of needles were often located in the same segments of innervation as the sites of the operations. In other instances, specific traditional acupuncture points were needled to produce analgesia in distal body regions, such as the Ho-ku point to produce analgesia in the mouth. Needling at various points on the ear was used to produce analgesia for 19 different operations, since there seems to be an inverted body image located in the earlobe, so that stimulation at specific sites on the ear produces analgesia in the corresponding body sites.

Although many patients were premedicated with a sedative or narcotic prior to surgery, patients were not heavily sedated. The anesthetists had been informed that hand stimulation of the needles was more effective than electrical stimulation. However, electrical stimulation (at either a low frequency, 120–180 per minute, or a high frequency, over 1,000 per minute) was used for more than two-thirds of the operations. For some operations, neither manual twirling nor electrical stimulation was employed; the needles were simply inserted and allowed to remain in place.

In addition, Spoerel was impressed by the patients' behaviors immediately after surgery. Not only were they wide awake and comfortable throughout the surgery, but they moved freely and exhibited no pain after surgery. For example, Spoerel described one patient as waving cheerfully after a gastrectomy and another as sitting up after a lung resection to have her picture taken with the surgeons. Patients were well prepared in advance of the surgery, and surgical procedures were strictly planned so that patients were prepared for all sensations they would experience. Although acupuncture was not used for procedures longer than 3 hours or for any emergency surgery, the many and varied operations in which good to excellent analgesia was obtained provided a substantial and provocative glimpse of acupuncture analgesia.

This glimpse, shared by many scientists and clinicians who toured China, gave renewed impetus to the scientific investigation of acupuncture analgesia, as evidenced by a dramatic increase in both clinical trials and laboratory studies of the quality, nature, and extent of the analgesia produced under varied needling conditions. (For comprehensive reviews, see Chaves & Barber, 1976; Melzack, 1984; Richardson & Vincent, 1986; Vincent & Richardson, 1986.) Although studies differed in the method and site of stimulation, the type of pain evaluated, the measures used to assess pain, and the use of comparison control groups, several common findings emerged that provide new insight into the nature of acupuncture-induced analgesia.

Clinical studies suggest that approximately 50–70% of adults who suffer from chronic pain can obtain immediate pain relief through acupuncture, but that only a small number of patients continue to benefit from long-term pain relief (Fox & Melzack, 1976; Gaw, Chang, & Shaw, 1975; Ghia, Mao, Toomey, & Gregg, 1976; Richardson & Vincent 1986). However, the long-term efficacy of acupuncture for reducing chronic pain has not been generally monitored, so that accurate data for different types of pain or for different acupuncture techniques are not available. Basic studies of acupuncture, which usually consist of inducing experimental pain in healthy adult volunteers before and after acupuncture induction, show that acupuncture reduces acute pain perception (Bakke, 1976; Lynn & Perl, 1977; Mayer, Price, & Rafii, 1977; Price, Rafii, Watkins, & Buckingham, 1984; Reichmanis & Becker, 1977).

Although the efficacy and the mechanism of acupuncture analgesia remain controversial despite well over a decade of research, many findings indicate the role of both an endogenous endorphin-mediated analgesia system and spinal inhibitory mechanisms in acupuncture (Clement-Jones et al., 1980; LeBars, Dickenson, & Besson, 1979; Mayer et al., 1977; Pomeranz, Cheng, & Law, 1977; Price et al., 1984; Sjolund & Eriksson, 1979; Willer, Roby, Boulu, & Boureau, 1982). The majority of acupuncture research consists of separate clinical or basic studies; however, a recent study examined the effects of acupuncture on the strength and unpleasantness of pain and compared analgesic efficacy for experimentally induced pain and chronic pain (Price et al., 1984). This study indicated that the pain sensations for both laboratory-induced noxious heat pulse pain and chronic low back pain were reduced in an internally consistent manner. However, they demonstrated that the electroacupuncture (acupuncture induced by low-frequency, high-intensity electrical stimulation through the needles) produced central inhibitory analgesia in some patients and direct or indirect origin-specific analgesia in others. The central inhibitory component was a general effect, in that areas within and remote from the site of acupuncture stimulation were changed to a similar extent. However, the initial origin-specific component was a localized effect, in that only the site near the region of patients' lower back pain was changed.

Price et al. (1984) propose that the central analgesia may have relieved the pain, but not necessarily the cause of pain. Several days after acupuncture treatment, there was a residual pain reduction that was origin-specific. Thus, the initial analgesia, whether central inhibitory or origin-specific, may have allowed a greater range of movement or increased activity in pain patients. The greater movement was therapeutic and contributed to the longer-lasting and origin-specific pain relief. The authors also report that the maximal analgesic effect was delayed, usually occurring 1–2 hours after treatment and sometimes as long as 24 hours afterward. The electroanalgesia lasted for several days. The long delays to maximal effect may partly account for some of the inconsistent results obtained in studies on experimental pain, in which the analgesic effects are usually measured within minutes after treatment.

The spatial and temporal patterns of analgesia, the long delays to maximal effect, the generalized spatial extent of the analgesia, and the long duration of the effects are all consistent with a neuromodulatory mechanism of action underlying acupuncture analgesia. This interpretation is also supported by studies demonstrating that endorphins in cerebrospinal fluid increased after electroacupuncture and during analgesia (Clement-Jones et al., 1980; Sjolund & Eriksson, 1979) and studies showing that naloxone can antagonize or reverse acupuncture analgesia (Chapman & Benedetti, 1977; Mayer et al., 1977).

Although acupuncture has been used for children at the discretion of physicians, the children themselves, and their parents, there are few clinical reports about its application or efficacy. In fact, only one published controlled trial examined the effects of acupuncture on sore throat symptomatology in children (Gunsberger, 1973). Children in the two acupuncture conditions had significantly better pain relief than the control groups, but serious methodological flaws in the research design limit the scientific validity and interpretation of these results. Much more research is needed to understand the feasibility and efficacy of acupuncture as a pain intervention in Western society for both adults and children.

Summary

Although several surgical, anesthetic, and physical therapy techniques have been used to reduce pain in adults and children, the majority of clinical and basic research studies that have objectively evaluated the efficacy of these interventions for various types of pain have been confined to adults. It is possible to extrapolate some of the observations from adult studies to pediatrics, but much research is necessary to decide which interventions are most effective for infants and children according to the nature, intensity, and duration of their pain problems, as well as to the relevant situational, emotional, and familial factors that modify their pain.

In general, physical interventions control pain because they directly block the transmission of nociceptive input along peripheral or central pathways, modify neuronal processing at spinal and supraspinal levels, or activate descending endogenous pain-suppressing systems. Surgical techniques and anesthetic blocks prevent normal nociceptive processing. Surgery, in which sensory pathways are physically interrupted or brain sites destroyed, has been used to control chronic pain in adults when the pain is not relieved by other approaches. Anesthetic blocks temporarily prevent nociceptive conduction and have been used more frequently than other physical modalities to control acute pain in infants and children.

Pressure, massage, thermal stimulation, electrical nerve stimulation, and acupuncture share some physiological mechanisms. They activate low-threshold primary afferents that modify the effects of primary nociceptive afferents on second-order afferents at spinal levels. In addition, the analgesia induced by low-frequency TENS and by acupuncture is reduced by administration of the narcotic antagonist naloxone, indicating the role of an endogenous opiate system in the pain reduction. Although the specific nature of the physiological mechanisms responsible for the analgesia produced by these physical interventions has not yet been elucidated, research indicates that both peripheral and central mechanisms are involved. (The physiology of nociceptive systems and endogenous pain control systems has been described in Chapter 3.)

Behavioral Methods

Behavior therapy is used widely in medical practice to modify those symptoms that interfere with an individual's adaptive functioning. Clinical data about the patient's behaviors are collected and evaluated, so that individual treatment programs can be designed to promote adaptive behaviors. (See Melamed & Siegel, 1980, for a comprehensive review on the theoretical and empirical foundations of behavioral medicine and applications of behavior therapy to health care.)

Since the perception of pain depends on many physical, familial, emotional, situational, and behavioral factors, it should be possible to alter children's pain by modifying each of these factors. Behavioral techniques for reducing pain typically consist of methods that are targeted either for the children themselves or for the adults who respond to them when they experience pain. The primary objectives are to modify any behaviors on the part of either the children or the adults that may initiate, maintain, or exacerbate the children's pain.

Children who tense their muscles or restrict their behaviors because they fear that they will develop pain or increase their pain may actually initiate or increase their pain as a *consequence* of the physical changes associated with their altered behaviors. Pain perception is determined by activity not only in nociceptive pathways, but also in non-nociceptive pathways, with the result that abnormal sensory input due to abnormal physical restrictions can exacerbate pain. In addition, parents, teachers, physicians, or nurses may inadvertently respond to children in such a way that their anxiety, fear, distress, and pain are increased. Children may be rewarded for their pain complaints when they receive special attention, reduced expectations for achievement, and permission to stay home from school; as a result, their pain complaints may be maintained. A recognition of the manner in which the behaviors of children and adults may influence children's pain is essential for the optimal management of any acute, recurrent, or chronic childhood pain (Gross & Gardner, 1980; Thompson & Varni, 1986; Varni, 1984). Several methods may be used to modify behaviors to reduce various pain problems for children, such as physical exercise, operant conditioning, biofeedback, modeling, art therapy, and play therapy.

Exercise

The benefits of physical exercise for promoting general health and alleviating stress have been well documented. Special attention has been focused on the mental and physiological advantages of exercise, and, more recently, on the potential benefit of pain reduction associated with regular exercise. Exercise programs, which may include walking, calisthenics, or swimming, are frequently incorporated into comprehensive multistrategy pain management programs for patients with chronic pain. The objectives are to restore as many of patients' normal physical activities as possible in order to provide them with enjoyment, increase their participation in other events beyond their pain, and help them to reduce stress.

The exercise may reduce pain because of both its psychological and its physiological consequences. Generally, patients improve their physical health and mental outlook. They become more involved in the world and less preoccupied with their pain. In addition, a regular exercise program can alleviate some of the depression that may accompany pain by increasing serotonin production or beta-endorphin release. Exercise also normalizes some of the abnormal sensory input that may actually exacerbate existing pain states, when patients continuously alter their posture or restrict their body movements to prevent increases in their chronic pain.

Although formal exercise programs have not generally been integrated into the management of children's pain, physiotherapy and rehabilitative movement exercises are used for the overall management of childhood diseases in which mobility is restricted and pain is a prevalent symptom, such as arthritis. Recently, exercise has been used to reduce anxiety in children who are scheduled for regular painful medical procedures. When children participate in enjoyable physical sports the day before their medical appointments, they are more naturally relaxed (mentally and physically) the night before, so that their anxiety and fear is lessened. As described more fully in Chapter 7, exercise and play are important behavioral methods to alleviate distress and acute pain.

Exercise has also been used to promote relaxation in children with recurrent pains, who may limit their participation in normal childhood activities because they are afraid that physical activities will trigger new pain episodes. As a consequence of their withdrawal from all activities that require exertion, these children lack the normal emotional release and outlet that total mental and physical concentration can provide. In fact, adolescents with recurrent pains who are also depressed benefit emotionally and physically from a moderate exercise regimen as part of their pain management program (see Chapter 8).

Operant Conditioning

"Operant conditioning" refers to a specific type of learning in which an individual's behaviors are determined by the effects of those behaviors on other people in the environment. The behaviors that lead to positive outcomes will continue to occur, while the behaviors that lead to negative outcomes will decrease. The behaviors of adults or children who experience pain are inevitably shaped by the reactions of significant others in their environment. Certain overt behaviors, such as crying, seeking reassurance, grimacing, or withdrawing from other family members, may be rewarded by increased attention, empathy, and comfort, or by reduction of work and performance expectations. These positive outcomes, whether implicitly or explicitly communicated, will lead to repetition of the behaviors that elicited the favorable responses of others.

Thus, some pain behaviors represent learned or conditioned behaviors rather than natural spontaneous pain-evoked responses. These conditioned behaviors may lead not only to exaggerated pain symptomatology, but also to increased pain levels for patients with chronic pain. Children with acute, recurrent, and chronic pains may develop conditioned maladaptive pain behaviors that actually increase their pain. When parents reward children's acute pain complaints during necessary procedures or their chronic pain by increased attention, with the parents assuming full responsibility for helping the children to cope by relying on them or medication, they also increase the children's passiveness, decrease their control over the situation or disease, impair their ability to learn independent methods for reducing pain, and increase the aversive relevance of the procedure or disorder. These situational factors should increase children's anxiety, distress, and pain.

Children with recurrent pain are at risk for developing exaggerated pain symptomatology, because they experience frequent episodes of strong pain in the absence of a well-defined organic etiology that requires medical treatment. The usual reassurance that "nothing is wrong" despite the recurrent pains may lead to the development of more symptoms or increased pain complaints, as children attempt to convince their parents that the pain is real and requires attention. Children whose parents do not respond consistently to their pain complaints often have many conditioned pain behaviors that are directly related to the intermittent responses of their parents. These parents generally vary in their responses, either providing excessive emotional and physical support or indicating that they do not have time to assist the children. The implicit message that many children receive from these inconsistent messages is that their pains or pain complaints need to be stronger to convince their parents that they need the same level of support that they sometimes receive.

Children with recurrent pain syndromes are also susceptible to the development of conditioned pain "triggers," environmental stimuli or situations that can initiate a painful episode. The longer these otherwise healthy children experience frequent headaches, abdominal pains, or limb pains in the absence of a well-defined stimulus, the more likely they are to develop beliefs that the environmental stimuli that are associated in time or place with the pain episodes are the true triggers for the pain. Some foods, weather conditions, and social situations may of course lead to pain; however, the usual cause is not an environmental factor, but the parents' and children's anxiety about that factor. As more fully described in Chapter 8, conditioned pain stimuli are a major problem for the effective control of recurrent pain syndromes.

Special attention has been focused on the role of operant conditioning in maintaining pain behaviors and invalidism for adults with persistent pain. Even if their pain was initially caused by injury, the subsequent therapy of rest, medication, and individual care may facilitate the pain persisting beyond the usual time period required for healing. Fordyce (1976a, 1976b, 1976c, 1978) provides a comprehensive and practical description of how the general behavioral principles of operant conditioning are relevant for adults with chronic pain. The relevance of these principles for children with chronic pain are reviewed by Masek, Russo, and Varni (1984). Essentially, the use of operant conditioning to reduce pain and pain behaviors is similar for adults and children. It is necessary to identify all pain behaviors (verbal and nonverbal); evaluate the responses of significant persons (familial, medical, school, work, peer) to the patient's pain; and then modify the responses of these significant persons in order to minimize the occurrence of maladaptive pain behaviors and to maximize the occurrence of adaptive behaviors that reduce pain. Children's pain behaviors are often inadvertently reinforced by concerned parents and medical staff, when children perceive that the special attention they receive is contingent on their needs for pain relief and comfort. Behaviors that lead to immediate increased child–staff or child–parent interactions will generally increase, even if the behaviors themselves prolong disability and reliance on parents or medication.

The application of operant conditioning for pain management in children requires a systematic program to monitor and modify both parents' and children's behaviors. First, a thorough assessment of a child's pain and pain behaviors, and of the relevant emotional, situational, and familial factors, is conducted. Next, the most disruptive or pain-increasing behaviors are targeted for modification. Positive coping behaviors are selected according to the child's age, sex, and pain problem. A reward system is designed that will effectively motivate the child, such as stickers, points to be applied toward a treat, special time with parents, or increased social activities with peers.

Both parents and medical staff (if appropriate) must agree to follow the program consistently, with rewards contingent on the child's fulfilling well-defined behavioral criteria. The selection of behaviors and rewards is critical to the success of the program. The child must be able to achieve the positive behavioral criteria. Only one maladaptive behavior at a time should be targeted for reduction, with other behaviors added after the child has consistently modified previous behaviors. It is essential that the parents and child understand the objectives of the program, so that parents do not reward the targeted behavior and thereby reduce the efficacy of the intervention. Similarly, such a program should not be used indiscriminately with all children with similar types of pain: Not only should the behaviors and rewards be selected for each child individually, but, more importantly, the same overt pain behaviors (e.g., stalling, withdrawing, and screaming during an injection) may represent very different levels of fear, anxiety, emotional distress, and learning for different children. These differences necessarily indicate that different combinations of cognitive and behavioral programs are required for optimal pain control. The programs should be designed to meet the needs of each child and family. Although specific program goals will differ among children, the general principles and goals are consistent. The use of operant conditioning in a multistrategy program to control acute pain is demonstrated by the behavioral contracts shown in Figures 5.1 and 5.2 for a child with diabetes.

Although operant conditioning is usually one of the components of an integrated cognitive-behavioral approach to pain control, it may be the only approach required for children whose pain complaints are related solely to familial or environmental reinforcers. Operant conditioning has been successfully incorporated into several multistrategy pain management programs to reduce children's acute, recurrent, and chronic pain. The application of operant conditioning to reduce specific pain problems in children is described further in Chapters 7, 8, and 9.

Relaxation

Many behavioral interventions include procedures to facilitate physical and mental relaxation, in order to minimize pain increases resulting from physiological changes correlated with tension and anxiety. Progressive muscle relaxation, yoga, meditation, and biofeedback are now widely used to alleviate anxiety, distress, and pain for both adults and children. (Biofeedback is discussed in more detail below.) The physiological changes associated with a relaxed state, "the relaxation response," are consistent with a general decrease in sympathetic nervous system activity (for reviews, see Benson, Pomeranz, & Kutz, 1984; Linton, 1982; Richter, 1984). Decreased oxygen consumption, respiratory rate, and respiration rate are accompanied by increased skin resistance and production of alpha waves. However, the precise mechanisms by which the relaxation response reduces pain is not yet known.

I, (child's name), agree to follow this contract as part of my Get Better Needles Plan.

Finger Pricks

Goals: 1. Do it myself.
              2. Reduce how long it takes.

If I do my own finger pricks, I get points. If Mom has to do it, I get no points. At the end of the week, I get a prize for getting a certain number of points. At the end of the day, I get Bonus Points for getting a certain number of points. Bonus Points are added up for a Grand Prize.

Weekly prizes must be decided on at the beginning of the week. The Grand Prize must be decided on before this contract starts.

Points:
      10 minutes or less   = 2 points
      11 to 15 minutes   = 1 point
      After 15 minutes, Mom does it = 0 points

      Week 1: 2 points per day = 5 Bonus Points. 12 points per week = prize.
      Week 2: 4 points per day = 5 Bonus Points. 25 points per week = prize.
      Week 3: 6 points per day = 5 Bonus Points. 39 points per week = prize.
      Week 4: 6 points per day = 5 Bonus Points. 42 points per week = prize.
      Week 5: 6 points per day = 5 Bonus Points. 42 points per week = prize.
                    150 Bonus Points = Grand Prize

If I do not record my points or Bonus Points, then I do not get any points for that day, regardless of whether I earned them.

Signed: _____ (child's signature) _____   Date: _____

Witness: _____ (pain therapist's signature) _____   Date: _____

FIGURE 5.1.   Get Better Needles Plan: Contract for finger pricks.

Various relaxation techniques have been incorporated into treatments to alleviate children's burn pain (Wakeman & Kaplan 1978), acute pain from necessary cancer treatments (Jay, Elliott, Ozolins, Olson, & Pruitt, 1985; McGrath & deVeber, 1986a, 1986b), sickle cell anemia (Zeltzer, Dash, & Holland, 1979), headaches (Diamond, 1979; Larsson & Melin, 1986; P. J. McGrath, 1983; Williamson et al., 1984), arthritic pain in hemophilia (Varni, 1981a, 1981b; Varni, Gilbert, & Dietrich, 1981), and dental pain. The most common techniques for assisting children to relax are deep breathing exercises and progressive muscle relaxation. Children learn to breathe calmly and deeply to relax their bodies during painful procedures or when the pain from their disease is strong. The slower and deeper their breathing, the more their bodies seem to relax naturally. The specific suggestions used to teach children about the pain-reducing effects of relaxation depend on the child's age, cognitive level, and pain source. In general, children younger than 7 require concrete examples and coaching assistance when they use relaxation to reduce pain.

I, <u>(child's name)</u>, agree to follow this contract as part of my Get Better Needles Plan.

Injections

Goals:　1. Alternate sites; inject in new sites.
　　　　2. Reduce how long it takes.

Points:

I get points based on where I give the needle and how long it takes for me to do it.

Time	Area				Bonus Points
	Buttocks	Stomach	New site: legs	Same site	1-2 points/day = 5 Bonus Points 3-5 points/day = 10 Bonus Points 6-10 points/day = 15 Bonus Points 11-15 points/day = 20 Bonus Points 16 or more " " = 25 Bonus Points
10 minutes or less	15	10	5	2	
11-15 minutes	10	5	2	1	
16 minutes or more	5	1	2	0	

After each needle, calculate points by where you gave it and how long it took. At the end of the day, add the points for each injection and figure out how many Bonus Points you get.

For example:
　Injection 1—stomach at 11 minutes　　　 =　5 points
　Injection 2—new site on legs at 8 minutes =　5 points
　At end of day, calculate total　　　　　 = 10 points
　　　　　　　　　　　　　　　　　　　 = 15 Bonus Points

If I do not record my points daily, then I do not get them.

500 Bonus Points = Prize

Signed: _____(child's signature)_____ Date: _____

Witness: _____(pain therapist's signature)_____ Date: _____

FIGURE 5.2.　Get Better Needles Plan: Contract for injections.

Progressive muscle relaxation is a specific training procedure, in which children are taught to tighten and relax various muscles, progressing gradually from concrete whole regions (e.g., the legs, feet, toes, and fists) to more abstract and specialized areas (e.g., temporalis muscles for tension headaches). Many of the progressive relaxation procedures used for children are revisions of the technique developed for adults by Jacobson (1938), in which adults can eventually recognize and control even slight muscle contractions. Usually children receive some concrete cognitive suggestions to assist them, such as imagining themselves in a past situation where they felt completely relaxed. There have been no studies evaluating the efficacy of relaxation training alone to control children's pain. Yet it is probable that relaxation in the absence of an overall cognitive-behavioral approach has limited value for children.

Biofeedback

Biofeedback, in which the nonobservable electrical activity of the body is amplified and translated into observable auditory or visual signals, is a very useful technique for pain management (for reviews, see Jessup, 1984; Stroebel & Glueck, 1976; Turk, Meichenbaum, & Berman, 1979; Turner & Chapman, 1982). Biofeedback is especially appropriate in pediatrics, because children can receive immediate and direct feedback about the state of their bodies. Thus, biofeedback is a concrete tool that assists children to distinguish easily between relaxed and tense body states and facilitates training in how to achieve relaxed states. Whereas biofeedback has been used to treat many pain conditions in adults, it has been primarily used to treat headaches in children. Electromyographic (EMG) activity in the frontalis muscle is monitored to provide patients with feedback about the efficacy of different muscle relaxation strategies.

A 15-year-old girl who received biofeedback as part of a multistrategy program to reduce her recurrent headaches is shown in Figure 5.3. Surface electrodes, attached to the skin overlying her temporalis and frontalis muscles, monitored electrical activity. Baseline levels were recorded at the onset of a pain management session, and activity was monitored throughout the session. Her objectives were to reduce levels throughout the session, using varied cognitive coping strategies, as well as to reduce baseline levels gradually over the duration of the 8-week program. Figure 5.4 illustrates the pattern of biofeedback reductions achieved in one session

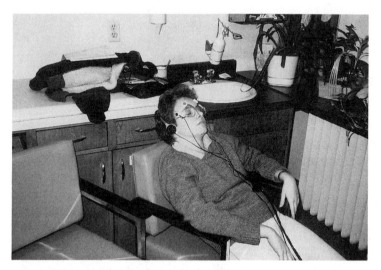

FIGURE 5.3. A 15-year-old girl with recurrent headaches is shown receiving biofeedback. Surface electrodes were attached to her forehead; the EMG activity was displayed on a screen to enable her to monitor her muscle tension.

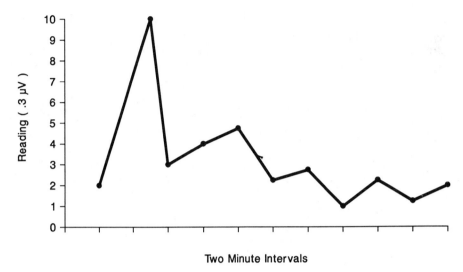

Two Minute Intervals

FIGURE 5.4. A pattern of biofeedback reductions achieved in one session by another child with recurrent headaches.

by another child with recurrent headaches. For both children, the biofeedback was used in an integrated cognitive-behavioral pain control program.

The rationale of the program was to teach these young people about the relationship between their emotions and their internal physiological states by using biofeedback. The visual feedback demonstrated clearly that there were sources of unrecognized anxiety for these children. For example, another 15-year-old girl with recurrent headaches earned excellent grades, had good peer relations, and reported no anxiety about school, social activities, or family relationships. Yet the results of her pain assessment indicated that she failed to recognize and to resolve stress-inducing situations in her life. (The specific assessment procedures for children with recurrent headaches are described in Chapter 8.) When she used biofeedback during a session, she could clearly observe that her muscle activity differed depending on the topics discussed, such as typical adolescent conflicts (peers, parental expectations) or more neutral topics (the family pets). In this manner, she gradually came to realize that her body was responding to stressful situations, even though she did not apparently recognize these situations as difficult. The recurrent headaches were due in part to her stress. However, biofeedback alone would presumably have been inadequate for pain relief, because the primary causative factor in her headaches was her failure to identify and resolve sources of stress in her life. She also required intensive counseling, in which she learned age-appropriate problem-solving skills.

Biofeedback is particularly appropriate for use with children whose pain is caused by or exacerbated by physiological changes associated with a stressed or tense state. Attanasio et al. (1985) cite eight advantages for biofeedback with children in comparison with adults: (1) Children are more enthusiastic; (2) children learn more quickly; (3) children are less skeptical about self-control procedures; (4) children have more confidence in special abilities; (5) children have more psychophysiological ability; (6) children have had fewer failures with treatment; (7) children enjoy the practice sessions; and (8) children are more reliable at symptom monitoring. My own observations from the use of biofeedback for patients referred to the Pain Clinic at the Children's Hospital of Western Ontario support these advantages.

Although children's relatively brief attention spans, their limited understanding, their potential fear of the electronic equipment, and the lack of standardized sites for electrode placement have been cited as potential disadvantages for the use of biofeedback, these difficulties are not insurmountable (Attanasio et al., 1985). Biofeedback may be used successfully even with very young children, who may be able to understand the rationale if the rationale is presented to them as a special game rather than a specific therapy. The major contraindication for biofeedback-assisted pain reduction is for children whose pain is related to their expectations for unreasonably high levels of performance in all their activities. They can become more stressed by their need to achieve dramatic reductions in their EMG levels, with subsequent increases in the intensity or frequency of their pain.

Modeling

"Modeling" refers to observational or vicarious learning in which children observe an individual's behavior in a particular situation. They learn by imitating the observed behaviors, without receiving direct instructions about the reasons for the model's actions. Modeling procedures have effectively reduced many fears and avoidance behaviors. As an example, one child may observe another receiving a painful procedure. The child model remains calm and uses simple pain-coping strategies throughout the procedure. The observer child may be less anxious and fearful after watching the manner in which the model has successfully coped in a potentially aversive situation (Melamed & Siegel, 1980; Melamed, Yurcheson, Fleece, Hutcherson, & Hawes, 1978).

Much research has been conducted to identify the critical components of modeling that ensure optimal learning. A powerful approach, "participant modeling" or "modeling with guided practice," consists of guided practice with the observer after children have watched the model (Bandura, 1976). It is a graduated and structured intervention in which children practice the modeled behaviors in progressively more realistic circumstances. The therapist provides consistent encouragement and assistance as a child attempts to imitate the model's performance. Modeling is quite valuable in reducing pain for children requiring invasive medical and dental procedures, particularly young children, retarded children, and children who do not understand English. Most admissions preparatory programs for children's hospitals include modeling procedures using films, puppets, and active teaching sessions with child life or psychology staff.

Modeling can reduce the anxiety, fear, overt distress, and pain associated with finger pricks, injections, lumbar punctures (LPs), bone marrow aspirations, porta-catheter care, and dressing changes. However, as with other behavioral interventions, the specific efficacy of modeling alone has not been adequately demonstrated. Instead, modeling is often used in conjunction with operant conditioning principles and desensitization techniques; it also includes a cognitive focus in which children receive a more realistic and accurate understanding of the pain source. More research must be conducted to identify the best models for children in terms of their similarity to the children themselves, the numbers of behaviors modeled, initial anxiety level of the models, and the general effectiveness of the modeled coping behaviors. The best model for teaching a child how to reduce pain presumably depends on the child's age, sex, cognitive level, previous experience, fear, and anxiety, as well as on the nature of the pain.

Desensitization

"Desensitization" is a procedure in which individuals are gradually exposed to an anxiety-producing object or situation in a progressive sequence, so that their anxiety eventually decreases. The anxiety-arousing stimulus is systematically paired with a response that is incompatible with anxiety, such as relaxation (Wolpe, 1982). Children who develop conditioned fears and anxiety about pain related to repeated invasive treatments benefit from systematic desensitization.

During an initial pain assessment (which ideally includes structured interviews with parents and child and an observation of the child receiving the treatment), the specific anxiety-producing components of the treatment are identified. Then a program is structured to expose the child gradually to the less anxiety-provoking components while teaching him/her some coping strategies to increase relaxation, control, and understanding of the treatment, and to reduce the aversiveness of the situation. The child learns to relax and cope with each aspect of the procedure. Progressively more realistic practice sessions that include a successively greater number of the identified anxiety components are scheduled, as the child learns to adjust to each one.

As an example, Mary, a 3-year-old girl with leukemia, developed excessive fear and anxiety about the LPs that she required every 3 months, according to her treatment protocol. She had also developed allergic reactions to each of the sedatives that had been administered, so that her parents requested a nonpharmacological approach for anxiety and pain control. Assessment showed that the primary anxiety-inducing component, which Mary rated as extremely painful, was the ethyl chloride spray used prior to the administration of a local anesthetic and the insertion of the spinal needle. Consequently, as part of her pain control program, systematic desensitization was used to counter her fears of the spray.

At first, Mary did not allow the bottle to remain in the treatment room. She needed to know the purpose of the spray, which was to slightly freeze her back and numb the area where the needle would be inserted, and to understand that the sensation was "cold and stinging" rather than "hurting." She then became interested in the appearance of the spray on skin, so that she eventually watched the therapist spray her own (i.e., the therapist's) hand, observed the whitened frost-like appearance, touched the skin, and felt that the sprayed skin was slightly cooler than the surrounding skin. She then carried the spray home to use on her stuffed animals, brothers, and parents. Within four sessions, the spray was applied to her back as part of a realistic LP practice in which she actively used simple pain-coping strategies, such as squeezing a hand in proportion to pain, visual imagery (imagining that the cold spray was a "kiss from a polar bear" and that the prick of the needle was its "tooth" as the local anesthetic was administered), and distraction during the withdrawal of spinal fluid. The program consisted of approximately six 30-minute sessions at weekly intervals. She successfully used all coping strategies during her next LP.

As indicated by the brief description of Mary's pain program, desensitization represented only one component of a broad cognitive-behavioral intervention that included operant conditioning, education about internal pain control systems, relaxation, participant modeling, and specific cognitive strategies or suggestions for alleviating pain. Desensitization procedures should be incorporated into all pain control programs when children are afraid, anxious, or distressed by specific aspects of the pain-inducing treatment or the situation in which the pain occurs.

Art and Play Therapy

The general use of art and play for alleviating children's distress during hospitalization or prior to invasive treatments has evolved into specific therapeutic interventions for anxiety and pain reduction. Art therapy provides a method for assessing children's emotional states by interpreting their drawings (e.g., color selection, subject choice, or relationships among figures). The therapist can guide children to express themselves through their art so that their problems may be identified and managed. Artwork also provides a comfortable and natural release for all young children who are waiting for scheduled hospital treatments. Their active mental and physical absorption or concentration in their drawings and paintings limits their development of anxiety related to the upcoming treatment. The art provides relaxation and enjoyment and reduces stress.

Similarly, play is used for both assessment and therapy to help children cope with their stress, anxiety, fear, and pain. Play represents a natural outlet for children's emotional expression, provides an opportunity for positive mental and physical activity that reduces their anxiety, serves as a means of teaching children how to cope with pain by modeling, and facilitates mutual peer support that alters the aversiveness of the situation. Play therapy, supervised by appropriately trained personnel and augmented by volunteers, is an important service that should be offered in all children's hospitals.

Art and play therapy have special roles in pediatric pain management, because they provide natural and familiar contexts in which essential information may be obtained about children's emotional reactions to pain-inducing procedures or painful diseases. In addition, they can facilitate an evaluation of children's coping abilities and can provide a convenient method for improving children's understanding of their disease and their ability to cope during painful treatments. Children who are actively playing prior to a painful procedure benefit from decreased stress, anxiety, and pain. Children with chronic painful diseases will benefit from regular play periods interspersed throughout their daily routine. In fact, many hospitalized children report that they have significantly less pain during active play in the child life program than at any other times.

Summary

Behavioral therapies increase adults' physical activity levels, decrease their medication use, and reduce their pain behaviors (for review, see Turner & Chapman, 1982). Although the specific analgesic efficacy of exercise, operant conditioning, relaxation, biofeedback, modeling, desensitization, and art or play therapy has not been studied comprehensively for children, these behavioral therapies can increase children's physical activity, decrease their fear and anxiety, decrease their reliance on medication or parents for pain relief, reduce maladaptive pain behaviors, and reduce their pain. Most behavioral therapies may be used to control pain for children of all ages, from toddlers to adolescents. However, the selection of a particular method depends on the age of the child; the nature of the child and family's behaviors; the child's pain-coping abilities; the child's emotional state; and whether the pain is acute, recurrent, or chronic. Method selection is based primarily on clinical practice, since there have not yet been systematic evaluations of which behavioral methods are most effective for children according to the relevant factors that influence their pain. Table 5.2, which lists the various behavioral methods that are commonly used with children, indicates which methods have been most beneficial for the children referred to our pain clinic.

In general, play therapy is the only behavioral method that is restricted to younger children. All other methods may be used with children of all ages, from toddlers to adolescents. Yet, as shown by the ++ symbol in Table 5.2, certain behavioral methods seem most appropriate for different age groups. Similarly, certain methods are more appropriate when children exhibit overt distress during painful treatments or painful episodes, when parents have unintentionally reinforced maladaptive pain behaviors or pain complaints, or when children have developed a variety of learned pain stimuli. The type of pain per se is insufficient to determine a particular method for pain intervention. For example, although desensitization is usually used only for acute pain, several other behavioral meth-

TABLE 5.2. Behavioral Methods Used at the Pain Clinic, Children's Hospital of Western Ontario

Variable	Exercise	Operant conditioning	Relaxation	Biofeedback	Modeling	Art, play	Desensitization
Child's age							
2–7	+	++	+	+	++	++	++
7–12	++	++	++	++	+	+	++
12–16	++	+	+	++			+
Behavioral factors							
Child's overt distress	++	+	+	+	++	+	+
Parents reward pain behaviors		++					
Learned pain triggers		++		++			
No pain-coping ability		++			++		
Fear, anxiety	+	++	+		+	+	++
Pain category							
Acute	+	++	+		++	+	++
Recurrent	++	++	++	++		+	
Chronic	++	+	++	+	+	+	

Note. Plus signs indicate clinical impression that method is appropriate (+) or very appropriate (++) for category.

ods are equally beneficial. Therefore, there are no simple rules that determine which method is best for which child on the basis of age or pain complaint. Instead, method selection is guided by a careful and thorough assessment of the situational, familial, emotional, and behavioral factors relevant to a child's pain, to determine which of the available methods will modify those factors and reduce pain.

In summary, the various behavioral interventions constitute a versatile array of tools that can be incorporated into pain management programs for children who experience all types of pain. Many of these methods are alike in that children's physical activity increases, their pain behaviors decrease, parental responses become more consistent, children's fear and anxiety are reduced, and children's control increases. Children become more physically and mentally relaxed. Thus, although children's behaviors are specifically targeted for modification, there are concomitant positive changes in children's attitudes, expectations, and control. Pain reduction is probably achieved by a combination of physiological mechanisms resulting from increased physical activity, reduced postural restrictions, decreased muscular tension, and altered cognitive factors.

Cognitive Approaches

Many different cognitive interventions have been used successfully to reduce acute, chronic, and recurrent pains (for reviews, see Anderson & Masur, 1983; Chapman & Turner, 1986; Meichenbaum & Turk, 1976; Sternbach, 1980; Turk, 1978; Turk & Meichenbaum, 1984). These interventions include simple distraction and attention, visual imagery, thought-stopping, hypnosis, music therapy, and psychotherapy. Most cognitive methods share a primary objective—having patients become completely and selectively focused on a thought or image, so that they are unable to attend to or perceive sensations (such as pain) at their usual intensity. Patients' selective mental concentration blocks or lessens their perception of pain. Cognitive methods reduce pain by activating endogenous opioid and nonopioid pain-suppressing systems. Although there is considerable overlap among the different cognitive interventions, each method has unique characteristics.

Children have effectively used cognitive coping strategies to reduce acute pain evoked by the normal bumps and scrapes of childhood, acute pain evoked by invasive medical or dental treatments, recurrent headaches, abdominal pains, limb pains, phantom limb pain, arthritic pain, and cancer pain. The particular cognitive intervention selected depends, of course, on a child's age, cognitive level, previous pain experience, and history of pain control, as well as on parental attitudes and the nature of the pain. Although many cognitive methods are necessarily limited to children who are able to communicate verbally and express their ideas, other methods may be used with infants in all situations in which they are distressed.

Distraction and Attention

Distraction is the most common cognitive method used to alleviate children's suffering. When an infant is hurt and cries in pain, parents provide comfort and reassurance after attending to the cause of the pain. They then attempt to distract the infant and divert attention away from the pain. When young children fall, bump their heads, or scrape their knees, parents usually try to focus their children's attention on an interesting topic or game after they have medicated the wound and comforted the child. Distraction does not passively divert children's attention away from pain, but actively alters their perception. The more absorbed they are by an event, the more their pain will be reduced. The common distraction strategies children use are as follows:

- Singing
- Describing a favorite place, toy, or cartoon
- Playing video games
- Watching a special cartoon
- Describing a novel object (auditory or visual)
- Deep breathing
- Coughing (during injections)
- Hand-squeezing

The scientific reason why distraction reduces the intensity and unpleasantness of children's pain has only recently been recognized. Cognitive interventions may directly attenuate the neuronal impulses evoked by a noxious stimulus. The child's active absorption or concentration may be the key factor for triggering an internal pain-suppressing system to block pain. Distraction has been incorrectly perceived as a simple diversionary tactic in which a child is passively placed in a situation where he/she does not attend to the presence of a pain. The implication is that the pain is still there but the child is momentarily focused elsewhere. However, distraction, particularly when the child's attention is actively involved in an area or topic other than his/her pain, is a very active process that can actually reduce the neuronal responses to a noxious stimulus. Children do not simply ignore their pain, but are actually reducing it. This interpretation is based on animal studies in which the neuronal activity evoked by a constant noxious stimulus varied, depending on the animal's attention.

The essential feature for producing pain relief by distraction is the child's ability to attend fully to and concentrate on something else besides his/her pain. Therefore, the choice of a distraction is critical to the success of this cognitive intervention. The distraction will necessarily vary according to children's ages and interests. Infants and young children require concrete external events or objects to absorb their attention, such as interesting toys with complex visual, auditory, or tactile dimensions. The more intriguing the object, the more likely it is that children will be attentive to it.

Older children can be distracted by both physical and mental activities; the specific activities should be selected according to the children's normal interests and hobbies. As an example, distraction was used to assist several children who experienced difficulties during weekly intravenous chemotherapy. These children developed anxiety about scheduled treatments with particular drugs, identifying days as "good" or "bad" treatment days. They had sleeping, eating, and behavioral problems prior to the "bad" days and experienced much more nausea, vomiting, and pain during those treatments. Although some of the nausea was a side effect of the type of drug being used, there was a possibility that the children's heightened anxiety contributed to some of their pain and distress. A trial program was designed in which children were encouraged to play video games, which required their complete attention during the 3-4 hours in which the intravenous drugs were administered, in order to earn points. This program was quite successful for 10- to 12-year-old boys. They were not allowed to play until they were already "hooked up" for treatment. They then played as long as they wanted, even though they might vomit intermittently. Their weekly high scores were recorded on a large poster in the clinic, along with the times at which they played. Several prizes were allocated monthly.

Children became less anxious about treatments, vomited less during treatments, and resumed more of their normal activities after treatments than before the introduction of the video distractions. Children and parents recorded objective information about their progress and were guided to understand that the children's concentration, not the games, had truly reduced their distress and pain. The optimal use of distraction requires a creative and imaginative approach, so that the most interesting available object or situation is chosen for each child. Because of the current reasonable costs for microcomputers, and the diversity of games and educational programs for children of all ages, an extensive repertoire of innovative and interesting distractions is available for children.

Imagery

"Imagery" refers to the process in which an individual concentrates on the image of an experience or situation. The image is not a flat description of an event, but a rich recall of and immersion in the sensations and perceptions associated wtih the experience. Although the term "visual imagery" is used synonomously with "imagery," true imagery should encompass more than visual perception. Imagery has been used frequently with children and adolescents to alleviate pain. Often, children are guided to recall and vividly describe previous positive experiences. They are asked to describe specific details of the experience—the colors, sounds, tastes, and feel of the experience. They are asked about the reactions of others and are guided to become as immersed in their image as if it were occurring in the present situation.

Imagery, then, can be considered a specific method for distraction and attention. Yet imagery can also be considered a specific method for producing physiological changes to relax the body. It is difficult for patients, whether adults or children, to control their physical state (heart rate or skin temperature) by simply concentrating on changing their state, as if they were moving a limb. However, imagery can be used to induce these changes. For example, the vivid image of a frightening experience will accelerate heart rate. Similarly, the vivid image that one's hand is placed against a hot surface can produce increases in skin temperature and blood volume. Even very young children can use imagery to produce dramatic physical changes. (See McCaffery, 1979, for detailed description of the uses and effects of imagery for pain control.)

The manner in which imagery reduces pain or alters physiological systems is not yet understood. But the efficacy of imagery depends on the ability of the individual to select an appropriately vivid image consistent with the objectives of relaxation and pain relief, and to concentrate fully on that image. Children generally have rich imaginations, so that a diverse repertoire of potential images are available. Most of the images that are currently used in our pain program have been developed by the children themselves. A young girl with cancer invented "magic sparklies," an invisible air to breathe in deeply prior to invasive procedures. The air helped to relax her and lightly numb her skin before medical treatments. Many children, including a 13-year-old boy, have chosen to imagine sparklies. They have been described variously as gold, silver, white, small stars, sunbursts, and speckles of rainbow.

A 4-year-old boy who had difficulty maintaining a curled body position during lumbar punctures and a straight body position during bone marrow aspirations imagined that he was a different fruit or vegetable for each procedure: He became a "big, fat, rounded watermelon" during lumbar punctures and a "tall, thin carrot" during bone marrows. Other children imagine that they have super-hero characteristics, that they are on a special trip (a new trip each treatment), or that they are playing with their pets to assist them with painful procedures. More sophisticated images are used by adolescents with chronic or recurrent pain to help them to relax and prevent tense musculature and body states. Imagery is a powerful tool that children approximately 3 years of age and older can use to alleviate some of their pain.

Thought-Stopping

Thought-stopping is a process in which children who anticipate pain related either to medical procedures or to diseases learn to substitute positive thoughts for their negative ones. D. M. Ross (1984) developed this process for children to reduce their anticipatory anxiety and to increase their control during painful treatments. Children collect information about both the positive aspects of the feared event and the reassuring aspects associated with the event. This information is condensed into simple statements that can be memorized easily by children. Whenever children begin to think about the event, they are required to stop any activities and repeat all the positive statements. Thought-stopping has been used successfully to reduce anxiety in 6- to 9-year-old educable mentally retarded children during dental treatments, and in hospitalized children who require repeated blood tests (D. M. Ross, 1984).

The procedure encourages children to develop some independent coping strategies. Children should always receive some positive and reassuring information about painful procedures or painful disorders, regardless of which pharmacological or nonpharmacological interventions are selected. Thought-stopping may be a particularly useful therapy for children whose fear and anxiety represent conditioned emotional reactions, and for children who lack insight into the nature of their pain or their disease.

Hypnosis

Since Mesmer's first magnetic treatments in 1794, the use of hypnosis for pain relief has gained both scientific credibility and popular appeal. A vast number of research studies have been conducted to identify the critical features in hypnosis and to explain how hypnosis can produce such diverse effects, from curing warts to reducing chronic pain (for reviews, see Fromm & Shor, 1979; Hilgard & Hilgard, 1983; Olness, 1981a, 1981b; Orne, 1980, 1983; Thompson, 1976). Although some contradictory and controversial findings have emerged from the myriad of research on hypnosis, much knowledge has accrued about hypnotic analgesia in adults and children.

The earliest descriptions of hypnosis in children are included in the writings of Franz Mesmer (1734–1815), who reported how "magnetism" had helped several children and adolescents (Bloch, 1980). Mesmer's hypnosis or magnetism consisted of a procedure in which patients held iron rods as they sat around a "baquet," a tub filled with water and iron filings. The rods supposedly transmitted the magnetic influence to cure the patients. Although Mesmer's magnetism was eventually discredited by the scientific community, the power of the patients' imagination and the influence of suggestion gradually emerged as critical features of the process that were worthy of scientific study. James Braid (1795–1860), the English surgeon who first described the procedure as "hypnosis," theorized that the hypnotist directs vital forces within the patient's body to produce dramatic changes. The acceptance of his theories contributed to the increasing study of hypnosis. Although there are many references to the clinical efficacy of hypnosis for children interspersed throughout the recorded history of hypnosis (Olness, 1981, 1981b), the scientific study of hypnosis for relieving children's pain is relatively new.

It has long been recognized that people differ in their responsiveness to hypnosis, despite the similarity of the hypnotic procedures. Standardized tests that assess an individual's "hypnotic susceptibility," or ability to be hypnotized, have shown that hypnotic susceptibility rises rapidly from when children are 4 and 5 years old to reach a maximum at 8–12 years of age (London & Cooper,

1969). Scores then decrease gradually with age. Yet there are some individuals who remain highly susceptible throughout their lives, while others remain non-susceptible.

Hypnosis can successfully relieve pain associated with burns, cancer, child-birth, surgery, dental procedures, hemophilia, and arthritis (for reviews, see J. Barber, 1979; T. X. Barber, 1963; Hilgard & Hilgard, 1983; Orne & Dinges, 1984). The major application of hypnosis in pediatrics has been to control acute pain related to invasive procedures for children with cancer. Several clinical studies have demonstrated unequivocally that hypnosis reduces the anxiety, discomfort, and pain evoked by chemotherapy, injections, LPs, and bone marrow aspirations for children and adolescents (Ellenberg, Kellerman, Dash, Higgins, & Zeltzer, 1980; Hilgard & LeBaron, 1984; Katz, Kellerman, & Ellenberg, 1987; Kellerman, Zeltzer, Ellenberg, & Dash, 1983; LaBaw, Holton, Tewell, & Eccles, 1975; Olness, 1981b; Olness, Wain, & Ng, 1980; Zeltzer & LeBaron, 1982). In addition, hypnosis has been used as primary or adjunctive therapy for children with burns (LaBaw, 1973; Schafer, 1975), migraine headaches (Olness & MacDonald, 1981), hemophilia (LaBaw, 1975; Varni et al., 1981), and sickle cell anemia (Zeltzer, Dash, & Holland, 1979), as well as for children receiving anesthesia (Antitich, 1967; Cullen, 1958; Daniels, 1962; Gaal, Goldsmith, & Needs, 1980).

Although many studies have shown clearly that hypnosis reduces pain, there is no clear understanding of the mechanisms responsible for hypnotic analgesia. In fact, there are two general and contradictory views of the hypnotic process. According to the traditional viewpoint, hypnosis represents an altered or special state of consciousness, often referred to as a "trance state." In this state, the hypnotized person becomes both an objective observer of his/her behavior and also the initiator of that behavior. During a hypnotic state, an individual is extremely susceptible to suggestions. People who are hypnotized may describe the experience as though they were aware that they were responding to certain suggestions (e.g., that they raise their arms), but that they perceived their arms as lifting without their conscious control. Proponents of this theory argue that the physiological state of a hypnotized subject is qualitatively different from other conscious states, such as the alert, sleeping, or unconscious states (Hilgard, 1973).

However, there are no consistent behavioral or physiological reactions associated with a hypnotic state that distinguish a hypnotized individual from a nonhypnotized individual. Consequently, several other explanations of hypnosis have been proposed that may be summarized under the rubric of an "alternative paradigm," a term coined by Barber (1963). The behavioral changes after hypnotic suggestions, whether arm levitation or decreased pain reports, are due to subjects' behaving in accordance with their attitudes, motivations, and expectations about hypnosis. Subjects respond because they share positive attitudes toward the hypnotic experience. Their behavior is consistent with their beliefs about hypnosis and reflects their individual expectations about what hypnosis can do. In this alternative viewpoint, patients are not fakers or malingerers per se; they are simply behaving as they perceive they should.

Despite the major differences between the traditional and alternative-paradigm theories of hypnosis, many aspects of hypnosis are common to both viewpoints. There is usually a hypnotic induction procedure, often involving relaxation exercises, in which the subject's attention is gradually focused on the hypnotist and his/her suggestions. The induction is a simple procedure, which varies according to children's age and dev"lpmental level as well as to their interests. Children can be guided into a hypnotic state by instructing them to vividly imagine their favorite television shows, movies, books, or cartoon characters (Olness & Gardner, 1978). As they imagine an activity, scene, or character, they can gradually receive suggestions for relaxation, reduced anxiety, increased control, and pain reduction. The therapist provides consistent positive suggestions, rather than authoritative commands. The emphasis is on the child's own natural abilities, as in this sample suggestion: "Notice that your back feels sleepy and my touch seems lighter than before. It seems as if you don't feel the hurt as much as before. You are doing well at turning off the pain switch."

Children become relaxed and concentrate progressively on certain aspects of the situation, while ignoring other aspects. As an example, a 5-year-old girl whose veins are difficult to locate for needle insertion may be asked to focus on how she can control a sense of numbness in her hand. (Most children have experienced the sensation of having an arm or leg "fall asleep" because of its position, so that they are not surprised that localized body regions can be selectively numbed.) As she becomes more relaxed, she can begin to notice that one hand seems a bit duller and less responsive successively to touch, to heavier pressure, to a light prick, and finally to the needle insertion. She may use progressive muscle relaxation, deep breathing, and visual imagery in order to achieve this numb state in her hand. The therapist slowly introduces more specific suggestions for analgesia, such as this: "When you are relaxed like this, the feelings in your hand are less intense. You seem less anxious and afraid. The more you breathe the magic sparklies, the deeper your ability to relax becomes, and the more control you will have over your hand. You may notice that it is becoming slightly less sensitive to the air and to pressure. In fact, when I touch your hand, your left hand does not feel my touch as well as your right hand does."

The more children concentrate on breathing the "magic sparklies" and relaxing, or imagining that they are their favorite cartoon superhero, the more they will be able to relax and lessen their pain sensations. In essence, then, hypnosis, even if it is not a different state of consciousness, is a method that provides both relaxation and cognitive pain-coping skills for children. The responsibility for the success or failure of subsequent pain reduction is shared, in that a child's ability to reduce his/her pain is enhanced by the hypnotic process and not dependent solely on the child himself/herself. The assistance provides the child with more mastery, so that ultimately he/she can use self-hypnosis confidently without relying on a hypnotist.

Hilgard and Hilgard (1983) describe three general classes of procedures in hypnosis that may be used to reduce pain: first, suggesting directly that the pain is reduced; second, altering the aversiveness of pain, even though the pain itself persists; and third, directing attention away from the pain and its sources. Direct suggestions for the reduction of pain include many simple statements that the painful area is getting numb so that children will no longer feel any pain or any other sensations. These suggestions may be made more concretely by asking children to imagine that their arms have fallen asleep. Sometimes children imagine that there is a switch that will turn sensations in a particular body part on and off. "Transferring" is a practical approach that has been used successfully by young children to reduce pain during lumbar punctures. Transferring is described by Hilgard and Hilgard (1983) as moving an area of numbness and insensitivity from an anesthetic hand to the body site where pain is located, in order to transfer the anesthesia. The transfer of pain can also occur when a patient localizes a widely diffused and poorly localized pain into a smaller and smaller area or into a distant body area where the pain is more tolerable.

Young children can easily transfer their pain during LPs, as part of a multi-strategy pain program for children with cancer (described in Chapters 6 and 9). They move their pain from their lower backs at the site of the spinal needle up along their spinal columns, down their arms, and into their hands, where they put the pain into someone else's hand. They are instructed to squeeze the other hand (that of an assistant, a nurse, or a parent) in proportion to the strength of any pain that they feel. After the pain has accumulated in the other person's hand, the children ask that the person shake that hand and drop the pain on the floor.

Although transferring may seem at first to be an irrational or somewhat silly approach, it is based on sound reasoning. Clearly, all humans have the ability to activate different internal systems that can modulate pain suppression. Since some of the key features for activating these systems are concentration, expectation, and attention, then the use of an age-appropriate transfer tool is logical. These suggestions can concretely assist children to improve their control and alter their expectations so that endogenous pain-suppressing systems are activated. Ingenuity is required in designing the most appropriate suggestions and tools to achieve hypnotic analgesia for children. The same methods will not be applicable for all children, and the same child probably requires a repertoire of tools. (A variety of hypnotic techniques and approaches for children are reviewed by Gardner & Olness, 1981.)

Hypnotized children are not passive, but actively participate in controlling their own behavior. It is important with children to let them know that learning hypnosis is like acquiring any new skill, such as riding a bike or swimming. The manner in which children learn hypnosis may be slightly different from the manner in which their siblings or friends learn the technique. A bike-riding, swimming, or sports analogy is useful for teaching children that the effects of hypnotic pain relief may vary slightly, depending on other circumstances related to their treatment: "Some days, you will ride with more energy and stamina than others, swim longer or better, hit a ball farther, and so on." It is important to ensure that children's confidence in hypnosis remains high; they must realize that some methods of hypnosis will be very effective for other children, but not necessarily for them, and that some days may be better for them than other days. The children themselves work with the therapist to search actively for the best tools to induce a hypnotic analgesia state.

The specific physiological mechanisms responsible for hypnotic analgesia are not known. Evidence indicates that naloxone does not consistently reverse analgesia produced by hypnotic suggestions (Barber & Mayer, 1977; Frid & Singer, 1979) and that many differences exist between opioid-mediated and hypnosis-mediated analgesia (Price, 1988). Probably several complex mechanisms are responsible rather than one single mechanism.

Music Therapy

Music therapy, which promotes relaxation, mood alteration, a sense of control, and self-expression, has been used in multidisciplinary programs to treat pain in adults. Recent studies have documented the beneficial physiological and psychological effects of music (for review, see Bailey, 1986). Patients are encouraged to play musical instruments or to listen to their favorite musical recordings. A therapist guides patients in selecting music that will help them to refocus their attentions from their pain to pleasant auditory stimulation. The music is used not only to calm and soothe patients, but also to facilitate emotional expression and therapeutic counseling.

Although music therapy has not been studied to date with children, this therapy may be useful for young children and infants who are hospitalized, in helping to promote a soothing or more natural environment. Music may be also used in conjunction with relaxation and biofeedback to assist children in learning how to relax and to maintain a relaxed physical and mental state.

Summary

Many cognitive interventions, such as hypnosis, visual imagery, distraction, and thought-stopping, involve common principles of pain management. They modify relevant situational factors that have been shown in animal behavioral studies and human psychophysical studies to alter nociceptive responses and human pain perception. As described in Chapter 1, situational variables are the particular psychological and contextual factors that exist in a given pain situation. These variables do not depend solely on an individual's sex, age, culture, or previous pain experiences, but depend on the unique interaction between the individual experiencing pain and the context in which that pain is experienced.

Situational variables include children's expectations about the type and intensity of pain that they may experience during a medical procedure, their expectations about receiving adequate pain relief from different treatments, their understanding of the disease or disorder causing pain, their perceived control in a painful situation, and the significance or relevance of the pain source to their lives. Differences in the context or situation in which children experience identical noxious stimuli can produce significant differences in the strength or unpleasantness of the pain that is evoked by those stimuli.

Many nonpharmacological interventions (not only cognitive approaches) provide patients with accurate information and realistic expectations about the noxious stimulus, improve the patients' perceived control over a noxious stimulus by teaching them specific coping strategies (relaxation, imagery, hypnotic suggestions, physical exercise), and reduce the aversive significance or meaning of the noxious stimulus.

Multistrategy Programs

The majority of physical, behavioral, and cognitive methods for alleviating children's pain are used in conjunction with one another, rather than independently. In fact, the term "cognitive-behavioral" is gradually evolving as the most appropriate descriptor of most comprehensive pain management programs. Cognitive-behavioral interventions consist of a wide range of treatment strategies and techniques that are provided according to a specific sequence. Patients learn to understand that their pain is a multidimensional experience involving much more than the sensory aspects. They gradually learn to modify their attitudes, expectations, and emotional distress as they become more active individuals rather than "pain patients." They learn specific skills to cope with their pain so that they can lead more productive and satisfying lives (for reviews, see Turk & Meichenbaum, 1984; Turk, Meichenbaum, & Genest, 1983).

Although the majority of research on cognitive-behavioral and multistrategy pain programs has been conducted with adults, simliar programs have been developed recently for children. Multimodal strategies, in which physical, behavioral, and cognitive methods are integrated, have a special role in pediatrics because children are continuously changing as they mature. Their physical and cognitive development requires that a consistent approach to pain management be applied in a flexible and versatile manner. The wide variety of nonpharmacological methods provides a comprehensive source for selecting those age-appropriate interventions most beneficial for a particular child. Multimodal strategies need not represent a kitchen-sink approach; rather, they can represent a careful integration of all the tools necessary to reduce a child's pain when the methods are selected on the basis of their unique contribution to modifying situational, psychological or sensory components of the patient's pain experience.

For example, at our hospital, children with cancer who required repeated invasive procedures as part of their medical treatment (e.g., LPs and bone marrow aspirations) often developed fear, anxiety, and distress behavior, with concomitant increases in the pain produced by the treatment. Selection of the appropriate pharmacological or nonpharmacological methods for reducing the acute pain evoked by their treatment first required an identification of the relevant factors contributing to the pain in addition to the objective source of noxious stimulation (the spinal needle). Several situational factors influenced all children's perceptions of acute pain from LPs, regardless of their sex, age, number of years on treatment, or prognosis (McGrath & deVeber, 1986a). These included a general lack of control prior to and during the LP, a frustration at feeling held or constrained in the fetal position during the LP, inaccurate expectations about the nature and purpose of each part of the LP, the lack of any pain-coping strategies, and an extremely fearful and anxious attitude towards the treatments.

A multistrategy program was designed that incorporated relaxation training, hypnotic suggestions for analgesia, desensitization procedures (in which children practiced receiving painful procedures using several coping strategies), operant conditioning, and cognitive restructuring. There were significant reductions in pain, anxiety, and distress behavior for subsequent LPs after children participated in this program (described in greater detail in Chapter 7). Although questions may be posed as to the relative contribution of each of the separate approaches for the pain reduction, these methods were integrated from a consideration of both the pain source and the situational factors relevant for the children in order to improve patient control, provide accurate age-appropriate information, teach simple coping strategies, and reduce the fear associated with treatment.

Similar multimodal approaches have been developed for children with recurrent pain syndromes and children with chronic pain who are referred to our pain clinic. The specific combination of nonpharmacological and pharmacological approaches that will be used depends on the individual child, his/her coping abilities, the family, the school environment, and the pattern of the child's pain. When learned or exaggerated pain behaviors are present, an operant conditioning program is also used to reduce pain complaints. Although much research, including cross-sectional and longitudinal studies, must be conducted to establish clear criteria for selecting the most appropriate interventions, the recent trend in clinical research toward systematically selecting a nonpharmacological intervention or combination of interventions after a careful evaluation of the pain, in relationship to the patient, is an important and necessary step in establishing these criteria.

The focus of many pain management programs for children has been on the integration of several nonpharmacological methods, rather than the administration of only one pain intervention. The recognition that pain is a multidimensional perception, regardless of its etiology, has led to a multidisciplinary approach to pain management. In fact, as shown in the previous descriptions of specific cognitive and behavioral interventions, there is considerable overlap among the various techniques. Most methods provide accurate information about the pain source; improve patient control; minimize anxiety, fear, and distress behavior; and provide a repertoire of pain-coping strategies.

Peterson and Shigetomi (1981) demonstrated that children were more calm and cooperative during hospitalization for elective tonsillectomies after they had been taught coping skills and viewed modeling films than when they received information, coping training, or modeling alone. Similar cognitive-behavioral interventions have been found to be effective in decreasing disruptive behavior, anxiety, discomfort, and physiological arousal for children during dental prophylaxis and restoration (Nocella & Kaplan, 1982; Siegel & Peterson, 1980, 1981). Elliott and Olson (1983) have documented a significant decrease in observed frequency of behavioral distress for children receiving burn treatment, following training in relaxation, deep breathing, and imagery. Their observation that a live therapist coaching children was necessary suggests that more active, ongoing intervention may be needed for frequently repeated invasive procedures. The efficacy of cognitive-behavioral coping strategies, including cue-controlled deep muscle relaxation, controlled breathing, pleasant imagery, and positive self-talk, has been well demonstrated for children receiving cancer treatments.

Guidelines for Method Selection

When one considers the diverse array of nonpharmacological interventions available for controlling pain, method selection becomes a special concern. The choice of a method for pain control has often been based on the particular biases of individual health professionals, rather than on well-defined criteria. In fact, there has been a tendency to view pain as an entity distinct from the patient. As a consequence, certain interventions become matched to certain types of pain, without attention to the patient who is experiencing the pain. For example, children with recurrent headaches often receive biofeedback and relaxation-based therapies for reducing the frequency and intensity of their headaches. However, usually no attempt is made to distinguish children on the basis of the relevant familial, situational, and emotional factors that contribute to the pain. Children are lumped together with the same pain diagnosis, "recurrent pain syndrome." Thus, the diagnosis represents the problem that requires treatment, rather than the pain in relationship to the child and the context in which he/she is experiencing it.

This tendency has naturally evolved from the medical conception of pain as a symptomatic problem associated with disease. The treatment of a disease, or medical management of a physical disorder, is consistent and usually determined solely by the disease or disorder and its characteristics. However, when pain is not a symptom of an underlying disease, then the causative factors for the pain must be identified and managed to ensure optimal and long-lasting pain control. Although all children with recurrent headaches may be generally labeled as having recurrent pain syndrome, they may form special subgroups whose headache etiology is primarily emotional, primarily situational, or some combination of the two.

Even when pain is a symptom of an underlying disease or is related to a well-defined noxious stimulus, the appropriate pharmacological or nonpharmacological interventions should be selected on the basis of the contributing factors, not simply on the basis of the pain type. More recently, attention is being focused on how to select a method for reducing pain, based on a careful evaluation not only of sensory attributes of the pain (quality, intensity, location, duration, and frequency), but also of its psychological and situational attributes for the patient. Investigators are attempting to identify the relevant factors that may affect the patient's pain, in order to select the method or combination of methods that most adequately modifies those factors to attenuate pain. Table 5.3 summarizes the frequency with which the major categories of nonpharmacological methods are used for different types of pain and for different age groups of children; however, there are few established, black-and-white guidelines. Children as young as 2 years old may benefit from a cognitive approach, and adolescents with recurrent pain syndrome may benefit from a behavioral approach. Selection of the appropriate methods begins with a thorough and comprehensive pain assessment and the identification of all the factors that contribute to children's pain experience. An integrated multistrategy program is generally the most effective approach, because it provides a multidimensional modification of the many factors that are relevant to children's pain.

In summary, there has been an increase in research on, and in the clinical application of, nonpharmacological interventions for controlling pain in children. Recent developments include a shift in the nature of research questions from general inquiries as to whether or not these methods are effective, to specific considerations of how they affect the multiple dimensions of children's pain experiences and to elucidation of the responsible physiological mechanisms. More research is being focused on identifying the components of individual methods critical for analgesia and on integrating several methods in well-controlled multistrategy programs. Method selection is a special concern, in that choice of an intervention is gradually being based more on a consideration of the pain in relationship to the patient than simply on the physical diagnosis. However, definitive answers to several crucial questions about nonpharmacological methods still remain unanswered. What are the key or active ingredients of the various approaches? What criteria should be used to select an appropriate intervention? What is the long-term efficacy of the various methods? Studies on the comparative efficacy of different methods often have shown equivalent posttreatment results,

TABLE 5.3. Nonpharmacological Interventions Commonly Used for Children

Type of pain	Infants and toddlers			Children under 7			Children over 7		
	Phy.	Beh.	Cog.	Phy.	Beh.	Cog.	Phy.	Beh.	Cog.
Acute	S	S	N	S	U	S	U	S	U
Recurrent	NA	NA	NA	N	U	S	N	S	U
Chronic	S	S	N	S	U	S	U	S	U

Note. U, usually; S, sometimes; N, never; NA, not applicable.

but will one method prove significantly more effective at long-term follow-up? And, finally, what are the specific physiological mechanisms that are responsible for the analgesic effects of various nonpharmacological interventions?

In order to answer these questions, future research must integrate basic psychophysical investigations on the effects of nonpharmacological methods for reducing different dimensions of experimental pain with controlled clinical investigations on the therapeutic efficacy of the same methods. These research designs can be used in combination with anatomical and physiological studies to elucidate the mechanisms responsible for the pain-reducing effects of nonpharmacological interventions.

6

Suggestions for an Integrated Pain Management Program

Although some of the interventions reviewed in the preceding two chapters are ideally suited for use with certain types of acute, recurrent, or chronic pains, many interventions should be integrated into all clinical programs for children, regardless of the specific source of noxious stimulation. The serious challenge in pediatrics is how to apply these available pain control methods consistently in standard clinical practice within hospital wards, recovery rooms, intensive care units, critical care units, emergency departments, ambulatory clinics, and physicians' and dentists' offices. Since pain is not determined solely by the nature of the noxious stimulus, adequate analgesic prescriptions administered at regular dosing intervals must be complemented with a cognitive-behavioral approach to ensure optimal pain relief. The challenge of pediatric pain control requires a dual emphasis (1) on appropriate analgesic selection and administration, in relation to the intensity and source of the pain; and (2) on selective modification of the primary situational, emotional, behavioral, and familial factors that can exacerbate pain, regardless of the pain source.

In order to meet this challenge, it is essential to address the typical problems that health professionals encounter as they attempt to design, implement, and evaluate integrated treatment programs for infants and children in different clinical settings. Common difficulties arise in selecting a pain-coping strategy for children, teaching children how to use the strategy with clear age-appropriate instructions, encouraging children actually to use the strategy when they experience pain, assisting parents to allow their children more independence or more control, objectively evaluating the efficacy of an intervention, and deciding when interventions are not effective. Unfortunately, few explicit guidelines are available for resolving these problems, because of the lack of research on pain in children. Yet the results of studies from behavioral medicine, psychology, nursing, and dentistry on reducing children's anxiety, fear, and distress and on improving their treatment compliance are relevant for pediatric pain management and provide some empirical solutions for common pain problems.

This chapter provides a critical foundation for applying the information about various pain interventions (detailed in Chapters 4 and 5) to the control of specific pediatric pains (described in Chapters 7, 8, and 9) by addressing the typical questions that confront health professionals. Special emphasis is placed on the need for a consistent cognitive-behavioral approach throughout a hospital, a description of practical pain control strategies for all types of pain, and the design of age-appropriate instructions for teaching children how to reduce their pain. Valuable insights that have accrued from children, families, and staff in the Pain Clinic at the Children's Hospital of Western Ontario are presented, along with practical suggestions and empirical observations derived from research in several disciplines.

A Cognitive-Behavioral Approach throughout a Hospital

Commitment to Pain Control

The undermedication of infants and children for almost all types of pain represents a critical problem, which has recently generated much controversy and public attention in Canada, the United States, and the United Kingdom. As a consequence both of a public outcry for adequate pain management for infants and children and of the continually increasing efforts of researchers and health professionals, improved recommendations and specific guidelines for analgesic prescription and administration will be established in pediatrics throughout the next decade.

In the interim, the general guidelines that exist for pain control in children should be followed more consistently. A primary pharmacological therapy (non-narcotic, narcotic, or adjunctive drugs prescribed according to the criteria for analgesic administration outlined in Chapter 4) or a primary physical therapy (e.g., transcutaneous electrical nerve stimulation [TENS], acupuncture) should be selected as the main intervention to control most moderate to strong childhood pains associated with disease, accidental trauma, and invasive medical procedures. A complementary cognitive-behavioral approach should be included to ensure optimal pain control, even when children receive potent narcotics. A primary psychological therapy should be selected as the main intervention for children with recurrent pain syndromes or chronic pains, when psychological factors have been identified as relevant to the etiology or the maintenance of the syndrome.

As described in the two preceding chapters, many interventions are available to reduce children's pains. The major problem in providing adequate analgesia to infants and children arises not from a lack of analgesic methodology, but from a lack of consistent application. At present, there is no evidence that children feel less pain or require fewer analgesics than adults. Consequently, the first step in pediatric pain management is the recognition by all health professionals that infants and children require adequate analgesia, selected on the basis of the nature and source of noxious stimulation, children's pain level, and the situation in which they experience the pain.

Within a pediatrics ward or a children's hospital, it is very common to observe many different approaches to inserting intravenous (IV) instrumentation, pricking a finger for blood, administering an intramuscular injection, cleaning a dressing, or preparing children for invasive procedures. The approaches vary in the extent to which children receive preparatory information about the sensations that they will experience, hear the words "pain" or "hurt," are active, have choices, use pain-coping strategies, or are physically restrained. Naturally, some of these differences can be attributed to differences among children in age, personality, overt distress, expectation, fear, and anxiety. However, many differences in approach are due primarily to differences in the attitudes of the adults who conduct these procedures. They often base their approach on a general subjective impression about what is best for children—an impression that may not be based on objective facts. Some adults may believe it is best to surprise a child with a noxious procedure so that he/she cannot become overly distressed ahead of time, or to reassure a child that it will not hurt, even though the procedure will probably cause some pain. Some adults may assume that it is best for all children to be distracted, whereas others may advocate that children should participate in any procedure when possible.

Although more research is needed to clarify the optimal approach for administering a medical procedure that will cause pain for a child, much is already known about the situational, emotional, and behavioral factors that generally increase pain. Inaccurate expectations about what will happen during a treatment, little perceived control during noxious procedures, heightened fear and anxiety, lack of a simple pain-coping strategy, parental fears and anxiety, and behavioral restrictions can all increase children's pain and distress. This knowledge alone provides the foundation for a cognitive-behavioral focus in pediatric pain management to control the primary contextual factors that can exacerbate children's pain.

Although our knowledge of how situational and emotional factors can modify pain is relatively new, many of the principles of pain management based on this knowledge are not new. Providing children with an accurate understanding of procedures and encouraging them to participate actively have long been advocated to reduce their stress, fear, and anxiety during dental or medical treatments. Yet individual adherence to these recommendations usually varies widely, for several reasons. First, individuals differ with respect to the importance they attach to these recommendations. Their differences arise not only from their personal beliefs, training, or previous experiences, but also from the fact that pain control in pediatrics has been a secondary concern until recently. As a result of the fact that medicine's primary concern is disease management, insufficient attention has been devoted to pain management. Pain has been regarded as a correlating symptom of disease that is naturally alleviated as the disease is managed.

Second, there has been a general reliance on pharmacological interventions for pain control, even though drugs have not been adequately prescribed or administered to children, so that health professionals do not know about many of the nonpharmacological interventions that are available. In addition, responsibility for providing pain control has been diffused among many disciplines, with no clear interdisciplinary guidelines to ensure that all infants, children, and adolescents are treated in accordance with consistent principles of pain management. Few hospital libraries contain any books on pain management, except for drug handbooks and pharmacological texts. In fact, few hospitals subscribe to any of the three major pain journals (*Pain*, the *Journal of Pain and Symptom Management*, and the *Clinical Journal of Pain*), so that opportunities to learn about the new advances in pain control are quite limited. As a result, approaches to pain control usually vary among disciplines, so that medicine, nursing, psychology, social work, and child life may inadvertently work against one another to exacerbate rather than relieve children's distress.

Third, the time demands required to provide medical care to many children, varying in age, sex, health status, and anxiety, impose constraints on the staff's ability to devote additional time specifically to pain management. Yet many general principles of pain control can be applied consistently without lengthening the time required to administer a treatment, particularly for children who are already anxious and distressed. Even if a child requires more assistance during the first invasive procedure, it is likely that subsequent procedures will require *less* staff time, since children will gradually become less apprehensive and more cooperative. The physical environment of different settings within a hospital can impose additional constraints on optimal pain management for children. For example, an emergency room or critical care unit, with the corresponding demands of such a unit on health professionals, constitutes a dramatically different environment from a general ward or an ambulatory clinic. It is more difficult to develop a consistent cognitive-behavioral focus in a pediatric emergency area than in an ambulatory clinic, but it is not an impossible task.

Program Development

After adequate pain control for all infants and children is recognized as a primary objective for any children's hospital or pediatrics department, an integrated pharmacological and nonpharmacological approach can then be developed to meet the specific requirements of different acute, recurrent and chronic childhood pains. Because all disciplines have a role in pain management, a cohesive program requires an interdisciplinary approach. Such an approach can be achieved when each discipline (e.g., medicine, nursing, pain, psychology, social work, child life, and volunteer services) is represented in the initial development and subsequent maintenance of a comprehensive hospital-based, rather than a discipline-based, pain control program. The interdisciplinary composition of a committee whose sole mandate is the provision of adequate pain control will facilitate the recognition of any pain problems in all hospital environments and the design of appropriate interventions integrating the skills and expertise of each of the disciplines. Each member should serve as principal liaison between the pain program and all other members of the profession, to ensure communication, consistency, and cooperation among all the individuals who share responsibility for children's care.

A typical pain management program evolves from a theoretical perspective in which a child's pain is regarded as a complex perception, usually initiated by tissue damage but always modified by situational and emotional factors. A thorough assessment is conducted to identify the factors that intensify pain from the perspective of all those involved—the child, the parents, the physician, the nurses, and any other relevant health professional, because each person has a unique perspective on a child's pain problem. When the primary source of noxious stimulation is known (e.g., an injection, postsurgical trauma, or a burn), situational factors may be assessed during brief structured interviews and procedural observations. When the source of noxious stimulation is not known (e.g., pain complaints in the absence of clear-cut tissue damage), systematic diagnostic investigations should be conducted concurrently with pain interviews.

Analgesic or anesthetic recommendations for children are based on medical guidelines within the hospital, in conjunction with the dynamically revised recommendations based on controlled clinical trials with infants and children. Any medication problems are reported and reviewed by the committee, or a subcommittee consisting of a physician, nurse, pharmacist, and pain therapist, which then makes recommendations to the medical advisory board. Nonpharmacological interventions should also be included for optimal control of childhood pains. After the typical factors that contribute to children's pain experience have been identified, the pain control committee designs a program to modify these factors and reduce pain. The general objectives for a cognitive-behavioral program are listed in Table 6.1. The program must be practical, so that it can be easily implemented without encumbering staff. However, provisions must be made to monitor the efficacy of the program objectively and at regular intervals. In this manner, general pain control programs can be developed and implemented throughout the hospital for common pain problems. Children with special pain problems should be referred to an inter- and multidisciplinary pain clinic for individualized programs.

Evaluation of Pain Problems

The objective evaluation of either a child's specific pain complaint or a general pain problem within a particular medical setting begins with a structured interview. The purpose of the interview is to describe the sensory dimensions of the

TABLE 6.1. Objectives for a Cognitive-Behavioral Program

Pain assessment: Evaluate factors	*Behavor: Child, parent*
that contribute to pain	Increase coping behaviors
Situational	Decrease anxiety-increasing behaviors
Behavioral	Reduce overt distress behaviors
Emotional	*Clinic staff awareness*
Familial	Provide adequate analgesic medications
Education: Child, parent	Improve predictability
Nociceptive system	Minimize waiting period
Pain control strategies	Encourage children to use pain strategies
Treatment—equipment and rationale	Use consistent approach
Need for children's control	Encourage active play before procedures

child's pain (when the child is able to communicate his/her perceptions) and to identify the situational, behavioral, and emotional factors that affect their perceptions. The assessment strategies are similar for all types of pediatric pain, but the focus naturally differs in accordance with the type of pain problem, the child's age, and the clinical environment (as reviewed in Chapter 2).

In order to illustrate how a consistent approach may be adapted to meet the needs of children in all clinical areas, three programs are presented that were developed in our pain clinic to address different pain problems from a cohesive framework: one for infants in the critical care unit; one for children with leukemia receiving repeated lumbar punctures in the ambulatory clinic; and one for children with recurrent headaches.

Infants in Critical Care

Recently, much attention has been focused on the special problems associated with the evaluation and control of pain in infants, particularly infants in intensive or critical care units. The design of an infant pain management program requires an initial survey of the professional staff to identify the specific pain problems they confront. Medical and nursing staff members should be interviewed independently by a member of the pain committee to ensure that they can freely express all their concerns without prejudice, and that the committee can identify all pain problems accurately. The committee then meets to establish priorities for addressing these problems and outlines several immediate and long-term objectives. Problem resolution usually involves a multidisciplinary approach with major support from the director and physicians of the unit, the head nurse and unit nurse, the psychologist assigned to the unit, and members of the pain program. Often, the problem requires a research component, because many interventions have not been evaluated objectively for infants and because few pain measures have been used with sick infants.

An initial structured interview developed in our pain program for nurses in the critical care unit is presented below. These questions may be easily adapted for each discipline within a hospital to survey potential pain problems in all areas.

What are the common invasive procedures performed on infants and children?

What are the most stressful procedures, for patients and for staff? Why?

Is there sufficient communication between the attending physician and the nurse in patient management?

Do you have freedom to suggest pain medications or interventions for invasive procedures?

What criteria do you use to start, maintain, and discontinue medication if it is prescribed p.r.n. (as needed)?

How do you determine whether an infant/child is in pain?
  a. What are your primary indications?
  b. What are some of the other considerations?
  c. Do you rely more on behavioral or on physiological parameters?
  d. Do you rely more on the condition of the child or the nature of the disease?

How does your approach to pain management for infants differ from that for children?
  a. At a personal level, how do you feel they are different?
  b. What are your own methods that you have personally acquired during your practice, and what are the methods you learned in training?

Is a local anesthetic or analgesic commonly used for infants? If not, why do you think this is so, and do you agree?

How do you help an infant or child cope with the various procedures performed?

If a patient is comatose, on Pavulon, or severely asphyxiated and unable to give overt responses to pain, what are your criteria for pain management?

How do you get parents involved in pain management?

How would you describe the pediatric critical care unit (PCCU), from the perspective of patients, nurses, and doctors?

What do you consider to be the major ethical concerns in the PCCU?

What questions do you have about how to reduce pain in infants?

If we conduct a study to better measure and control infants' pain, what area (age group, pain problem) do you think is most important?

This interview was designed to collect general information about nurses' attitudes on infant pain management, their perspective on the common painful procedures for infants, and their specific pain concerns. A similar interview was conducted with physicians. The interviews were conducted over a 2-month period, during which a member of the pain program observed procedures in the unit. Several concerns were raised from interviews and observations, such as the following: Why

do some infants fail to respond during noxious procedures after prolonged hospitalization and repeated invasive procedures? How can staff minimize infants' distress
during invasive diagnostic and therapeutic procedures? When should infants
receive premedication for difficult procedures? Do infants react less (and presumably feel less pain) if IVs are inserted in a particular body site? Will cannulation
evoke less distress when infants receive a narcotic or when they receive a local
anesthetic?

On the basis of these and similar questions, several areas were selected for
development. First, a workshop was designed to inform staff members of the recent
developments in pain management for infants receiving invasive procedures and
for infants after surgery. A lengthy discussion about analgesic prescription, application of TENS, and the use of standardized counterstimulation procedures during
routine IV insertions followed the formal presentation. Second, important questions, such as which IV site produces less stress for an infant, whether a narcotic
reduces pain better than a local for a cannulation, and whether rubbing the
intended site vigorously prior to a heel prick reduces the stress of the procedure,
were chosen as the basis for brief randomized controlled trials to provide practical,
objective information for the staff. Third, larger-scale questions, such as what the
long-term effects of repeated noxious procedures are and whether the usual
physiological or behavioral infant pain measures are reliable and valid for sick
infants in the unit, led to the design of comprehensive cross-sectional and longitudinal investigations.

Although the infant program is still in the initial stages, enormous progress has
already been made, because all staff members are working together to identify and
resolve pain problems as they occur and to teach pain management skills as an
integral part of children's medical management.

Children with Leukemia

Special attention has also been focused on the management of acute pain produced during repeated medical procedures. Fear and anxiety may develop as a
consequence of repeated invasive medical procedures, with the result that the pain
experienced during such procedures is intensified. An increase in anxiety, with
concomitant increase in pain, is a potential problem for children with cancer who
require intensive and prolonged medical treatment. In fact, this problem developed
at our hospital several years ago for children with leukemia.

Twenty-five children (12 girls, 13 boys; 3–11 years old, mean age 9.1 years) who
were receiving treatment for acute myelogenous or acute lymphoblastic leukemia
participated in an initial research study to identify and modify the situational
factors that led to increased anxiety and pain associated with repeated lumbar
punctures (LPs). Parents and nurses used visual analog scales (VASs) to rate
children's anxiety and pain from their LPs. They also used a behavioral distress
checklist to record the occurrence of specific behaviors usually associated with an

anxious or fearful child (e.g., crying, stalling, flailing, withdrawing, or refusing treatment) or behaviors usually associated with a relaxed, nonanxious child (e.g., conversing, playing, watching television, or maintaining a calm disposition).

Each child had an average of six LPs during a 2-year period. Many children showed increased anxiety before procedures in their second year of treatment. In fact, 50% of children experienced a consistent increase in reported pain or behavioral anxiety during the first 2 years of treatment, regardless of age or sex. The increase in pain and anxiety was not evaluated statistically for each child, because of the lack of solid normative comparison data (by age, sex, treatment year) against which to evaluate these individual increases.

Since many of the nonpharmacological therapies that have been used to minimize anxiety and pain for children share the common principle of modifying expectations, perceived control, and the relevance or significance associated with a painful situation, a multistrategy program for the management of acute pain evoked by medical procedures was developed for children with cancer (McGrath & deVeber, 1986a). This program integrated a variety of cognitive approaches in order to modify situational factors in a consistent manner for children during repeated medical procedures. The principal objectives of the program were to provide children with accurate expectations about the source of noxious stimulation, to improve children's perceived pain control during noxious stimulation, and to alter the relevance of the aversive situation for children in order to minimize their fear and anxiety.

Fourteen children (9 boys, 5 girls; 3-14 years old, mean age 7.6 years) participated in the pain management part of the research study. The pain management program consisted of four 45-minute sessions (approximately 1 week apart) scheduled 6 weeks prior to the next scheduled LP. During the first session, children discussed the purpose for each part of the procedure with the therapist. They answered questions about the tools that they might have used during previous LPs to cope with pain, as well as those that they usually used in other painful situations (e.g., cut hand, headache, stomachache). This structured interview provided information about the children's perceived abilities to control their pain, their general attitudes toward the LPs and other cancer treatment procedures, and their expectations about future procedures.

After the structured interview, children received age-appropriate information about the LP, including the rationale for each stage of the procedure. Young children had an opportunity to play with stuffed animals in which the animal's back seam was more visible when it was curled into the same position as the children during an LP; older children had an opportunity to feel the therapist's back in both a straight and a curled position. In both instances, children were able to understand more concretely how their body position influenced the ease of inserting a needle into the spinal cord. Children received an introduction to the use of such tools as distraction and guided imagery to control their pain. Concrete examples included a discussion of specific examples from children's own experiences and general examples of how children who are absorbed in watching a TV show or a movie are often not aware of extraneous sounds, movements, or even pressure on their bodies. Since children often believe that a parental hug or kiss after they receive an injury decreases their pain, this information was used to remind children that there are simple methods to help reduce pain and discomfort. Finally, the therapist discussed how LPs are a normal part of treatment for childhood cancer, rather than the dreaded anxiety-producing situations that children might have described at the beginning of the session.

Based on the information derived from the first session, a program was developed for each child to modify expectations, perceived control, and the relevance of the procedure. The program incorporated desensitization procedures; guided imagery; hypnotic-like suggestions for analgesia; relaxation training; and cognitive information on the purpose of the LP and on the tools that the children could use to maintain the curled body position necessary for the LP, to relax throughout the procedure, and to minimize pain during the insertion of the LP needle. At the end of the fourth session, all children had an adequate understanding of the LP, several simple tools for pain and anxiety reduction, and a less negative (rather than extremely negative) attitude toward the procedure.

In summary, the general goals of the pain management program were to optimize understanding and control for children by providing information, by teaching them how to relax using guided imagery and progressive relaxation exercises, and by restructuring negative sensations so that they could be more positive and therapeutic. The specific goals for each child depended on age, sex, previous experience, and the major source of fear or anxiety.

The modification of children's expectations required accurate descriptions of the source of fear, anxiety, or pain from the children's own perspective. For example, the source of fear during a procedure was not always the insertion of the spinal needle; instead, many children identified the application of ethyl chloride spray as the most painful aspect. This perception was altered by teaching the children to describe the actual sensations produced by the spray ("wet, cold, tingling, like snow under your jacket when you're sledding") rather than reacting to their presumptions that it would be "painful." Children identified several factors as contributing to the aversiveness of the procedure: the need to maintain the rigid curled position necessary for the LP; fear of sedation by intramuscular injection of Innovar; frustration at losing a whole day for treatment (particularly for school-age children); and boredom from lying on their backs for several hours after the LP.

Control was maximized by allowing the children to choose whether they would prefer to be sedated or alert during the procedure, by allowing them additional time between successive parts of the procedure so that they were able to maintain the necessary body position comfortably, and by encouraging them to use simple pain control methods. The relevance of the situation was altered by requiring children to participate in realistic practice sessions using traditional desensitization procedures, while emphasizing the therapeutic benefits of the LP. Two children were unable to complete the multistrategy pain management program: a 3-year-old girl who was too young to understand the procedures, and an

8-year-old boy who was retarded. (Usually simple behavioral programs are benefi-cial for such children as these during less invasive procedures to ensure consistency and predictability in treatments, along with modeling by other children to mini-mize their fear and distress and to demonstrate some concrete coping strategies. However, they should receive sedation for more invasive procedures, such as LPs.)

Children used two direct self-report pain measures, a VAS and an affective facial scale, to rate the strength and unpleasantness of their pain for LPs and for all other necesary medical procedures during the same period (finger pricks, IV procedures, intramuscular injections, and bone marrow aspirations). The efficacy of the program was evaluated by comparing parent, nurse, and child responses obtained at the posttreatment LP with the mean pretreatment values. Children's anxiety and pain decreased significantly at posttreatment and at 3-month and 6-month follow-ups. The mean number of distress behaviors (the highest possible number was 5) observed during LPs decreased from 3.6 per child to 1.3 after participation in the pain management program.

These specific principles of pain management can be applied effectively to a heterogeneous sample of children experiencing acute clinical pain. A larger study, which is in progress, indicates that this pain management program alleviates acute pain for children with diabetes, growth hormone deficiency, and arthritis, as well as for children requiring invasive diagnostic procedures.

Children with Recurrent Headaches

Recurrent pain syndromes constitute a prevalent pain problem for otherwise healthy children and adolescents. Children may suffer from recurrent episodes of severe abdominal pains, limb pains, or headaches that are not due to an underlying disease. The primary concern for these children is pain management rather than disease management. Children with recurrent headaches represent the majority of outpatient pain referrals for our pain clinic. Consequently, a dual research and service program was initiated to develop an effective intervention for reducing the frequency and intensity of children's headaches.

Since no research study had yet evaluated the situational, familial, emotional and behavioral factors that might contribute to the onset or maintenance of recurrent headaches, the first stage involved a thorough assessment of these factors in addition to the sensory dimensions of children's pain (McGrath, 1987b; McGrath & Hinton, 1987). Pain assessments were conducted for 200 children from 5 to 17 years old who had been diagnosed with recurrent migraine or tension headaches. Structured interviews were conducted with children and their parents to obtain information about the children's pain history, pain behavior, parents' criteria for evaluating the presence and intensity of their children's pain, the number and efficacy of pain interventions used, and the parents' pain history. Children completed three standardized pain assessment instruments: the Child-hood Comprehensive Pain Questionnaire (CCPQ), consisting of generate and supplied format questions and quantitative scales; the Children's Pain Inventory (CPI); and a daily pain diary to complete for 1 month. (These measures are described in Chapter 2 and are included in the Appendix to this volume.) In addition, children completed some standardized psychological inventories to assess their anxiety levels and to describe their general personality characteristics.

Children's and parents' responses were analyzed as a function of age, sex, diagnosis, syndrome duration, and intensity and frequency of headaches. Several situational, emotional, familial, and behavioral factors were present for all children, but the extent to which they contributed to headache onset or severity varied among children. Contributing factors were similar for all recurrent headaches. Thus, a similar approach should be used for children with recurrent migraine or tension headaches. The only differences in pain profiles by diagnosis were for sensory dimensions of pain (location, intensity, quality, temporal pattern, duration of headache), which is not surprising, since these features are used in the diagnostic classification.

Children and parents had inaccurate expectations about the headache diagnosis and prognosis, with the result that their anxiety increased as their expectations for a favorable outcome decreased. Parents believed that painful episodes were caused predominantly by environmental stimuli (noise, loudness, temperature, physical activity); they often denied that internal factors (children's responses to these stimuli or their anxiety) were important or that stress and somatic complaints could be related. Children developed a variety of maladaptive pain behaviors to try to prevent their headaches—behaviors that may actually have increased pain by restricting their normal interests and emotional outlets. The longer children endured the headaches, the greater the number of environmental stimuli that they believed would trigger their headaches. Children lacked practical strategies for coping with painful episodes, often depending exclusively on parental intervention or medication. Finally, children did not demonstrate age-appropriate skills in responding to stressful situations. Although all factors were present for all children, they were not present to the same extent. Consequently, a pain management program should address each of these six factors, but in a flexible manner to meet the specific needs of a child and family.

Serious emotional problems have been cited as important for the development of recurrent pain syndromes. Yet these were not evident for all children. Approximately 50% of children were described as very anxious by parents or by themselves, while 75% had very high expectations for achievement (scholastic, familial, sports). Hypochondriasis, depression, or anxiety was noted for approximately 50% of the adolescents (significant elevations on subscales of the Basic Personality Inventory). Since this group had experienced the syndrome longer than younger children, these elevations may reflect the emotional consequences of the pain, rather than simply the fact that they were pain-prone adolescents. Only 10% of children and adolescents presented with recurrent pains due to a serious psychological etiology (e.g., masked depression or conversion reaction). Diagnoses were made by a psychiatrist to whom children were referred after pain assessment.

About 25% of children had drastically reduced their physical activities to prevent headaches, despite no clear evidence of a causal relationship between physical exertion and headache onset. Another 25% participated in an extremely high level of competitive sports; in fact, they were often very stressed by the competitiveness, so that they derived little enjoyment from their participation. Children who were in these minimal or excessive categories could often not describe any time periods when they felt mentally or physically relaxed.

The results of the assessment indicated that a combination of emotional, behavioral, situational, and familial factors contributed to the syndrome in these children. The findings suggested that nonpharmacological methods, with a cognitive-behavioral approach to modify situational factors and reduce pain by improving the children's understanding of painful episodes and increasing their control, should be useful for reducing the number of headaches. However, the specific cognitive or behavioral tools should depend on the extent to which each factor contributed to a child's pain. For example, the use of biofeedback or behavioral management would depend on whether a child's anxiety increased muscle tension, whether a child required concrete examples of how internal emotions can produce observable physiological changes, and whether a child's parents might have reinforced maladaptive pain behaviors. The preliminary study indicated that a multistrategy treatment program was necessary for the optimal management of recurrent pain syndrome.

Consequently, a cognitive-behavioral program with biofeedback was designed to address the factors common to most children with recurrent headaches, but in a flexible manner to meet the needs of individual children and modify the factors initiating pain episodes or increasing the painfulness or duration of headaches (as illustrated in Table 6.2). In general, children with recurrent headaches respond to stress-inducing situations (school, sports, peers, and family) with inappropriate coping strategies. Their inability to cope and reduce the stress seems to add progressively to their anxiety. They seem unable to recognize their anxiety, which might help them resolve a stressful situation. Instead, anxiety builds until a headache develops, which temporarily removes the child from the source of anxiety. Children experience musculoskeletal and vascular headaches that are affected by many situational and emotional factors. Parents may inform children that their headaches will occur throughout their lives, or that the headaches are caused by many external stimuli, so that children begin to develop headaches when they come into contact with the stimuli as a physiological conditioned response due to their expectations. Parents may provide inconsistent responses to children, alternating between ignoring them and smothering them with attention, so that children develop more exaggerated symptomatology to convince their parents to attend to them.

We developed our pain program by considering which available pain control techniques would best meet the needs of such children to modify the contributing factors. First, an educational component should present accurate facts about the syndrome: the multiple causative factors; the lack of a definite prognosis that

TABLE 6.2. Factors Identified in the Preliminary Study as Initiating or Exacerbating Recurrent Headaches

Factor	Percentage of children experiencing factor	
	Most (~ 80%)	Some (~ 33%)
Situational factors		
Inaccurate expectations regarding cause and cure	×	
Little perceived control	×	
Dependence on		
Medication		×
Parents		×
Self		×
Physical activity		
Minimum		×
Moderate		×
Excessive		×
Peer and social activities		
Minimum		×
Moderate		×
Excessive		×
Learned pain-inducing situations	×	
Emotional factors		
Anxiety and fear related to headaches	×	
Inability to relax	×	
General anxiety		×
Depression		×
Inability to identify and express emotions	×	
High expectations for achievement	×	
Inability to identify stressful situations		×
Outwardly mature beyond their age		×
Somatic expression of emotions		×
Familial factors		
Positive family history	×	
Family structure		
Natural parents		×
Single parent		×
Reconstituted family		×
Parental responses		
Reinforce pain behavior		×
Encourage independence		×
Relationship with mother		
Supportive		×
Emotionally enmeshed		×

children will inevitably continue to have headaches or, conversely, suddenly stop having headaches; and the ability to reduce the syndrome by identifying and modifying some of the contributing factors. Information is needed about nonpharmacological methods of pain control for children and endogenous pain-suppressing mechanisms that may be triggered by hypnosis, relaxation, and physical exercise. Finally, parents and children need to understand the effects of stress on their bodies.

Second, the children should learn simple and versatile techniques for pain management during headaches. Although 90% of our preliminary sample relied on rest and medication, they lacked other tools to use independently and conveniently throughout all the situations in which their headaches occurred. Physical and mental relaxation through progressive muscle relaxation is a practical and simple method for most children to use, particularly when it is combined with biofeedback so that they can have immediate feedback about their body states. (Biofeedback and relaxation have been shown to reduce headaches in children, but there are no data about their long-term efficacy.) Since relaxation-induced pain relief cannot be used in all situations, hypnosis-like suggestions for analgesia, visual imagery, and mental absorption in an activity offer more flexibility. Also, there are natural alterations in children's activities, both physical and social, that can promote a more relaxed state and may extend the time periods between headaches. Children should be guided to understand the relationship between their activities and the effects of their activities on their bodies. As an example, teenage girls in the preliminary study seemed to experience more frequent headaches at an age when teenage boys began to notice reductions in headache frequency. An obvious gender-related difference was noted, in that the boys were more physically active and seemed to have natural outlets for stress when they were concentrating during physical activities, followed by periods of mental and physical relaxation. The role of physical exercise for alleviating stress in adults has been well documented. Children with headaches may benefit from a moderate exercise program. Children with excessive activities (some children actually have difficulty in scheduling a pain assessment because of their extracurricular activities) may gradually reduce them if they are stressful, whereas those with little or no exercise may take up a moderate program.

Third, children require some basic assistance to recognize potential stress-inducing situations, to cope in an age-appropriate manner, to minimize stress, and to reduce the likelihood of developing stress-related headaches. Such assistance does not require intensive counseling, but a problem-solving approach to teach children practical responses in typical school, sports, and familial situations that are stress-inducing. Children and parents can learn to set more realistic goals for the children, if they have been attempting to accomplish impossible tasks.

Fourth, a simple behavioral management program should be included to encourage children to use pain control techniques, to use problem-solving skills, and to prevent parents from reinforcing maladaptive pain behaviors.

This program incorporates the same principles of pain and syndrome management for all children, but the specific application depends on age and cognitive level. For example, 6-year-old children learn different suggestions for hypnotic analgesia than do adolescents. Children select suggestions that best assist them to relax and reduce pain. Although the program goals are similar for all children, there are differences in how these goals are achieved. For example, some children increase their activity, while others decrease it. The rationale for a flexible cognitive-behavioral management program to reduce pain in adults is not new, but this approach is quite new for the management of recurrent headaches in children and adolescents. (The specific program for recurrent headaches is described in Chapter 8.) This program has successfully reduced headaches for children and adolescents. However, a randomized controlled trial to objectively evaluate the efficacy of this program in comparison with other treatments is now in progress.

In summary, a consistent cognitive-behavioral approach can be adapted within a hospital for the management of all pains in infants and children, when there is an integrated emphasis on a comprehensive pain assessment, on the consistent application of available pain control methodology, and on an objective evaluation of treatment efficacy. The model depicted in Chapter 1 (see Figure 1.7) provides a framework for evaluating the primary factors that determine children's pain. After the relative contributions of these factors to a pain problem are assessed, a consistent management program can be developed to minimize a child's pain, regardless of the nature of the pain or the age of the child. Specific interventions are selected according to the type of pain and the assessment results. The efficacy of the intervention must then be objectively determined.

Practical Strategies for Reducing Pain

Children, even very young children, can easily learn and successfully use a variety of practical strategies to reduce their acute, recurrent, or chronic pain. In fact, children seem more adept than adults at using nonpharmacological interventions, presumably because they are usually less biased than adults about the potential efficacy of nondrug therapies. However, because adults teach children how to use these interventions, the biases of adults (either parents or staff members) can weaken treatment efficacy. Therefore, it is essential to consider not only a child's capabilities and needs, but also the attitudes, beliefs, and motivations of the relevant adults, when selecting a pain-coping strategy. Optimal pain control requires a consistent, cohesive, and thorough approach to method selection, instruction, and evaluation, with an awareness of the common difficulties encountered in each area that can affect treatment outcome.

Selecting Pain Control Strategies

As described in the preceding section, method selection begins with an assessment of the pain complaint, the child, the parents, and the context in which the pain is experienced. Table 6.3 lists the common factors that influence children's pain. As children mature, they generally gain a better understanding of their pain, acquire more coping strategies, and exhibit less overt behavioral distress; however, they may have learned exaggerated or maladaptive pain behaviors. Their emotions vary from situation-specific fear and anxiety related to the present or immediate effects of pain and treatment, to deeper fear, anxiety, or depression related to the future consequences of pain or disease on their health and ability to live normally. Parents' and siblings' responses to children's pain complaints shape the manner in which they express and cope with pain. Parents who encourage children to rely almost exclusively on them to alleviate their distress teach their children to be passive and inadvertently encourage them to adopt "sick" roles. Children may then exaggerate their pain complaints, or their pain may increase. Parents who respond inconsistently to their children's pain, alternating between providing excessive

TABLE 6.3.   Common Factors That Increase Children's Pain

Factor	< 7.0	7.0–12.0	> 13.0
Situational			
Limited control	U	U	S
Inaccurate information	U	U	S
Negative expectations	U	U	U
Few coping strategies	U	S	S
Behavioral			
Overt distress behaviors	U	S	R
Learned pain behaviors	U	S	S
Restriction of physical activities	S	S	S
Emotional			
Anxiety, fear regarding:			
Diagnosis	S	U	A
Treatment	U	U	S
Hospitalization	U	S	A
Physical appearance	S	S	A
Future implications	R	S	A
Depression	R	S	S
Familial			
Inconsistent responses	S	S	S
Excessive attention for pain complaints	S	S	S
Excessive protection	S	S	S

Note. Extent to which these factors are seen in each age group: A, always; U, usually; S, sometimes; N, never.

reassurance and ignoring them, also pose a serious challenge for pain management programs. Their children's pain or pain behaviors are very resistant to change because of the intermittent reinforcement the parents have provided. Research on learning has demonstrated that behaviors reinforced at unpredictable intervals are more often maintained and less likely to be reduced than behaviors reinforced consistently.

Pain control strategies must be selected according to the situational, behavioral, emotional, and familial factors relevant for each child. Most children under 7 years old require a behavioral management component in their pain program to reduce the number of overt distress behaviors and any learned pain behaviors; most adolescents require a counseling component to address the emotional effects of the disease, trauma, or syndrome causing their pain. All parents should learn how their behaviors affect their children's pain, their expression of pain, and their abilities to cope with pain.

The focus of this chapter is on the general selection, administration, and evaluation of cognitive-behavoral pain control strategies for children that are based on the principal factors that contribute to their pain problems, rather than on the specific diseases responsible for their pain. These strategies are used in conjunction with the medical treatment for any underlying disease and any prescribed pharmacological therapies. Obviously, the emphasis of the pain control program shifts according to whether the pain is acute, recurrent, or chronic, and the application of the program shifts according to a child's age, cognitive level, and familial support. Individual differences among children, their families, and relevant situational factors necessitate that all pain programs be flexible, so that they can be adapted to the special needs of each child, family, and pain problem. Yet general pain programs seem to evolve naturally for different types of pain as a consequence of the situational factors comon to them.

The factors listed in Table 6.3 provide a framework for a cognitive-behavioral program with four major objectives: (1) to provide children and parents with accurate information about the pain problem in relation to nociceptive systems and the factors that modify pain perception; (2) to alter the situational factors that usually increase pain—for example, to reduce waiting time for invasive procedures (acute pain), to decrease excessive reliance on parents or medication for pain relief (all types of pain), to increase regular physical activities (recurrent and chronic pains), and to reduce anxiety-related and conditioned pain behaviors (all types of pain); (3) to improve children's control by teaching them simple ways to cope with or to reduce their pain; and (4) to encourage children to be actively involved in pain management, using a positive and consistent approach from staff and parents, with appropriate support for parents.

The manner in which these objectives are achieved will depend on the pain problem, the child, and the family, as shown by the following case illustrations from our pain clinic.

Acute Pain Evoked by Medical Treatments

A 6-year-old girl, Cheryl, who was on a high-risk protocol for acute lymphoblastic leukemia, was referred for pain and anxiety management related to invasive procedures. Despite sedation, Cheryl became very distressed prior to and during treatments. In fact, she was withdrawn and unable to sleep the night before LPs and bone marrow aspirations (BMAs) because she was frightened. She seemed to fight the sedation and analgesia (Valium and Demerol), so that she often needed to be restrained during treatments, and she reported stronger pains than any other children. Because of her anxiety, her parents stopped telling her in advance when LPs and BMAs were scheduled, under the assumption that she would not become as anxious about her treatment. However, her father would take a day off work for LP and BMA appointments (unlike non-LP appointments, when only her mother would accompany her to the clinic), because her parents were apprehensive and believed that she would need their mutual support.

Cheryl had limited control during procedures, inaccurate information about what happened in LPs and BMAs, negative expectations about pain and being restrained, no positive coping skills, and no predictability for these treatments. Because she did not know when LPs and BMAs were scheduled (except by the fact that her father accompanied her to the clinic), she was wholly unprepared, so that her only possible reactions were crying, resisting, and refusing treatments. As described in Chapter 3, adults report less pain when a noxious stimulus is signaled or predictable than when it is not signaled. Also, signaling reduces the neuronal response (from wide-dynamic-range neurons) produced by a noxious stimulus in monkeys, presumably by activating an endogenous pain inhibitory system. Consequently, Cheryl's parents were asked to prepare her for LPs and BMAs, with the expectation that her preprocedural distress would gradually diminish as she learned some positive tools for pain and anxiety reduction. They were also asked to treat LP and BMA appointments as routinely as any others, to minimize their aversive significance for her.

Her age, fear, anxiety, and lack of coping skills were the main criteria in selecting specific pain control strategies for Cheryl's program. However, since her anxiety was exacerbated by LPs' lack of predictability because of her parents' concerns, strategies were also selected to facilitate her mother's and father's positive assistance and to reduce their anxiety. Pain-coping strategies are most effective when they are built onto children's existing framework for coping with pain or with treatments. Therefore, the first session of any program begins with a review of the least invasive procedure (from the child's perspective) to identify his/her positive coping strategies and the situational factors that promote coping. The child gradually reviews the most invasive or painful procedure to understand why he/she may not be able to apply these coping strategies to this situation, and to identify the situational factors that intensify fear, anxiety, or pain.

Although the least invasive procedure for Cheryl was the finger prick, it was evident during our review that she merely endured the procedure by bracing herself, but still felt anxious and frightened. Consequently, she first needed some simple coping strategies for the finger prick before she could develop more sophisticated strategies for LPs and BMAs. Young children require concrete explanations about blocking pain. They have all experienced the pain relief provided by a parental hug or kiss after an injury, so they understand that their pain can be truly modified by nondrug techniques. The role of the pain therapist is to introduce other techniques to them that will be as effective as a parental hug, building on their already positive expectations that their distress and pain can be reduced.

Since Cheryl was usually very passive during procedures, we emphasized the potential pain-reducing benefits of active participation and encouraged her to assist when possible. In a concrete practice session in which the therapist conducted a finger prick on herself, Cheryl learned the rationale for the procedure and the equipment used; she also learned how the pain can be lessened when children choose the finger, help to clean it with alcohol, rub it vigorously immediately afterwards, and even learn to prick their own fingers and smear the blood on a slide. She discovered that many children can lessen pain by squeezing someone's hand during the procedure, so that their squeeze communicates the strength of any pain that they experience. The emphasis is on actively communicating sensations, rather than simply squeezing as hard as possible.

During the first session, Cheryl was eager to try her own finger prick; she reported no anxiety or pain. At her next clinical appointment, she also conducted her own blood-sampling and reported no anxiety or pain. Her subsequent pain management sessions progressively focused on dressing changes, portacatheter injections, LPs, and BMAs. She learned that active play in the child life program prior to treatments reduced her anxiety and that simple pain control strategies during treatments reduced her pain. These sessions involved role play with puppets, desensitization with medical equipment, and practice at home with her parents and siblings. In light of her age and need for concrete tools for pain control, we encouraged her to squeeze her father's hand, take deep and regularly paced breaths, and use guided imagery to lessen her pain during LPs and BMAs. She used these strategies effectively, so that her anxiety and pain were reduced.

However, her parents were unable to regard her LP and BMA procedures as routine appointments. Her father still accompanied her, along with her mother and younger siblings. Cheryl was often pulled from child life activities in the ambulatory clinic to lie down in a darkened treatment room with one parent (while the other parent watched her brothers and sisters), to wait for the procedure. Her parents spoke in whispers and insisted on being present for the brief coaching session on pain management prior to the LP. They often interrupted, so that Cheryl's attention was diverted from the therapist. Her pain and anxiety during LPs and BMAs gradually increased slightly, but not to previous levels.

In sharp contrast to her usual pretreatment environment (children playing in the clinic waiting area with regular noise and light levels), the dark room, hushed voices, and excessive parental ministrations created an environment with a powerful impact for a 6-year-old girl. The implicit message was "The treatment today has a special significance," but the emphasis was focused on the aversive signifi- cance. Although we attempted to illustrate the impact of this situation for Cheryl, her parents believed that it was the best approach for their daughter, and they were unwilling to modify their behavior. Usually, we are able to demonstrate which approaches are best for children by objectively evaluating children's distress behav- iors and self-reports of pain and anxiety. We review this information with parents to document why we have selected a particular approach. Yet Cheryl's parents were reluctant to allow her to complete questionnaires regularly, so that we could not obtain information from her perspective. When we were able to interview her (in her parents' presence), her responses were often invalidated by their responses, such as "You don't really feel that way, do you?"

Cheryl's parents were not insensitive to their daughter's needs; they really believed that they were acting in her best interests. They were adjusting to her cancer and to her cancer treatments by providing her with the emotional reassur- ance, support, and protective attention that they judged necessary. The parents of any child who has been diagnosed with a potentially fatal disease face a prolonged and difficult adjustment. They must provide information and support for the ill child, their other children, grandparents, and perhaps other members of the extended family. The mother and father may differ not only in their coping abilities, but also in their perceptions of what their ill child needs from them. The anguish of watching their child endure invasive treatments adds incredibly to their emotional burden. As a consequence, even though the primary focus of the pain program is the child, it is necessary to consider his/her parents' own pain.

It is necessary to confront parents when their behaviors are adversely affecting their child. Yet it is cruel to confront them without understanding their perspec- tive. It is also foolish to confront them bluntly if the pain therapist is hoping to improve the situation for their child, since they may withdraw their child from pain management, insisting that the program is ineffective. This has happened for approximately 1 in 25 families of our oncology patients. The most sensitive approach also is the most sensible. It is beneficial to build upon the parents' needs to support their child by including them more actively in the program, so that they participate in some practice procedures to coach and encourage their child to use pain-coping strategies. They can provide a hand to squeeze or can coach their child to breathe deeply, relax, and use guided imagery. At the same time, these parents also require emotional support for themselves.

In recognition of the complex needs of children with cancer and their parents, many oncology services have developed multidisciplinary teams to assist the whole family. Hematologist/oncologists, nurses, social workers, psychologists, child life specialists, and art therapists form a cohesive group to provide family, parent, and child support. In our hospital, the oncology team routinely refers all newly diagnosed children to the pain clinic. However, even with the team's support, Cheryl's parents did not feel that further involvement with the pain program would benefit their daughter. They were reluctant to receive any assistance from the team for themselves. Although her fear, anxiety, distress behaviors, and pain decreased, Cheryl might have experienced even more reductions if her LP and BMA appointments had been treated more routinely.

Recurrent Abdominal Pain

A 7½-year-old girl, Peggy, had experienced recurrent episodes of dull, aching abdominal pain for 2 years. The frequency of painful episodes varied, but they often occurred daily during the week, with pain-free periods on weekends and holidays. Her pains occurred primarily in the morning or in the middle of the night. She usually felt nauseated when she had pain, but she never vomited. Her pain descriptions were atypical, in that she was unable to provide clear and consistent information about the sensory dimensions (the quality, location, strength, or duration) of the pain, in comparison with other children her age. She showed no evidence of emotional distress or fear related to the painful episodes, which is quite unusual when children suffer severe pain for a long period without obtaining satisfactory pain relief. Her parents responded to her pain complaints inconsistently, alternating between staying with her until the pain subsided or simply telling her to rest.

The results of the pain assessment indicated that stress, particularly stress related to maintaining her A grades in school, contributed to a generally high level of anxiety. However, her pain complaints were also exacerbated by a learned or conditioned behavioral pattern. Inconsistent parental responses and an inability to cope with school or peer stress led her gradually to exaggerate pain complaints, so that she received more parental reassurance and was able to stay home from school. She seemed to complain about pain without really feeling pain. It seemed to us that she might have suffered initial episodes of abdominal pain from a gastrointestinal virus or from stress, and that the positive benefits associated with her pain might have led to increased pain reports in the absence of an organic source.

Therefore, Peggy's pain program emphasized a behavioral component to decrease the positive benefits of her pain complaints and to promote healthy, pain-free behaviors, in addition to a stress reduction component. During the feedback session, she and her parents received general information about nociceptive systems; endogenous pain-inhibitory systems; and the relationships among emotional, situational, behavioral, and familial factors and children's pain complaints. Her parents were then informed that Peggy seemed to suffer more from learned pain behaviors than from stress-induced pains, so that she required a strict behavioral management program to decrease these complaints gradually. Her parents did not want to schedule a specific program for her, but preferred to follow our recomendations for behavioral management and stress reduction. The parents initiated a behavioral modification program in which Peggy received a gold star each morning when she did not wake during the night with abdominal pain. Her painful episodes stopped immediately.

The startling overnight success of a behavioral program may not be maintained indefinitely. If the pain complaints are primarily due to learned behaviors, then the behaviors should be reduced when parents adopt a consistent management approach. In Peggy's case, stress reduction was a necesary component to maintain pain reductions. Regular relaxation periods were scheduled into homework periods; weekly physical activities were planned; and she was encouraged to develop some nonacademic, noncompetitive hobbies. She developed better insights about how her body responded to stress, as well as about the need to incorporate more nonstressful activities in her life. Her pain complaints were dramatically abolished.

Few children present with recurrent pains that are due solely to learned pain behaviors. Instead, most children suffer pains as a consequence of true environmental and internal factors that must be identified and modified to provide long-lasting pain reduction. The dramatic results seen for Peggy are somewhat misleading with respect to the majority of children with recurrent pain syndromes. More often, an immediate and complete reduction in recurrent pains, particularly after a 2-year duration, indicates an abnormally high need for parental approval or a need to "get better" so that the children do not have to attend the pain management program. The latter case is common for adolescents who want to avoid confronting stressors in their lives, and for young children whose parents do not want to admit that stress underlies their children's pains. These children often spontaneously recover, only to relapse a few months later with the same pain complaint or similar aches and pains in other body sites. (Recurrent pain syndromes and interventions are described in greater detail in Chapter 8.)

Chronic Pain

A 14-year-old girl, Sandy, was referred for the management of chronic back pain due to mild scoliosis. She had experienced weekly episodes of mild, aching pain and dull, throbbing pain in her lumbar region for 1 year; these then progressed to a constant pain. She did not notice any decrease in the strength of her pain throughout the day, even though some natural pain reductions usually occur when children participate in physical activities, are concentrating on interesting events, are distracted, or are resting. She believed that physical exertion increased her pain. There seemed to be no obvious reason for the gradual increase in pain from weekly episodes to a continuous level, or for her failure to experience complete pain relief even when she rested, applied heat, and used aspirin. Yet Sandy reported minimal frustration, fear, and anger, and she did not appear overly concerned by pain strength or by the regular interruptions that pain caused in her life.

Her mother described Sandy as a nervous child who had difficulty expressing her emotions. She was an A student who strove to do her best in all academic, social, and physical endeavors; in fact, her mother described her as a "perfectionist." Her back pain had recently forced her to withdraw from physiotherapy, regular exercise, and school gym. Oddly, though, she was able to continue her dance classes (tap, ballet, and jazz) three times each week. This discrepant information alone suggested that physical exertion did not always increase her pain. Although Sandy had not reported any problems related to her parents' separation 3 years earlier, her mother explained that Sandy's father had not maintained close contact with her and neglected to visit her for many scheduled events that were important to Sandy. She had noticed that Sandy's pain complaints increased at these times, even though her daughter denied that she was hurt or angry.

Although Sandy's pain was due to her scoliosis, it was exacerbated primarily by emotional factors. The absence of any discernible variations in pain strength associated with daily activities, the lack of affect related to the daily frustration of living with pain, and Sandy's high expectations for achievement all led to the interpretation that her pain had strong functional components, regardless of the original etiology. Her inability to identify, express, and resolve her feelings had led to the gradual expression of those emotions in an existing somatic complaint, and thus to increased pain. The pain enabled her to withdraw from potentially stressful activities or situations and to seek comfort, sympathy, and reassurance without acknowledging that she was stressed or unable to cope with her feelings. She was not consciously using her pain to malinger; instead, her emotional distress actually exacerbated her pain.

On the basis of these assessment findings, a six-session pain management program was recommended for Sandy. The program objectives were as follows: to monitor her pain with daily diaries, with an emphasis on identifying situations, activities, emotions, and behaviors that led to increases or decreases in her pain; to teach her to recognize these events and increase those that decreased her pain, while modifying her responses to those that increased her pain so that they no longer adversely affected her; to teach her some independent strategies to reduce her constant pain; to assist her mother in learning how to respond to Sandy's complaints to minimize excessive pain behaviors; and to counsel both Sandy and her mother about the relationship between emotional factors and somatic complaints, so that they would consider a psychiatric consultation.

The need for a psychiatric referral was discussed at the feedback session, in which the results of the assessment were reviewed with Sandy's mother. She was initially hesitant to accept a referral, and her daughter adamantly refused one. This situation is common for many adolescents with recurrent or chronic pain when their pain has a strong psychological component. Previous experience has led us to recruit these children into brief pain management programs in which a major objective is to teach children and their families that real physical pain has psychological dimensions that can intensify and prolong suffering. The need for psychiatric or psychological counseling does not mean that the pain is not real, but that emotional factors are primarily responsible and must be resolved for optimal pain control.

Children and families learn about the relationship between mind and body in influencing pain, using illustrations of nociceptive inhibitory systems to show how situational factors modify neuronal coding, and using biofeedback to show concretely how the children's own bodies react to pleasant and stressful topics. This information is presented in the first three sessions, since the emphasis is on understanding and modifying all the factors (environmental and internal) that affect pain. Usually, by the end of a six-session program, the majority of families recognize that emotions can affect their children's pain; they are thus more willing to accept a psychiatric or psychological referral. Continued pain management is provided in accordance with the therapy program, often only to teach children specific pain-coping skills and to support parents in providing consistent responses when their children experience pain.

The focus of Sandy's first session was on reviewing the typical factors that create stress and can intensify pain for adolescents, such as school, relationships with peers or siblings, parental expectations, and personal expectations for achievement, and then on evaluating whether these were relevant in her own life. She was asked to complete a detailed pain diary, in which she also recorded daily events and her feelings about them. In the second session, the diary was reviewed. Her pain had intensified during the previous weekend, but she did not know why. She had been able only to record her activities, not her feelings about them. Sandy's mother completed a diary independently to monitor Sandy's pain from her perspective, as well as her own responses when Sandy experienced pain. She noted that Sandy was spending more time with her instead of with friends her own age; that she denied she was bothered when her former boyfriend asked her best friend to a dance (the dance coincided with the weekend during which Sandy's pain was inexplicably stronger); and that minor pain complaints occurred when Sandy felt that her brother received special treatment at home. At this point, Sandy's mother accepted (indeed, suggested) that psychological counseling might be needed to address some of Sandy's emotional problems. She realized that her daughter would probably refuse, but she felt confident that therapy was necessary.

During the third session, electrodes were attached to Sandy's forearm for a biofeedback session. The voltage levels fluctuated from 1.5 to 2.8 μV during normal conversation, but increased to the highest point on the scale (8 μV) when she was asked about school, her father, or her friends, even though she did not admit to any stress in these areas of her life. She was quite surprised that her body reacted involuntarily to these topics. We discussed the possibility that her body reacted to protect her from emotional issues, and that her pain probably reflected the intensity of these emotions and provided a warning signal that she needed assistance to understand her feelings. She then agreed to a psychiatric consultation concurrent with continuing her pain program.

Normally, when children comply with a referral as Sandy did, with a calm acceptance in front of the therapist, there is an intense delayed reaction with their parents. Reactions may vary from suddenly experiencing complete pain relief to complaining about a dramatic increase in pain or a reduction in their physical ability. We prepare parents for both extremes, since we cannot predict which children will react in which manner. Sandy became lethargic, reported increased pain, and spent the next 3 days at home lying on the couch. Prior to her appointment with a psychiatrist, she developed various somatic complaints for which no physical causes were established. She missed school throughout most of this period, although her mother had been encouraged to send her to school as much as possible. After Sandy was seen regularly by a psychiatrist, both her back pain and her other somatic complaints decreased.

In general, the optimal management of chronic pain requires both a pharmacological and a nonpharmacological approach to manage the pain induced by tissue damage, pain evoked by abnormal sensory input due to postural restrictions for fear of pain, and pain associated with psychological factors (as described in Chapter 9). Although all chronic pain has psychological consequences for children and their families, not all children with chronic pain require psychological counseling. When children's chronic pain is exacerbated primarily by emotional factors, as it was for Sandy, then they require psychiatric or psychological consultation and therapy.

Teaching Pain Control Strategies to Children

As stressed throughout this book, pain-coping strategies are selected for a child according to the type of pain; the child's age or cognitive level; and the situational, emotional, behavioral, and familial factors identified in the pain assessment. Several general interventions are taught to each child so that he/she can develop a flexible repertoire of pain-coping strategies. The same strategy will probably not be effective for all occurrences of a child's pain, since the strength, quality, extent, and unpleasantness of the same pain problem will undoubtedly vary somewhat. Consequently, the child and parents should learn several methods for reducing pain. Emphasis should be placed on the manner in which they are reducing the pain, rather than on the magical benefits of any one method. Children should not be encouraged to develop a false reliance on a particular pain-coping strategy; instead, they should learn some principles of pain management, so that they will naturally evolve their own techniques for reducing pain. Children must acquire a rationale for controlling their pain, based on the plasticity and complexity of their nociceptive systems.

Plasticity and Complexity of Nociceptive Processing

When a child is referred to our pain clinic, an assessment is conducted in which the parents and child are interviewed and complete some standardized inventories appropriate for the child's pain problem (acute, recurrent, or chronic). Each set of inventories provides quantitative, objective information about the main features of the pain and the primary factors that affect children's pain perceptions. (These inventories are described fully in Chapters 7, 8, and 9, and the pain questionnaires are included in the Appendix.)

The initial interview is conducted jointly with the parents and child to describe the Children's Pain Clinic and then to review briefly why the study of pain in general, and the study of children's pain in particular, represent new areas for clinical research. Then the family learns that the nociceptive system is plastic and complex, that pain is not simply and directly related to the intensity of a noxious stimulus, and that many environmental and internal factors can modify their pain perception. This information is presented in an accurate and thorough manner, but the emphasis is on the concept of the plasticity and modifiabilty of neuronal coding rather than on the specific terminology or mechanisms. Thus, parents learn that the dorsal horn is a major site for modifying nociceptive input, that opiate and nonopiate systems can be activated to inhibit pain, and that some of the factors activating these systems are known.

Several figures are used to illustrate information in a concrete and tangible manner. First, families are shown an illustration derived from the description by Descartes (1664/1972) of how people experience burning pain. Minute particles of energy triggered by the fire are conveyed along direct pathways from the limb to the brain, where pain is the inevitable result. The second figure consists of a single expression, "Noxious stimulus = Pain perception," to describe Descartes's view and the traditional concept of pain. Pain was traditionally regarded as the inevitable result of tissue damage, with the strength of the pain proportional to the nature or extent of physical damage. We then note that this concept is no longer tenable in light of our increased understanding of the nociceptive system, using a figure to illustrate that the dorsal horn is the location for a major pain gate to modulate nociceptive processing, as well as to point out the complexity of the possible interactions among arriving afferent impulses and descending messages. This general figure on the nociceptive system has already been shown in Chapter 3 (see Figure 3.3).

Two simple examples of pain modulation are also provided at this time. Children learn that rubbing their fingers after a finger prick can help to lessen pain, because they are activating nerves that can partially close the pain gate. The therapist demonstrates on the figure how the neural impulses for rubbing and pain are carried in separate pathways from the fingertip to the spinal cord, where one pathway can block the message carried by the other. Even very young children understand that messages (voices on telephones, pictures and sounds on television, sounds on radios) are transmitted along wires and that the transmission can be blocked by other signals. Parents and children are then reminded that they may not feel pain from an injury (e.g., a cut, scrape, or headache) when they are concentrating on something other than the injury (e.g., an interesting TV show, a conversation, a sports activity). They are asked to describe situations from their own experience in which this has happened, so that they can better understand why their pain was altered, while the therapist uses the figure to demonstrate how cognitive factors can modulate pain through descending inhibitory systems.

The term "situational factors" is then introduced to teach families about the tremendous potential impact of contextual and situational cues for modifying children's pain. A figure depicting a wide-dynamic-range neuron's response to the same noxious stimulus in two different contexts, signaled and nonsignaled, is used to demonstrate how situational factors may reduce pain (Figure 6.1). Another figure is shown to illustrate the pain reduction produced when noxious stimuli are signaled for adult volunteers (Figure 6.2). Parents and children are asked to describe the implications of this research for children's pain; this helps them understand that a main objective of the pain clinic is the practical application to children of pain management techniques based on research with adults, as well as evaluation of the success of these techniques. Finally, Figure 1.7 is shown to summarize our present knowledge of the relationship between a noxious stimulus and a child's perception of pain; this model also presents the rationale for the comprehensive assessment battery that children and families complete. With this format and these figures, information about the plasticity and complexity of the nociceptive system can be introduced within 20 minutes, so that families understand that their children's pain can be reduced by several methods in addition to altering the source of noxious stimulation.

Teaching Children How to Reduce Their Pain

Children can easily learn several methods for reducing their pain. The approach that has proven most beneficial in our clinic has been to teach children a few basic standardized methods, and then to encourage them to personalize these methods or to design new methods with their parents and families. Although some information about pain-reducing strategies is provided in the initial interview, children learn various pain control interventions in relatively brief pain management

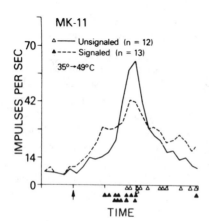

FIGURE 6.1. Peristimulus histograms comparing responses of four wide-dynamic-range neurons in monkey 11 on trials that were preceded by a warning signal (dashed line) to responses on trials that were not preceded by a signal (solid line). All thermal stimuli were 49°C. Open triangles indicate discrimination or escape latencies on unsignaled trials; filled triangles indicate panel release on signaled trials; *n* refers to the number of trials averaged in each histogram. From "Neuronal Activity in Medullary Dorsal Horn of Awake Monkeys Trained in a Thermal Discrimination Task: II. Behavioral Modulation of Responses to Thermal and Mechanical Stimuli" by R. L. Hayes, R. Dubner, and D. S. Hoffman, 1981, *Journal of Neurophysiology, 46*, p. 435. Copyright 1981 by the American Physiological Society. Reprinted by permission.

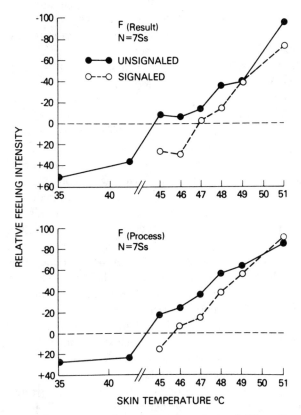

FIGURE 6.2. Mean affective magnitude evoked by thermal stimuli. The ordinate is divided into positive and negative scales coresponding to positive and negative affect. The upper graph shows the mean affective responses to the results of stimulation; the lower graph shows mean affective responses related to the pleasantness or unpleasantness of sensations. For both measures of affect the signal shifts the curve in a positive direction. Each point is the mean of at least 21 observations. From "A Psychophysical Analysis of Experiential Factors That Selectively Influence the Affective Dimension of Pain" by D. D. Price, J. J. Barrell, and R. H. Gracely, 1980, *Pain, 8,* p. 143. Copyright 1980 by Elsevier Science Publishers. Reprinted by permission.

programs (usually 4–12 sessions, depending on the nature of the pain). The sessions are structured to enable children to achieve definite objectives throughout the course of the program, beginning with the acquisition of standard pain-coping strategies and culminating in the design of a versatile repertoire of skills.

The sessions are scheduled weekly for children referred for acute pain management, if the children are currently receiving medical or dental treatments that evoke pain; sessions are usually scheduled biweekly for children referred for recurrent or chronic pain management. The weekly and biweekly schedules have evolved through our clinical practice. Outpatients who receive invasive procedures on a daily or weekly basis require a pain management program that enables them to learn, practice, and refine their pain control strategies in the normal course of their treatment. Inpatients may actually require daily sessions, depending on the factors affecting their pain or the number of invasive procedures they receive. Children with recurrent or chronic pain seem to respond to the program better when sessions are scheduled at 2-week intervals; this allows them sufficient time to practice management techniques and to complete assigned homework (the homework is to identify and modify pain triggers, as described in Chapter 8).

Table 6.4 lists the common strategies children learn during the course of their programs. Logical age-appropriate rationales as to why these strategies should lessen their pain are presented. Strategies that are easiest for all children to understand and use are taught in the first few sessions. Then more abstract methods are gradually introduced as children master the concrete methods. In general, the younger the child, the more concrete the methods selected must be. Children first learn to rub their fingertips deeply and continuously after a prick to shorten and reduce any pain, because all of them have already experienced acute pain from a finger prick. Most children remember that they have instinctively rubbed a painful body area to lessen the pain or that their mothers have massaged a painful site to reduce their discomfort. Pain reduction produced by physically rubbing the finger makes sense to them. They will understand that the pain reduction is due to the physiological mechanisms that were described to them. Adolescents benefit when the relatively simple mechanism of rubbing is compared to the more complex mechanisms of acupuncture, to illustrate that some physiological mechanisms are common to both.

Another physical intervention provides the second pain strategy for children. The pain-reducing potential of a relaxed body state is taught to children through

TABLE 6.4.   Pain-Coping Strategies

Rub body area deeply and continuously.

Take deep breaths and relax all your muscles.
   Imagine a relaxing situation.
   Listen to soothing music.
   Use progressive relaxation.

Concentrate on an interesting event.
   Tell a story.
   Converse with someone.
   Sing a song.
   Play a game.
   Assist with the procedure.

Make your pain disappear.
   Make your body numb.
   Move the pain.
   Imagine that the pain does not bother you.

discussion, progressive muscle relaxation, and biofeedback. Children easily distinguish between a tight, tense fist and a relaxed, open hand. They can visualize that it is harder to insert a needle (a concrete image for producing pain) into a tensed arm than a relaxed arm, with the probable result that the needle produces more pain in the tensed state. In fact, any type of pain can be intensified if the muscles are always tightened. Since fear or anxiety creates some body tension, children need to recognize when they are tense and to learn to relax. Again, the need for altering a physical state that can exacerbate their pain makes sense to children, so that they are motivated to learn how to control their bodies.

Biofeedback is an excellent tool for teaching children how their bodies react to pain-inducing stimuli or pain-arousing situations. Biofeedback is particularly useful for adolescents with recurrent pain syndromes who do not believe that there is an association between their painful episodes and their emotional reactions to stress. Children watch or listen to their body responses and use deep breathing, progressive muscle relaxation, guided imagery, or hypnosis to lower the amplified signals. Children learn which of these methods promote the most relaxed state for them. They then attempt to use the same method when they are in pain or when they expect pain (during medical procedures or at the onset of a headache).

Some cognitive interventions are introduced as children learn these concrete physical interventions. Special attention is focused on children's ability to reduce pain by controlling their minds in much the same way as they have learned to control their bodies. The most important feature is that they must concentrate fully on "something else"—an event (even the procedure or the sensation produced, without emphasizing the pain sensation), a distracting situation (a story, a conversation, a cartoon), or an activity (singing a song, playing a game, assisting with the procedure). The same event or activity will not be consistently effective for all children. Instead, children choose which techniques facilitate their complete mental absorption. Their full concentration is the critical component for pain reduction, not the particular method that they use to achieve it. Young children choose counting aloud; singing songs, particularly Christmas carols; squeezing a hand in proportion to the strength of any pain; and describing parties, cartoons, and trips as methods to absorb their attention during invasive procedures. Older children generally prefer conversations and hypnosis. Children with recurrent or chronic pain use primarily relaxation, induced by progressive muscle relaxation, guided imagery, music, and exercise, to lessen their pain.

The optimal use of cognitive pain interventions necessitates that children understand the importance of their full concentration. A practical auditory analogy has been useful in our program. Children are reminded that they often do not hear when their parents call them, because they are concentrating on television or actively playing a game. In a sense, they selectively tune out noises that are not interesting or relevant to what they are doing. At this point in the session, we usually remind them to listen to the hum of the ventilation system. They are aware that the sound has been present throughout the session, but that they really have not heard it throughout most of our discussion. They can learn to do a similar "tuning out" with pain. This sound analogy is also useful in teaching children how to use a cognitive intervention.

> "Imagine that you and I are watching a movie in a downtown theatre. Two people come in and sit in front of us. They are eating a jumbo box of popcorn and candies in crinkly plastic wrappers. They are making a lot of noise with their crunching and unwrapping. What if I told you to not pay attention to the noise that they are making, but to concentrate only on the movie?"

Most children respond that if they tried too hard to block out the noise of the people eating they would probably pay more attention to them than if they simply forgot them and watched the movie. We use this example to teach children that they should not constantly monitor how well their pain reduction technique is working; they should simply use it when they are feeling pain, and they can evaluate its efficacy with the therapist later.

The last cognitive interventions children learn are the more abstract methods of hypnosis or hypnotic-like suggestions for analgesia. As yet, there are no clear criteria for which children will benefit from these interventions according to age, sex, or pain type; instead, these techniques are introduced to all children. The common approach is to explain that their minds can move pain to different body areas, much as they can attend to and notice sensations in their arms, legs, or heads while ignoring sensations in other body areas. Children learn that this method is called "hypnosis"; adolescents receive more information about the hypnotic process and may participate in a standard induction procedure.

Most of the pain reduction children achieve with cognitive interventions derives from hypnotic-like suggestions for analgesia, rather than from a standard hypnotic induction procedure. The term "hypnotic-like" refers to the fact that the suggestions are similar to those used to induce analgesia under hypnosis. Two familiar sensations provide a framework for explaining to children how these suggestions can lessen their pain. They have usually experienced tingling sensations followed by numbness, either because of a lack of circulation while sitting or sleeping or because of a local anesthetic used at the dentist's. So children can readily accept that they will not feel pain as strongly when different parts of their bodies fall asleep. Similarly, many children have experienced nitrous oxide sedation, so they understand that a gas they can neither see nor smell can produce profound effects on their ability to feel pain. The loss of sensation associated with posture, Novocain, or nitrous oxide is a concrete experience that children remember. Their memories enable them to accept that physical pain reduction can be accomplished in an indirect and intangible manner, as well as in a direct and tangible manner.

They learn that they can imagine a magic gas with properties similar to nitrous oxide sedation, that they can numb a body region by imagining that it is going to sleep, and that they can even move the pain from one area to another.

Although it is probable that the children who easily follow these suggestions would test high on hypnotic susceptibility scales, we do not test children directly, but simply include a set of suggestions in all pain programs. The usual sequence for introducing these suggestions is described with typical instructions and coaching for a 5-year-old boy referred for acute pain management:

> "We know that your brain can shut off so that the injection won't hurt as much. But we don't know yet which method is best for you and the easiest for you to use. So let's practice some today, and we'll try them together during your next treatment. Okay?
>
> "First, you already said that you remember when the doctor froze your leg so that you wouldn't feel anything when he stitched your cut. Sometimes you can produce that same freezing or numbing feeling by yourself, just by thinking very hard about how it felt. In fact, you can make your hand go to sleep as if the doctor made it numb. Would you like to try it? It might feel as if you had played in the snow too long without mittens or as if you put your hands in very cold water. There's a funny sensation that feels different to different people. What does it feel like to you?"

The specific examples chosen depend on what types of numbness the child remembers from past experience. If the child does not have any memories of how pain may be blocked even when the skin looks the same and he/she is alert, the therapist may use a local anesthetic spray or cream to demonstrate a slight loss of pain sensation when it is applied. The anesthetic is placed on the therapist's hand so that the child can observe and touch the skin. The therapist reports that the child's touch feels different (usually less strong and distinct) on that hand and encourages the child to try it on himself/herself. This demonstration provides a more concrete image of pain reduction produced by a quick and noninvasive method.

> "Pretend that your hand is numb. It might help if you imagine that the doctor put some cream on it [the therapist should use the experience that the child has related]. You can also breathe the magic gas so that it will relax you and help make your hand numb so that it can't feel pain. Take deep breaths and imagine the gas. [If the child chooses to breathe the gas, he/she should be encouraged to describe it, because the more vivid the image, the more effective the gas is as a tool for inducing analgesia.] Notice that when I touch your hand, it might feel different than when I touch your other hand. Does it? How?"

Children generally describe the sensation as more fuzzy, blurred, or weak in comparison to that on the other hand. When a sharp object is gently placed on the skin, they may describe that it feels blunt, while the same object placed on the other hand may cause a startle response. The therapist coaches children who are responsive to these suggestions to try to numb another body part in the same way, or to move the numb area to a different area. The major goal is to enable children to numb the painful region. Another goal for young children is to encourage them to move the pain from the painful region to a neutral stimulus, such as the therapist's hand, where the pain can then be shaken off when enough has accumulated. Children tell the therapist when to shake it off, and sometimes to stomp on it after it has been shaken onto the floor.

Some children, both very young children and adolescents, respond almost immediately to these simple suggestions; other children are not able to adopt any of these suggestions for reducing their pain. Adolescents may benefit from a more adult approach, with a standard hypnotic induction technique and encouragement to activate their own natural endogenous pain-inhibitory systems.

These pain control strategies may be used by children above 5 years of age to modify their acute, recurrent, or chronic pain. The principles of pain management are consistent, regardless of children's age or the type of pain—that is, to identify and then modify the primary factors that affect pain perception. However, the particular methods for applying these principles naturally depend on the type of pain, children's ages, and parental support. Children from 3 to 5 years old benefit from a structured behavioral program in which their use of a concrete pain control tool (squeezing a hand, singing a song, conversing about a trip, breathing "magic sparklies") is rewarded to encourage them to use it, even if they do not understand the principle, and to encourage parents to assist the children to cope more independently. Older children and adolescents usually adopt and refine these strategies with minimal encouragement from parents and staff.

Summary

A consistent cognitive-behavioral approach should be used to control the situational, emotional, familial, and behavioral factors that can exacerbate a child's pain. As reviewed in Chapters 4 and 5, many interventions are available to alleviate pain in infants and children. Pain management problems in pediatrics arise not from a lack of analgesic methodology, but from a lack of consistent application. An integrated pharmacological and nonpharmacological approach can be developed to meet the specific requirements of different acute, recurrent, and chronic pains for all children.

A typical pain management program evolves from a theoretical perspective in which a child's pain is regarded as a complex perception, usually initiated by tissue damage, but always modified by situational and emotional factors. A thorough assessment is conducted to identify the factors that intensify pain from the unique perspectives of the child, parents, and relevant health professionals. A consistent management program can then be developed to minimize children's pain by selecting the treatments appropriate for modifying nociceptive input and for modifying the environmental and internal factors that modulate pain perception. Analgesic or anesthetic prescriptions for children are based on medical guidelines within the hospital, in conjunction with the dynamically revised recommendations based on controlled clinical trials with infants and children. Specific pain control strategies must be selected for a child according to the type of pain; the child's age or cognitive level; and the situational, emotional, behavioral, and familial factors identified in the pain assessment.

Several general interventions are taught to each child so that he/she can develop a flexible repertoire of pain-coping strategies. The same strategy will probably not be effective for all occurrences of a child's pain, since the strength, quality, extent, and unpleasantness of the same pain problem will undoubtedly vary somewhat. Consequently children and their parents should learn several methods for reducing pain. The emphasis should be placed on the manner in which they are reducing the pain, rather than on the magical benefits of any one method. Children should not be encouraged to develop a false reliance on a particular pain-coping strategy; instead, they should learn some principles of pain management, so that they will naturally evolve their own techniques for reducing pain. Children must acquire a rationale for controlling their pain—a rationale based on the plasticity and complexity of their nociceptive systems. Most children under 7 years old require a behavioral management component in their pain program to reduce the number of overt distress behaviors and any learned pain behaviors, whereas most adolescents require a counseling component to address the emotional effects of the disease, trauma, or syndrome causing their pain. All parents should learn how their behaviors affect their children's pain, their expression of pain, and their abilities to cope with pain.

Pain control strategies are used in conjunction with the medical treatment for any underlying disease and any prescribed pharmacological therapies. Obviously, the emphasis of the pain control program shifts according to whether the pain is acute, recurrent, or chronic, and the application of the program shifts according to a child's age, cognitive level, and familial support. Individual differences among children, their families, and relevant situational factors necessitate that all pain programs be flexible so that they can be adapted to the special needs of each child, family, and pain problem. Yet general pain programs seem to evolve naturally for different types of pain (e.g., acute pain evoked by medical procedures, recurrent headaches, chronic arthritis pain) as a consequence of the situational factors common to them.

The most effective programs are based on a thorough assessment of the factors that affect children's pain. Multistrategy programs, which incorporate several cognitive-behavioral approaches, represent flexible foundations for reducing children's pain in accordance with our present knowledge of the plasticity and complexity of nociceptive systems.

7

Acute Pains

Most children experience a wide variety of pains that differ in strength, quality, location, duration, and affective component. They suffer pains from bruises, cuts, scrapes, broken bones, stomachaches, headaches, toothaches, burns, and injections. Some children will also experience pain from major injuries and accidents, pain after surgery, and pain from diseases. Our ability to provide adequate pain relief for children depends, in part, on our ability to recognize the common and unique features integral to the myriad of their painful conditions, to identify the responsible mechanisms, and to develop the therapeutic interventions most effective for each condition.

The adoption of a common pain language with universally accepted definitions and the development of a classification system for specific pain syndromes have been important objectives of the International Association for the Study of Pain (IASP). Much progress has been achieved toward adopting a common language for understanding and controlling pain problems and toward developing a taxonomy of pain to distinguish among varied pain conditions. Although pain conditions have been described initially for pains experienced by adults, many descriptions as well as the overall classification scheme are relevant to children.

Classification of Pains as Acute, Chronic, Recurrent, or Cancer

Although the classification of pain as acute, chronic, or recurrent (many authorities now add cancer as a fourth category; see below) is relatively new, interest in classifying the diversity of pains into meaningful categories to facilitate communication, understanding, and therapeutic intervention has been evident throughout recorded history. The current classification system has evolved from a consideration of both physiological and psychological aspects of pain experience. Initially, pains were categorized in terms of their observable or easily reported attributes, such as whether or not they were associated with tissue damage, their assumed physical or spiritual origins, and their location (Bonica, 1953; Gruner, 1930; Tainter, 1948). Later categorizations emphasized the distinct sensory attributes of pain (the quality, intensity, duration, and location) corresponding to brief noxious experimental stimuli applied to different body regions, or the unique sensory characteristics associated with different clinical pain syndromes. However, as knowledge accrued about the plasticity and complexity of nociceptive processing and about the importance of situational, psychological, and emotional factors for modifying pain, pain classifications became more broad-based to recognize the tremendous impact of these factors on all pain experiences.

The present classification of pains as acute, recurrent, chronic, or cancer has emerged from a progressive consideration of the temporal characteristics of the pain condition; the presumed source of stimulation responsible for the pain; the major situational, emotional, and psychological factors unique to each type; and, more recently, the unequivocal demonstration of distinct physiological mechanisms underlying the pathology of acute versus chronic pain. (For reviews, see Bond, 1984; Bonica, Liebeskind, & Albe-Fessard, 1979; Devor, 1984; Melzack & Dennis, 1978; Sternbach, 1978; Ty, Melzack, & Wall, 1984; Wolff, 1980; Zimmermann, 1980.)

The usual attributes associated with the four pain categories are summarized in Table 7.1. Pains are classified according to their temporal duration, the source of noxious stimulation, their biological significance, the prolonged effects on the physical and psychological health of the patient, and the typical situational factors present. This classification system provides a general framework for understanding the principal multidimensional features of children's pain problems.

Acute pain has been traditionally defined as relatively brief pain, usually evoked by a well-defined noxious stimulus. The pain often has a rapid onset and diminishes progressively as an injury heals. Acute pains produced by tissue damage are the most common pains that infants, children, and adolescents experience. Since acute pain generally provides a warning signal that enables children to avoid physical harm, it has an adaptive biological significance. There is usually no prolonged emotional distress associated with acute pain, because the pain is explicable and can be controlled effectively.

However, because of the brief nature of the pain, the clear identification of the pain source, and the lack of adverse psychological consequences, there has been an implicit (albeit erroneous) assumption that the strength and quality of acute pain are simply and directly proportional to the nature and extent of tissue damage. Although nociceptive afferent input is proportional to the intensity of the noxious stimulus, the pain produced by an injury is modified by many factors in addition to the nature and extent of any tissue damage. Children's pain perceptions are affected by situational, emotional, and familial factors, so that even young infants' perceptions of acute pain produced by an intramuscular injection depend on the situation in which they receive that injection (Grunau & Craig, 1987).

TABLE 7.1. The Usual Attributes Associated with Pain Categories

Characteristic	Acute pain	Chronic pain	Recurrent pain	Cancer pain
Temporal duration				
Brief	U	N	S	S
Prolonged	N	U	S	S
Source of noxious stimulus				
Well-defined, single	U	R	R	S
Well-defined, multiple	S	R	S	S
Poorly defined	R	U	S	S
Biological significance				
Adaptive warning	U	R	S	R
No warning	N	U	S	S
Prolonged physical distress				
Fatigue	R	U	S	S
Sleeplessness	R	U	S	S
Restricted motion	R	U	S	S
Related somatic complaints, due to condition or treatment	R	U	S	U
Prolonged emotional distress				
Irritability	R	U	S	S
Concern for future health	N	U	S	U
Anger, fear, frustration	R	U	S	S
Depression	N	U	S	S
Hypochondriasis	N	U	S	S
Relevant situational factors				
Poor control	S	U	S	S
Inaccurate expectations	S	S	S	S
Relevance (life-threatening potential)	S	S	S	U

Note. U, usually; S, sometimes; R, rarely; N, never.

Chronic pain is defined as pain that persists beyond the usual time period required for healing or pain that develops and persists without obvious physical damage. The time period after which acute pains are regarded as chronic pains varies, depending on the nature of the original injury. As shown in Table 7.1, chronic pains may be distinguished from acute pains on the basis of several features in addition to their duration. The source of noxious stimulation is usually poorly defined. The pain generally has no positive biological significance as a warning signal. Patients often suffer prolonged physical and psychological distress, as evidenced by fatigue, sleeplessness, loss of motion, restricted physical abilities, additional somatic complaints, irritability, fear, anger, anxiety, depression, and a preoccupation with their health and physical symptoms. Situational factors may include an increasing reliance on medication as the only possible source of relief, inaccurate expectations about the diagnosis and prognosis, and concerns about the life-threatening potential of the pain source. Although chronic debilitating pain is a serious problem for adults, it is not regarded as a major health problem for children. However, there have not yet been any comprehensive studies on the prevalence of different chronic pains in children and adolescents.

Recurrent pain is a chronic-like condition in which otherwise healthy, pain-free adults and children experience frequent episodes of severe headaches, abdominal pains, or limb pains. Recurrent pain shares some of the attributes commonly associated with acute pain and some of the attributes common to chronic pain. Individual pain episodes are relatively brief, but the syndrome is prolonged and may persist throughout an individual's life. Painful episodes are frequently attributed to poorly defined causes, with the label "recurrent pain syndrome" applied more as a generic description of the pain problem than as a specific explanation. Pain episodes are triggered by a variety of environmental stimuli and internal factors, particularly stimuli that evoke stress. There seems to be no consistent biological significance for the pain, although for some children, the painful episodes provide a warning about an unrecognized stressor or underlying anxiety and depression.

Children can develop adverse physiological, behavioral, and psychological reactions from the unpredictable episodes of severe recurrent pain that interfere with their normal lives. In addition, children are at risk for developing additional "conditioned" pain triggers as they actively search for environmental stimuli that initiate their painful episodes. Although no prospective studies have been conducted on the incidence of recurrent headaches, abdominal pains and limb pains in children and adolescents, conservative estimates based on clinical referrals indicate that they constitute a major problem.

The management of cancer pain, both pain from metastatic disease and pain from necessary cancer treatments, is a serious health concern. Cancer pain is regarded by some as a subcategory of chronic pain (and is discussesd together with other varieties of chronic pain in Chapter 9 of this book); however, many now regard it as a special category of pain because of the unique constellation of emotional, physiological, and behavioral consequences of the diagnosis and subsequent treatment. Pain sensations may arise from multiple sources associated with the disease process, necessary medical treatments, or the psychological stress of living with a potentially fatal disease. Although the prolonged physical and emotional distress for patients with cancer pain is occasionally similar to that for patients with chronic pain resulting from nonmalignant disease or to that for relatively pain-free patients with cancer, the distress associated with cancer pain is much more profound. These patients generally experience more nausea, vomiting, and sleep disturbances, and develop more anxiety, depression, frustration, and somatic concerns, than patients with cancer who do not suffer from pain.

Cancer is a relatively rare disease in children. Yet it ranks second to trauma as a cause of death in children between 1 and 15 years old. Although the majority of children with cancer do not suffer the same chronic debilitating pain as adults with cancer, they do experience pain from the disease itself, from invasive treatments, and from psychological distress. There are no accurate estimates of the magnitude of these different pain problems for children with cancer.

In summary, the current pain classification system evaluates pain in relation to the patient experiencing it, rather than as an entity apart from the patient. As such, the system facilitates communication and understanding, and provides a general framework for evaluating the multidimensional aspects of a child's suffering; the adoption and widespread use of this system in pediatrics should improve pain control. Although each child with pain experiences a unique set of physical, psychological, social, and emotional changes, the classification system delineates the common profound factors associated with each type of pain that must be addressed if the pain is to be fully controlled.

A pain classification is not a succinct "label," synonymous with a specific pain diagnosis. Instead, it is a meaningful and useful code to describe a broad category of pains that have many common features but may differ with respect to the nature of noxious stimulus and the specific contributing factors.

Common Acute Pains during Childhood

Health professionals are becoming increasingly concerned about the management of acute pain for infants and children, since many studies have documented that undermedication is a prevalent problem in pediatrics. More attention is now being focused on previously neglected areas: pain assessment and control for neonates and infants, postoperative pain control for all children, and the management of multiple acute pains during prolonged medical treatments. There is increased recognition that children develop many coping strategies to lessen acute pain and that they can benefit from age-appropriate preparation for pain (Hillier & McGrath, 1987; McGrath & Unruh, 1987; D. M. Ross & Ross, 1985; S. A. Ross, 1984; Sehnert, 1980; Stevens, Hunsberger, & Browne, 1987; Tesler, Wegner, Savedra, Gibbons, & Ward, 1981).

As they mature, children naturally sustain a diversity of routine injuries, varying from superficial bumps, cuts, burns, and scrapes that cause minimal tissue damage to deeper wounds that cause moderate to severe tissue damage. All children also experience some brief pains from medical and dental treatments, such as immunization injections, blood-sampling, or local anesthetic infiltrations. Children who require intensive medical care after surgery or for treating a serious injury or disease will inevitably experience additional acute pains from many diagnostic procedures and therapeutic treatments. In general, then, children experience three types of acute pain: relatively brief, mild to moderate pain from common childhood diseases, routine injuries, or typical health treatments; more prolonged, moderate to strong pain caused by major disease, accidental trauma, invasive treatments, or surgery; and varying mild to strong pain from repeated invasive procedures. These acute pains represent separate categories, not simply because of their different temporal characteristics and intensities, but also because of the different situational and emotional factors unique to each context. When children experience pain associated with colds, the flu, mumps, measles, or minor injuries, they tend to perceive their pain more as an inevitable result of growing up than as something to fear. They have positive expectations that their pain can be alleviated and that it will not last long. Their parents show concern and empathy, and assist in providing pain relief, but they are not overly anxious about these acute pains. Although children's lives are temporarily disrupted by the disease or injury, the disruption is relatively brief.

By contrast, when children experience pain associated with serious injuries or major illnesses, they anticipate more prolonged pain and perhaps more intense pain. They may be uncertain about when or whether their pain will be wholly alleviated. Children are more disabled. Their daily routines are severely interrupted, so that they cannot participate fully in normal activities. They have little control over their pain, the time required to recover, and their lives in general. Depending on the nature of the injury or disease, children must rely more on their parents for physical assistance, entertainment, and medication, and may become isolated from their peers for long periods. Children and parents may become angry, frustrated, afraid, anxious, or depressed as they consider the future implications of their injuries. Physical disability, inaccurate expectations, little perceived control, and emotional distress can exacerbate their suffering.

Children who need prolonged medical or dental care will inevitably experience some pain from treatments that produce varying levels of tissue damage. Pain is usually brief, and the strength varies generally with the procedure—from mild pain for finger pricks, to moderate pain for intramuscular injections, and to severe pain for burn-dressing changes. Children typically receive anxiolytics, sedatives, or analgesics, depending on the procedure, their age, and overt distress. But children often feel that they have no control in a medical or dental situation; they may be uncertain about what to expect; they may not understand the need for a treatment that will hurt, particularly if they do not feel sick; and they may not know any simple tools to use to help them cope with their anxiety and pain. These factors can intensify children's pain, even though the pain source is constant and even though analgesics have been administered.

Pains Evoked by Brief Noxious Stimuli

Pains caused by mild tissue damage from superficial skin injuries are the acute pains children most frequently experience. In fact, cuts, scrapes, falls, pinched fingers and arms, insect bites, colds, burns, and stitches were the most frequent pains listed when 175 healthy children recorded all their pains on diaries for 1 month. Although their ratings of pain strength were roughly proportional to the presumed level of tissue damage, so that pains from a scraped knee were rated as weaker than pains from a cut knee, the same type of injury did not produce equivalent levels of pain in all children, or even in the same child at different times within the month. Even young children clearly noted distinct levels of pain and affect for similar noxious stimuli.

Differences in children's pain ratings for the same type of noxious stimulus do not reflect differences in how children used the rating scales, because children above 5 years old can reliably assess pain with visual analog scales (VASs). Instead, these differences indicate that children perceived pains differently as a result both of the particular stimulus and of the context in which they felt pain. Some children included information about how the context altered their pain by writing that "The pain didn't hurt much because I was playing," ". . . it was a friendly pinch," ". . . I was laughing," ". . . I was playing a game," and so on. Relatively brief pains caused by mild tissue damage are not frightening to children. They learn quickly that the pain dissipates when they are distracted or when their parents attend to the injury. Because they are not generally anxious, fearful, or apprehensive, their pain depends primarily on both the nature of the wound and the context in which they sustain the injury. As a result, these acute pains may be easily and effectively managed.

Routine superficial skin injuries require evaluation and appropriate medical treatment, which varies from a parental hug and kiss to cleansing, bandaging, or applying a topical anesthetic cream to the wound. Children need realistic reassurance about the pain source—that the damage is mild, the wound will heal, and the pain will gradually lessen. After children receive reassurance, minor pains often disappear immediately. Most children naturally rub painful skin areas. Adults should encourage them to massage the painful area when it will not interfere with healing. As described in Chapters 3, 5, and 6, their rubbing will activate large non-nociceptive afferents, which can reduce pain by inhibiting activity in the nociceptive nerves triggered by the tissue damage. Similarly, cold compresses should be applied to a wound to reduce inflammation and lessen pain.

In addition to physical interventions, parents often naturally try to divert children's attention away from their pain. Distraction, absorption, relaxation, and guided imagery are valuable tools for parents when their children are distressed or in pain. Their ultimate objective should be to assist the children to concentrate fully on something else besides their pain. Music, lights, colored objects, toys, and other children can be effective "attention-grabbing" stimuli for infants and toddlers. Conversation, play, games, and an exciting television show can be effective diversions for older children. The main objective is to select an interesting event or activity that can sustain children's full attention so that their pain is truly blocked. In general, the younger the child, the more concrete the diversion, and the more absorbed the child, the more effective the diversion.

Fowler-Kerry and Lander (1987) evaluated the efficacy of music distraction, with and without suggestions for pain relief, for reducing pain caused by routine diphtheria–pertussis–tetanus (DPT) immunization injections. Two hundred children (4.5–6 years old) were randomly assigned to receive music distraction, suggestion only, distraction with suggestion, or no intervention prior to their injections. Using a 4-point rating scale, children reported significantly less pain when they listened to music than in the other conditions. Although not systematically evaluated for children of all ages, many of the cognitive-behavioral interventions described in Chapter 5 can be used to minimize injection pain (Eland, 1982; Field, 1981).

Children should be taught that they, with their parents' assistance, can help to lessen the pain produced by simple injuries. They should learn a few simple physical and cognitive techniques, and parents should encourage them to use these techniques independently. Children enrolled in pain programs in our clinic generalize what they are learning in the clinic to other situations and to different pains. They are quite proud when they have created a new pain control method or revised a method to meet their own needs better. For instance, a 2½-year-old boy was excited when he decided that singing Christmas carols was more effective than singing ordinary songs. Although he sang carols during invasive medical procedures, he also began to sing when he hurt himself playing at home, and he suggested that his father try it for his own headaches.

Children with colds, the flu, mumps, measles, chicken pox, or sore throats suffer with general body aches and pains, as well as some specific sites of pain and tenderness. Pains are symptoms of the underlying illness and gradually lessen as children recover. Medications are administered to treat the illness and to provide symptomatic pain relief (for a review of guidelines on analgesic use, see American Pain Society, 1987). However, parents do not rely solely on analgesic medications. Instead, they comfort their children to help them get more rest; they massage their aches and sore spots; and they distract them with games, television, and interesting activities to alleviate their pain. Their natural approaches to reducing children's pain are identical to the physical and cognitive-behavioral approaches described in the preceding two chapters. Parents are directly modifying nociceptive input by physical stimulation and by altering relevant situational and emotional factors.

When children are scheduled for medical or dental appointments in which they will have procedures that damage tissue, they may feel pain. They do not always feel pain, even from injections; their expectations, their perceived control, their understanding of the procedure, their fear, and their parents' anxiety all influence the nociceptive activity initiated by the tissue damage. In a sense, the actual strength of their pain evoked by an invasive treatment falls within a flexible range of pain strengths, as depicted in Figure 7.1. Their actual pain is the result of a complex gating process involving ascending and descending sensory systems (see Chapter 3 for review) that modulate their pain perception. Although the range of children's pain reports for different medical procedures is generally proportional to the level of tissue damage, as shown in Figure 7.1, the pain for each procedure may be minimized or enhanced by emotional and situational factors. The pain ratings for two procedures in Figure 7.2 were made by 10 children at different times in their pain management programs. Their first ratings were made before they started the program, when they were anxious, frightened, and had inaccurate expectations and no coping strategies; subsequent ratings for the same procedures (conducted in the same manner) were made during and after completion of the program, when the children's anxiety and fears were reduced and after they had learned some pain-coping strategies.

NOXIOUS STIMULUS

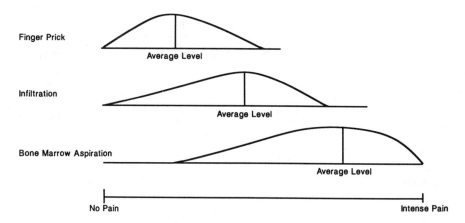

RANGE OF PAIN SENSATIONS EVOKED BY PROCEDURES

FIGURE 7.1. A model depicting the range of pain sensations produced by noxious stimulation. Three treatments causing different levels of tissue damage are shown with proportionally larger ranges of pain produced by these stimuli.

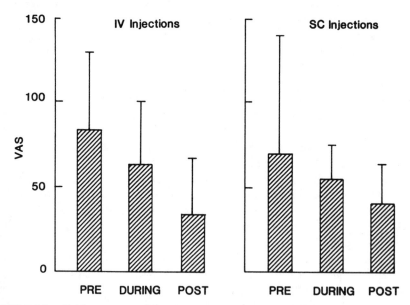

FIGURE 7.2. Children's reports of pain during intravenous (IV) and subcutaneous (SC) injections. Ten children with leukemia used VASs to rate their pain prior to, during, and after receiving individual pain programs.

Consequently, children's pain from invasive medical and dental treatments can be altered by modifying situational and emotional factors. Children should know what will happen during treatment. They should learn about the equipment to be used, the clinic room, the number of people present, and the sounds that they will hear. If they will be receiving treatments that do not require sedation or analgesics, then they should be prepared for the sensations that they will experience. If the procedure may hurt (even slightly), then children should be told, "It sometimes hurts a little, but it doesn't always hurt, I am not sure what it will feel like for you. Some children say it's a quick prick; some say it's a cool prick. I wonder what it will be like for you?"

Emphasis should be placed on what sensations children will feel—the warmth, coolness, or pressure associated with the procedure, rather than the frightening label "pain." At the same time, children should be reassured that even if it hurts, they can help to lessen the pain. They should be offered some techniques for coping, according to their ages and interests. A few suggestions that children can be offered are as follows:

1. Rub the injection site before and after the injection.
2. Squeeze someone's hand during the procedure to tell him/her how much it hurts.
3. Keep distracted.
   Talk about an interesting event.
   Count or sing during the injection.
   Do not think about the needle.
4. Use "magic sparklies" to relax and make the site numb.
5. Take deep breaths or pant to keep busy and relax.
6. Stay happy and try not to be afraid, because how you feel influences how much pain you have.

When possible, children should choose whether to see the equipment or to practice with it ahead of time. Young children should be encouraged to bring a favorite doll or stuffed animal with them, so that they can conduct the procedure on the toy. Children should actively participate as valuable assistants rather than as passive patients. These approaches will minimize children's fears (and parental anxiety), and will create a situation that should minimize the pain from the procedure.

Staff members should conduct procedures consistently, giving children some choices and allowing them time (if necessary) to recover their composure and use a coping strategy during invasive procedures. Yet staff members must set clear limits for children, so that their distress behaviors are not rewarded by postponing the procedure. Often children's overt distress behaviors are not due to anxiety about a procedure; rather, they have been shaped by the responses of the adults who have conducted or tried to conduct previous procedures. Children may develop various delaying tactics—trips to the bathroom, 5 more minutes of playtime, or a drink of water. Since the delays can increase their anxiety and reduce their ability to cope positively, parents and staff must set reasonable limits. Children require firm, consistent, and supportive approaches, with staff encouraging their active participation rather than their fearful acceptance.

Some children will require physical restraint. But even they can be allowed some choices, whether they want to lie down or sit on their mothers' laps during injections. They may cry and flail throughout the procedure, yet staff members should still respond encouragingly. After a difficult procedure (in terms of either technical care or children's distress), children should be reassured and calmed— and not simply by telling them, "It's all over; no more needles today." Such statements emphasize the aversive significance of the needles, so that children will approach their next "needles" with more apprehension. Instead, once children have been calmed they should be encouraged to describe what it felt like and why they cried, and the staff member should explain how to change the situation so it will be better in the future. This postprocedure discussion is not common for children requiring isolated medical treatments (though it is quite common for children receiving repeated treatments); however, it is extremely beneficial for all children, particularly young children whose pain attitudes are forming.

A cognitive-behavioral focus is critical to optimal pain control for all children for acute pains produced by minor trauma. However, children who have already developed excessive fear of physicians or dentists require special assistance to overcome their anxiety. They should be referred to outpatient pediatric pain clinics or to psychologists who specialize in behavioral medicine. A primary cognitive-behavioral focus is obviously restricted to children who can understand the necessary concepts, whether demonstrated in role-modeling, play therapy, or conversations and demonstrations. Yet infants, toddlers, and handicapped children should receive many of the same pain management approaches, but in a manner appropriate to their cognitive level.

Infants can be distracted during invasive procedures with colored mobiles, toys, and vivid sensory stimulation. For injections and blood-samplings, their skin can be rubbed deeply prior to treatment and the contralateral body site rubbed during treatment. Topical anesthetic creams can also be used. The primary interventions are physical, but cognitive methods of distraction and concentration should also be used. Similar approaches should be used with toddlers. They should see the equipment before the procedure, and perhaps observe a sham procedure conducted on a parent or toy. Parents can demonstrate by counting aloud to show children when (at what number) the procedure will start, and then demonstrate how to respond. Parents may say "ouch" throughout the sham procedure, hold children's hands, or express interest about what is happening to stimulate the children's curiosity. The objective of parental modeling is to prepare children without frightening them. Although much research has been conducted in behavioral medicine and dentistry on the efficacy of role-modeling to reduce anxiety and fear, there have been no specific studies examining which type of modeling (peers, puppets, or parents) is most effective for reducing pain. In our clinic, we use all three types of models for children, depending on their ages and interests. Some children prefer to see procedures conducted on other children (particularly of the same sex and age), whereas other children prefer to look only at photographs. We have several scrapbooks (one for each invasive procedure) with pictures of children during each part of a treatment, so that children can be prepared accurately for what will happen.

Mentally handicapped children require special attention to prepare them for invasive treatments. Often it is not possible to communicate to them what will happen, why it is happening, or how they can cope. They become excessively frightened, so that any pain produced is probably maximal. Although these children may require sedation for lengthy diagnostic procedures, they should still be introduced to the clinic environment, and perhaps should observe other children receiving treatments. No research has yet been conducted to identify the most effective approaches for reducing pain for handicapped children (or adults). Yet how often are these children treated inadvertently in a manner that exacerbates their fear, anxiety, and pain? Even a simple immunization may be a terrifying experience for them. More effort must be extended into designing programs for alleviating acute pain in handicapped children. In the interim, appropriate physical, cognitive, and behavioral interventions should be applied consistently to reduce their distress, improve the predictability of pain, and increase their coping ability.

Pains Evoked by Major Trauma

Although pains evoked by major trauma are classified as acute pains, since the noxious stimulus is known and the pain should diminish progressively as the injury heals, their unique sensory, situational, emotional, and behavioral features distinguish them from other acute pains. Pains evoked by serious injuries are stronger and more prolonged than acute pains evoked by minor trauma. Children require medical treatments that may also produce pain. Children's or parents' anxiety, fear, sadness, anger, frustration, or guilt about an injury can exacerbate pain. Children and their families may be uncertain about when the injury will heal, about possible disfigurement or loss of function, and about how to cope with the added emotional stress resulting from hospitalization and separation. As a consequence, the potential aversive impact of these situational and emotional factors must be modified to manage children's pains effectively.

Lacerations and fractures are common sources of acute pain for children admitted to emergency departments. Pain management is critical for simple wounds and breaks, to reduce both pain from the injury and pain from treatments (e.g., sutures, casts). Children hospitalized for more serious and complicated injuries require extensive care and many invasive treatments, with pain management a special concern throughout a prolonged period because of the different pain sources (injury, treatments) and fluctuating pain intensities (as the injury heals, from emotional distress, from postural restrictions, or from temporal variations in analgesic efficacy). Similarly, surgical pain requires consistent management of variable levels of pain for a more prolonged duration. The principles for controlling acute pain are the same, regardless of the severity of the injury. Yet the nature of the injury, the particular medical treatments required, and the anticipated strength and duration of pain shape the choice of interventions for children. The most common childhood acute pains caused by moderate trauma are lacerations and fractures, burns, and surgical pain.

Lacerations and Fractures

Injuries to the extremities are the most common complaints for children visiting emergency rooms. Rivara, Parish, and Mueller (1986) reviewed the medical records of 189 children aged 1–15, who were seen with a total of 209 extremity injuries. The most common causes of injuries were sports (29%), falls (21%), pedestrian–motor vehicle collisions (11%), and bicycle-related incidents (9%). Children sustain a number of injuries and lacerations that require sutures; local anesthetics should be administered to alleviate their pain during suturing. Similarly, fractures are common painful injuries that require anesthetics. Children are usually very distressed on admission to an emergency department, particularly if they have seen a gaping wound or a distended bone, have bled profusely, or are frightened by the reactions of their parents and other adults who have seen the injury. They require calm emotional support and reassurance about the physical injury. They should be prepared for anesthetic administration and encouraged to use one of the coping strategies described in the preceding section. Beales (1979b) observed 100 children, 43 girls and 57 boys from 3 months to 16 years of age, during treatment in the emergency department of a large children's hospital. When children's attention was primarily focused on their injuries, either because of lack of effective distractions or because of the comments of medical staff about the extent of the injury, they often complained about pain during treatment, even though anesthetics had been administered and they had not felt the first few sutures.

Although Beales's observations suggest that all children should not look at their wounds during suturing, our own clinical experience indicates that some children prefer to watch the physician intently and observe the procedure. Frequently children are advised by emergency room staff or parents to look elsewhere, with an implicit message that what is happening is too horrible to view. Yet children do not necessarily share these pain attitudes and biases. Instead, children may be intrigued by the fact that a quick needle seems to embody them with superhuman powers, so that their skin does not feel touch or pain. They may choose to watch simple sutures even if they need to use a mirror to see the body region. The emphasis shifts in these cases from trying to focus the children's attention away from an aversive and potentially painful procedure (when they will be continuously monitoring "Is it over yet?" on some level) to allowing them to see how wounds are healed.

In fact, a child may be asked to rate a suturing or bone-setting procedure as to how even the stitches are, how fast suturing is completed, how few/many stitches are counted, how many times the material is wound to form the cast, or how quickly the cast hardens. Some children are not able to have all of the attention of attending adults (pain therapist, nurse, physician, parent) focused on their ability to use a pain-coping strategy. They feel too much pressure to succeed, which makes them more anxious and frightened. So, with the cooperation of medical and nursing staff, children's attention can be focused away from conscious attempts to use a particular strategy and subsequent self-monitoring as to how well or poorly they are using it. Instead, the staff members facilitate children's unconscious use of distraction–concentration by asking them to attend to some concrete aspect of the procedure—an aspect that diverts their focus (and parents' focus) to a less aversive component and to someone else's proficiency. Naturally, the staff chooses an aspect that does not focus attention on the physician's competency, on a technically difficult aspect, or on a potentially frightening aspect (e.g., how hard the physician pushes the needle to get it through the skin). Children can receive rewards for coaching, counting, or learning how to sew so that they can repair their dolls or animals after their suturing or bone-setting; thus, the emphasis is more on the positive features of healing than on the aversive features of treatment.

Beales's (1979b) clinical observations are very important, but children's pain complaints probably reflect many factors other than effective distractions in the emergency department. Children who looked at their wounds in Beales's study may have been more frightened by the sight of the injury and the needle piercing their skin. But what might have happened if children had been prepared for the procedure with concrete information and taught simple coping strategies? It is the children themselves who have taught the staff in our pain clinic that they prefer having a choice about observing and participating (when possible) in their medical treatment. At present, we feel that children should be asked whether they want to watch and not routinely instructed "Don't look," unless their injuries clearly would frighten them. Unfortunately, there are no consistent guidelines as to what constitutes a frightening injury. Deep wounds and profuse bleeding frighten parents and children initially; after the emergency staff begins to work with children, however, their fears should subside, so that they are more able to decide for themselves how to respond during suturing or bone-setting. Generally children above the age of 5 can choose whether they want to watch the treatment—in the case of suturing, both the infiltration and the subsequent sutures. Very young children's attention should be distracted away from their injury because they will not understand reassurance from staff, but will only react to the blood and wound.

The management of pain evoked by infiltrations, sutures, and fractures has not been well studied. However, the few published reports indicate the benefits of a cognitive-behavioral approach. Alcock, Feldman, Goodman, McGrath, and Park

(1985) evaluated the efficacy of a child life intervention, consisting of emotional support, procedural information, and specific coping strategies, for reducing children's distress during suturing in the emergency room. After this intervention, children displayed less anxiety during procedures. Andolsek and Novik (1980) used hypnotic techniques to alleviate pain in four children (3–4 years old) who were receiving emergency treatment for injuries and lacerations. Children improved their control during procedures and used visual imagery to alter the aversive component. For example, a child popped a balloon and then imagined that the physician was popping a balloon on her hand when he drained an abscess. She was able to reduce her pain when she visualized the balloon. The concrete image diverted her focus from the fact that the needle was piercing her skin, and allowed her to become less afraid and anxious and to feel less pain.

Johnson, Kirchoff, and Endress (1975) examined whether children who heard a preparatory message that detailed the physical sensations produced by orthopedic cast removal displayed less distress than children who did not receive the information. A total of 84 children (6–11 years old) were randomly allocated into one of three information groups: (1) sensory information, in which they learned about the specific sensations they would feel during cast removal; (2) procedure information, in which they learned about the technical aspects of cast removal; and (3) control, in which they did not receive any sensory or procedural information. Investigators then observed children's overt distress during cast removal and recorded their pulse rates at four intervals throughout the procedure.

Children who knew about the sensory aspects of the procedure—the vibrations, tingling and warmth that they would feel; the noise of the saw that they would hear; and the scaly, dirty-looking appearance of their skin—had significantly less distress than other children. Mean pulse rates were significantly higher for children in the control and procedure groups during cast removal, but not for children in the sensory group. The children who admitted that having a cast removed was frightening had higher behavioral distress scores and were more frightened during the actual cast removal than children who were not frightened prior to the procedure.

This research supports clinical observations that children should be prepared for what will happen to them so that they are not unduly frightened. Staff members should assist children by using distraction techniques and by encouraging them to use simple coping strategies. More research should be conducted to establish strict guidelines for which types of preparation (puppets, live or filmed modeling, practice with equipment) and which interventions (distraction, active participation, hypnosis) are best for which children (age, sex, injury, anxiety level, parents' anxiety level). At present, we should continue to apply the principles of acute pain management consistently, by modifying the situational factors that can intensify children's pain. Perhaps the simplest approach is to ask children whether they would like to watch the suturing or whether they prefer to look at something else, without relying on their parents to decide for them. Information about the procedure and how the children can cope should be relayed by staff in a reassuring, matter-of-fact tone. Children respond to a confident approach, particularly when staff members do not seem overly concerned about the sight of their injuries (as parents often do), but emphasize the mending aspect rather than the damage aspect. Attention is immediately focused on how the injury is healed, just as when their dolls or superheroes are hurt. Simple choices and suggestions (e.g., "Which chair would you like to sit in? Do you want the puppet to have the same thing? What method do you want to use during the injection? Isn't it amazing how your skin now has superhuman powers, so that you can't feel the needle? Wait until you tell your friends about it") can effectively alter the significance of the situation for a child, so that he/she is less anxious, less worried, and more focused on positive aspects—all of which will reduce pain.

Many cognitive attention and/or distraction interventions are beneficial for children receiving emergency treatment for injuries requiring sutures. Children can be asked to describe details of the physical environment, perform mental arithmetic, imagine pleasant physical scenes incompatible with pain, or use hypnosis to reduce sensitivity in specific body regions. The younger and more frightened the child, the more concrete and practical the strategies for distraction. The person responsible for alleviating children's distress must also help parents to recognize that children will feel better when they know what will be happening to them and are reassured that they will receive medication to reduce their pain. Parents can inadvertently increase their children's anxiety when they are anxious, particularly if they regard the procedure as aversive and painful.

A cognitive-behavioral approach complements the pharmacological methods used to control pain during suturing and bone-setting. Although children who need only one stitch or who do not experience pain from a simple fracture may not need anesthetics, most children will require a local infiltration or narcotic administration, depending on the severity of their injury. Fracture pain, arising from the periosteum and the surrounding damaged soft tissues, can be severe and may require narcotic analgesia. Pain may be aggravated by movement or by reflex muscle spasm. Once a fracture is stabilized, pain is rapidly reduced. Until then, pain can be managed effectively with a local infiltration, nerve block, or narcotic analgesic (Berry, 1977; Tondare & Nadkarni, 1982). Intravenous regional anesthesia, 0.5% lignocaine (10–30 ml), was used routinely to treat 50 children with forearm fractures, supracondylar fractures, and elbow dislocations (Fitzgerald, 1976). The mean time from injection to adequate anesthesia varied from 1.5 to 8 minutes (mean, 3.5 minutes); the time for full recovery from anesthesia varied from 2 to 5 minutes (mean, 4 minutes). The investigator had assumed that children would not cooperate with the injections. However, there were no difficulties in administering anesthetics when time was taken to explain the procedure and when a parent was present.

Burns

Most children experience some slight burns from touching hot objects, eating hot foods, or staying in the sun too long. Their pain is usually relieved by applying cold compresses or topical anesthetics, because tissue damage is often superficial. Severe burns, however, cause major tissue damage and can produce intense pain for prolonged periods as the skin and underlying tissue heal. Children's pain depends on the extent and depth of their burns. Generally, first-degree burns are painful; second-degree burns are very painful; and third-degree burns are initially not painful or only slightly painful because sensory nerve endings have been destroyed. Third-degree burns may not begin to hurt until separation of the eschar and debridement begin. The longer it takes to remove the dead skin and gain initial skin coverage, the more difficult the pain (for reviews, see Khan, 1983; Nover, 1973; Perry, Cella, Falkenberg, Heidrich, & Goodwin, 1987; Wagner, 1984; Yurt & Pruitt, 1983).

Pain management for children who sustain serious burns with extensive damage over much of their bodies constitutes a special challenge. Their burn pain is exacerbated during the multiple treatments necessary to cleanse the tissue, prevent infections, and promote the growth of healthy tissue. Thus, children who have suffered severe burns may experience repeated episodes of intense, acute pain, superimposed on a background of constant pain as they endure the lengthy hospitalization, isolation in bacteria-controlled tents, and regular treatments required for healing. Like most types of pain that children experience, pain from pediatric burns has not been managed consistently. In 1982, Perry and Heidrich surveyed U.S. burn units and reported that a much higher proportion of children than of adults received no narcotics or analgesics for the debridement of burns, even when their pains were judged as comparable. Schechter (1985) reported similar findings for a large teaching hospital: The children hospitalized for treatment of moderate burns ($<$ 20% of surface area) received an average of 1.3 doses of narcotics per day, whereas adults with similar burns received 3.6 doses.

The burn-dressing change (BDC) is one of the most painful procedures for children. The BDC begins with the unwrapping of the many layers of gauze bandage that protect the injury. The innermost layers often adhere to the wound surface, so that their removal is difficult and exceedingly painful. Exposure to the air, debridement of the burned areas, and any necessary manipulations of the region may further intensify the pain. Even rebandaging may cause additional pain. Although children should receive an analgesic beforehand, the BDC is still usually an anxiety- and pain-producing ordeal that children must endure regularly. In an elegant study, Szyfelbein, Osgood, and Carr (1985) assessed 15 children's pain during BDCs. They correlated children's self-report pain ratings with a physiological index, plasma beta-endorphin immunoreactivity. Children used a thermometer-like 0–10 rating scale (shown earlier in Figure 2.3). They reported slight pain at the removal of the outermost layer of gauze (1.5), strong pain at the detachment of the innermost layer of gauze (8.6), moderate pain when silver nitrate was poured on the wound or bandage (4.10), and moderate pain when salve was applied to the skin (3.2). Their pain scores also reflected differences in sensitivitiy when they were sleepy (1.1), eating or drinking (1.4), shouting because of pain (8.3), or screaming in pain (10.0). Children's mean pain scores varied inversely with their plasma beta-endorphin levels (as described in Chapter 2).

Children require potent analgesic medication during painful treatment procedures, as well as analgesics to control any relatively constant pain from the burn. Since the strength of their pain is not simply and directly related to the nature or extent of their burn, but is also related to many salient emotional and situational factors, children's pain control must include nonpharmacological interventions to decrease any fear, anxiety, and depression and to increase their control and ability to cope. Psychological problems may arise as a consequence of the burn, the associated pain, and the difficult situation children endure as they are separated from family, friends, and daily activities during their prolonged medical care. Depending on children's ages and understanding of their injuries, they may become anxious about future disfigurement and continued impairments. They require reassurance, emotional support, and counseling to help them cope with both physical pain and emotional suffering.

Kavanagh (1983a, 1983b, 1983c) developed a method for assisting children to cope with BDCs—a method that modifies many of the situational and emotional factors typically present for children with burns. Her approach is based on the "learned helplessness" model, which describes the negative effects of uncontrollable and unpredictable aversive events on individuals. Cognitive, affective, and somatic disturbances result from exposure to unpredictable and uncontrollable aversive events, particularly aversive events that are intense, frequent, or prolonged. Children hospitalized for burns can develop this stress-induced condition and exhibit a variety of symptoms, including agitation, anxiety, lethargy, depression, eating disturbances, and learning impairments.

Kavanagh reasoned that a young child whose painful dressing changes were predictable and included age-appropriate patient control would adapt more positively to the stress associated with the burn and its treatment than a child whose treatment was less predictable and controlled wholly by staff. The emphasis switched from children's adopting passive patient roles to children's assuming active responsibilities in assisting with necessary procedures. Children helped to change their own dressings and sometimes assisted in the actual debridement. To improve predictability, nurses debrided burns only when they were wearing red aprons and only at predictable times. When the nurses were not in red, children were assured that these painful procedures would not take place, and they could relate to the nurses in a more natural and less apprehensive manner. Although Kavanagh did not use any objective measures to assess the efficacy of her experimental approach, all children showed less distress behavior, anxiety, and pain when predictability and children's control were increased during the dressing change. In addition, medication requirements also decreased.

Other programs for alleviating acute pain in burned children consist of multistrategy interventions to improve predictability, reduce anxiety, decrease distress behaviors, and increase control. Burned children have used visual imagery, relaxation, systematic desensitization, active participation, hypnosis, and distraction to cope with the pain from treatments (Galdston, 1972; Ravenscroft, 1982; Savedra, 1976; Stoddard, 1982; Weinstein, 1976). Wakeman and Kaplan (1978) used progressive muscle relaxation, guided imagery, dissociation, and specific suggestions for analgesia as adjunctive analgesics during the routine care of burns for children and adults. Children and adolescents were able to use hypnosis significantly better than the adults, as demonstrated by a reduction in their medication requests. Turk (1978) recommended attention concentration, relaxation, deep breathing, and visual imagery. He provided detailed analogies to teach children to imagine that they were in a different environment (one incompatible with pain); that they were unable to feel pain (because their burned parts had an abnormal insensitivity or superhuman powers); and that the intense stimulation from treatment was caused by a more positive and exciting stimulus (an injury sustained when they were heroes helping someone in an accident). Burned children should adopt a flexible repertoire of these difficult coping strategies to use during their treatments.

Elliott and Olson (1983) evaluated the efficacy of a stress management package for four boys (5–12 years old) with second- and third-degree burns. Children spent approximately 45 minutes with a therapist to learn four stress reduction strategies: attention distraction (focusing on the environment, mental arithmetic); relaxation (deep breathing); emotive imagery and/or reinterpretation of the context of the pain (interpretation of pain as caused within a heroic or relaxing context); and reinforcement for using these strategies during procedures. Children's behavioral distress during subsequent burn treatments was assessed by trained raters using a Burn Treatment Distress Scale, a behavioral pain scale adapted from the Procedural Behavior Rating Scale (described in Chapter 2). Although children were not asked how much pain they felt, their overt distress behaviors were reduced by the program. In addition, children showed less distress during procedures in which the therapist was present to coach them than when the therapist was not present.

Shorkey and Taylor (1973) applied behavioral modification techniques to the management of a 17-month-old girl suffering from second- and third-degree burns on 37% of her body, involving both legs, the perineum, the buttocks, and both hands and wrists. After 4 weeks of treatment, she became extremely distressed by any approach from the nursing staff, even comforting behaviors at nontreatment times. The investigators taught her to discriminate between technical nursing and nonmedical supportive care so that she would be distressed only during treatment times and could receive comfort, nourishment, and adequate rest at other times. The ward environment was changed so that the child received treatments from nurses dressed in green isolation gowns with the white room lights turned on. Staff members dressed in red, sterilized bags with armholes when they entered the room to provide emotional support or play with the child; red floodlights were turned on at these times. Nurses massaged the infant's neck and top of her shoulders (which had not been burned) to reduce muscle tension and promote relaxation. The child was fed after the massage. The increased predictability for treatments, coupled with specific supportive periods, reduced the child's overall stress. On the second day of the program, she cried less during the nontreatment period and began to watch quietly as staff members entered the room. She smiled for the first time in the hospital 2 days later. Her behaviors during treatment remained unchanged, but at least she was able to benefit from some positive emotional support at nontreatment times.

Several narcotic analgesics, sedatives, and anesthetics, and various nonpharmacological methods (including hypnosis, relaxation, distraction, and guided imagery), have been used to relieve children's burn pain and BDC pain. All these methods can be effective for managing children's burn pain, but few specific guidelines exist for selecting which methods to apply for different children or at different times. Clinical studies must be conducted to critically evaluate the efficacy of the available interventions and then to develop more stringent criteria for their application according to burn severity and location, as well as according to children's ages, attitudes, and pain-coping abilities. In the interim, both the general principles of analgesic administration and the modification of relevant situational and emotional factors should be consistently applied to all children. Children should receive appropriate types and doses of analgesic medication to control their pain. Analgesics should be administered prior to painful procedures, to ensure that maximal pain relief coincides with presumed peak pain during the treatment. When narcotics are chosen, they should be administered intravenously, since intramuscular injections may not be uniformly absorbed in the immediate postburn period.

The primary interventions for burn pain include appropriate analgesic medication during anticipated peak pain periods and adequate psychological preparation to modify situational, emotional, and familial factors that exacerbate the steady burn pain and the episodes of acute treatment-induced pain. Procedures should be scheduled and performed as consistently as possible, to provide children with accurate expectations about the technical aspects and to increase the predictability of all potentially aversive situations. Schedules of procedures can be drawn by children (when they are physically capable of doing so), or drawn by parents, siblings, or child life staff to the color, size, and shape specifications of the children, to help them to follow their "healing" programs actively. The emphasis should be on the positive aspects of healing and how much the children's skin is responding, rather than on the negative aspects. Treatment should be as routine as possible; children should learn at an age-appropriate level the names for equipment and the purpose of each part of treatment, and should be encouraged to assist as much as physically possible. A favorite doll or stuffed animal should be used to help teach children what is happening, why it is necessary, and how beneficial treatments will be.

Children should be taught that there are simple tools to use for reducing their pain and that they can use them in all situations. Children should learn a small repertoire of age-appropriate nonpharmacological interventions that they can use consistently with all nursing and medical personnel. Concrete goals should be established to reward children for participating in procedures or for using visual imagery, distraction, relaxation, or hypnosis. Young children can be rewarded in simple operant behavior programs by earning daily stickers; older children can earn points toward the acquisition of a special excursion or gift. The objectives of the program are to encourage children to improve control and reduce anxiety, fear, and distress, which will lower their pain. In addition, children and families should receive regular supportive counseling from nursing and social work, with referral to psychology or psychiatry as needed.

Many burn clinics consist of a multidisciplinary health team—a psychologist, a social worker, a child life worker, and a physical therapist, in addition to medical and nursing staff. Although each member of the team has a special role in helping the child or family to cope with the stress of hospitalization, the pain of the injury and treatment, and the future consequences of the burn, all members should assist children in pain management in three critical areas. First, a concrete pain control program should be developed for each child, based on a thorough assessment of the burn injury, familial factors, and the child's age, emotional state, expectations, and coping abilities. Second, the program should be followed as consistently as possible, regardless of personnel changes or unexpected physical complications, with both the child and the family receiving appropriate psychosocial support. Third, the efficacy of the program should be evaluated objectively. Program evaluation does not require that a burn unit adopt a major research focus; rather, it requires a commitment to ensuring the best possible service for each child in the unit and all future admissions. A major reason why children are still undermedicated has been the lack of documentation that they do feel pain and that their pain can often be relieved in a relatively simple and straightforward manner. Thus, it is essential to record objectively and quantitatively the pain-reducing success (or failure) of any therapeutic intervention, so that information based on fact, rather than on assumption, hearsay, or myths, can be communicated among all health professionals to benefit all children.

Surgical Pain

Many surgical procedures are performed on neonates, infants, and children. Although the amount of pain and distress varies according to the particular operation, infants and children require analgesics during surgery and postoperatively. Yet recent publications indicate that infants do not always receive adequate pain control during surgery and that children do not always receive adequate pain control after surgery (Anand, Sippell, & Aynsley-Green, 1987a, 1987b; Beyer, DeGood, Ashley, & Russell, 1983; Eland & Anderson, 1977; Mather & Mackie, 1983; Schechter, Allen, & Hanson, 1986). Despite the fact that most health care professionals believe infants feel pain at birth, analgesic prescription and administration within hospitals seem guided more by a general collective reluctance to admit that

children, particularly neonates and infants, experience pain from the same operations that cause pain for adults and therefore require similar analgesics. The
current procedures for providing pain control to infants may be based more on
what was believed true in the past than on what is true today, with respect to our
present understanding of pharmacokinetics and improved medical care for at-risk
infants.

Concerns, doubts and anxieties about adequately controlling pain in infants
and neonates are evident in many hospitals throughout the world. It is quite
interesting to discuss the analgesic needs of infants and children with members of
the medical and nursing staffs within a hospital. Their attitudes about the lack of
pain relief during common surgical procedures (e.g., circumcision) typically range
from "They don't feel the pain because they are distracted by the physical
restraints to immobilize them" to "I refuse to participate in the procedure unless
analgesics can be used." Lumbar punctures (LPs) may be routinely performed on
neonates without local anesthetics because "it's easier for the infants to just
perform the LP than to infiltrate the site first with a local." Other invasive
procedures (e.g., cannulations) may be performed with or without anesthetics
according to the attitudes of the medical staff, rather than according to need based
on the amount of tissue damage that will be caused.

The routine use of anesthesia or analgesia in neonates has been limited by the
real concern that most infants who require surgery are critically ill and may be
harmed by cardiovascular or respiratory depression from the anesthetics. Yet, in
spite of advances in anesthesiology so that neonates may be safely anesthetized
during surgery and their postsurgical pain controlled, students in some hospitals
continue to learn that infants should not be anesthetized, or that children do not
need the same potent analgesics after surgery as adults. Medical practices that
seemed appropriate in the past are perpetuated, even though available research
indicates that they are outdated. There has been more uniformity in educating
students about the technical aspects for surgical procedures in pediatrics than in
educating them about pain control.

Circumcisions have been performed on healthy newborn males for centuries.
Several behavioral and physiological indices of distress are apparent when infants
are circumcised without analgesia. They cry loudly and try to pull away from their
physical restraints; their blood pressure, heart rates, and cortisol levels become
significantly elevated; and their transcutaneous oxygen pressure levels decrease.
Anyone who watches a circumcision perceives that the infant feels pain. All
available research indicates that infants feel pain. Yet circumcisions continue to be
performed without adequate analgesia; instead, infants are immobilized by having
their arms and legs strapped to a standard restraint board. Medical students are
often taught that it is easier for infants when the procedure is performed quickly
without a local infiltration. They learn that the pain of the infiltration is worse
than the pain of the circumcision, despite the absence of unequivocal supporting
evidence. Until research conclusively demonstrates that the distress evoked by
circumcision without anesthesia is less than that evoked when infants are anesthet-

ized, we should not assume that it is easier or less painful for infants when they do not receive anesthetics.

Adequate pain control is essential during surgery and in the postoperative period for all infants and children, not only to prevent any needless suffering or distress, but also to promote their physical recovery after surgery. Pain causes more physiological stress, which impedes their optimal recovery (Anand, Brown, Causon, et al., 1985; Anand et al., 1987a, 1987b; Williamson & Williamson, 1983). Surgical trauma initiates a major endocrine and metabolic stress response in neonates, as evidenced by catecholamine release and by the inhibition of insulin secretion (Anand, Brown, Bloom, & Aynsley-Green, 1985). The thoracotomy for ligation of a patent ductus arteriosus (PDA) is one of the most commonly performed surgical procedures in the preterm neonate. Anesthesia has often been provided by nitrous oxide, oxygen, and *d*-tubocurarine, which does not prevent a major stress response for infants (Anand & Aynsley-Green, 1985). Anand et al. (1987a) evaluated hormonal responses in preterm infants after PDA surgery. Infants were randomly allocated into two groups: a usual-treatment group, who received nitrous oxide and curare; or an experimental group, who received the usual treatment plus an intravenous narcotic, fentanyl. The primary hormonal stress responses to surgery were significantly greater for the infants who did not receive fentanyl. In addition, these infants were more likely to develop postoperative circulatory and metabolic complications and to have a clinically unstable course. The investigators postulated that fentanyl's prevention of the usual massive stress response during surgery improved infants' clinical outcome after surgery.

Ethical concerns and increasing publicity about the lack of analgesia for infants during surgical procedures (Fletcher, 1987; Richards, 1985; Yaster, 1987) have led to a dramatic upsurge in clinical research to document objectively how infants respond to surgery and how anesthesia affects their postsurgical outcome (Bryan-Brown, 1986; Friesen & Henry, 1986). Robinson and Gregory (1981) administered high-dose fentanyl with pancuronium to 10 premature infants during PDA surgery. There was no evidence of hypotension or tight-chest syndrome, and respiratory depression after surgery was easily managed. Collins et al. (1985) investigated the pharmacokinetics and hemodynamic effects of a fentanyl bolus (30 μg/kg) for induction of anesthesia for PDA surgery in nine preterm infants. Their observations indicated that a higher dose (50 μg/kg) or continuous infusion of fentanyl may be necessary to reduce stress.

Unfortunately, anesthetic practice has often been based on recommendations that as light an anesthetic as possible should be administered to neonates (Bennett, Ignacio, Patel, Grundy, & Salem, 1976; Bush & Stead, 1962; Downes & Raphaely, 1973; Neuman & Hansen, 1980). In fact, in some centers, major surgery has been performed on premature neonates under the influence of muscle relaxants alone. Parents assume that their infants are adequately anesthetized so that they do not feel pain; instead, infants may be paralyzed so that they cannot react to pain. The metabolic response to surgery for preterm neonates is very different from that for full-term neonates, and there are specific differences in stress responses among neonates anesthetized by different techniques (Anand, Brown, Bloom, & Aynsley-Green, 1985; Anand, Brown, Causon, et al., 1985). Continued research is needed to describe the stress responses related to different surgical, anesthetic, and analgesic techniques in neonates and infants, and to identify the most effective interventions for minimizing their distress and presumably their pain.

Significant attention is now being focused on the alleviation of children's postsurgical pain, with the recognition that children should receive narcotic analgesics for noxious surgical procedures. The pharmacological guidelines established for the management of acute pain in adults have been extended to children, as evidenced in the recent *Principles of Analgesic Use in the Treatment of Acute Pain and Chronic Cancer Pain: A Concise Guide to Medical Practice* (American Pain Society, 1987). Starting doses of narcotic analgesics for postoperative pain are selected after consideration of a child's age, weight, and prior narcotic experience. Then doses are titrated to obtain analgesia with minimal side effects. Children develop tolerance during prolonged narcotic treatment and may require larger doses to relieve their pain adequately.

There is insufficient information available as to how well children's postoperative pain is controlled. Published surveys on the disparity in the prescription and administration of analgesics between adults and children, as well as discussions with clinical investigators, suggest that pain in the immediate postoperative period is adequately controlled. However, problems may develop when children are transferred to hospital wards from recovery rooms and intensive care units. The relative lack of continuous, immediate supervision for each child by physicians, nurses, and physiological monitors on the wards, in comparison to the intensive, specialized care environment immediately after surgery, probably contributes to a switch from potent narcotic analgesics to less potent non-narcotic analgesics. In addition, drugs that may have been administered through continuous infusion after surgery, are later administered orally or through subcutaneous injections. Thus, pain problems may develop for children because of inappropriate analgesic selection, administration route, and dosing interval. Although drug selection has been based explicitly on children's needs for pain medication, it is also based implicitly on assumptions about children's needs for postoperative pain medication. Assumptions as to the comparative efficacy of non-narcotics versus narcotics, intravenous versus intramuscular versus oral administration, and continuous infusion versus single doses must be objectively verified for children from a developmental perspective according to the type of surgery.

Much research has already been conducted on how to minimize the stress and anxiety children experience when they are admitted to the hospital for surgery. The efficacy of different hospital and surgical preparation programs has been evaluated by physiological, behavioral, and self-report ratings (for review, see Auerbach, 1979; Melamed, 1980; Melamed, Robbins, & Graves, 1982; McCue, 1980). Most of the preparation procedures provide information about what will happen to children during hospitalization, with emphasis on the periods prior to, during, and after surgery. The mode of preparation (e.g., modeling, verbal instructions, desensitization) and interventions differ according to children's ages, cognitive levels, and the type of surgery they require, as well as their general anxiety levels, source of anxiety (separation, fear of pain, lack of concrete understanding, parental anxiety), coping abilities, and parents. A child's preparation should be based on the same general principles of pain modification described in Chapter 6, but applied in an individual manner to meet his/her specific needs.

Phantom Limb Pain

The term "phantom limb" was first used by Mitchell (1871/1965) when he described Civil War veterans at the "Stump Hospital" in Philadelphia. The veterans suffered from painful sensations in amputated body parts; these sensations were so vivid that patients felt as if the limbs were still present. Phantom limb pain may begin immediately after amputation or develop many months or years after surgery. Vivid sensations probably develop in the absent limb after most amputations in adults and children, but not all sensations became painful. As noted in Chapter 1, children do experience phantom limb pain, but there is little information about the prevalence and nature of their pains. In fact, whereas phantom limb pain is often regarded as a chronic pain problem for adults (and is discussed again briefly with other types of childhood chronic pain in Chapter 9), it might best be regarded as an acute postsurgical pain problem for children. Children do not generally develop the chronic, intractable phantom limb pain that afflicts a proportion of adults with amputations. However, there have been no comparative studies on the incidence, severity, and chronicity of phantom limb sensations or pains for adults and children with similar amputations.

Most children with amputations experience some vivid phantom sensations, described variously as tingling, itching, pricking, or fluttering. Simmel (1962) interviewed children, and adults who had had one or more limbs amputated as children, to evaluate the incidence of phantom limb pain in childhood. Phantom pains were not generally experienced by children who lost limbs before the age of 4, but one child (4.3 years old) had had phantom foot sensations since a below-knee amputation when she was 6 months of age. The incidence of phantoms increased with children's age at amputation, so that all children above 8 years old reported phantom sensations. Some children reported pain; others described just "normal" sensations similar to those from other limbs. Since children will probably experience some phantom sensations after amputation, it is important to prepare them for what they may feel and to help them cope with these sensations. Because little information is available about phantom limb pain from the child's own perspective, it is useful to encourage a child to assist staff members in learning more about the phenomenon. The child becomes active in the postsurgical treatment plan, so that any fears due to unexpected limb sensations are prevented. The benefits to staff are enormous.

As an illustration, a 15-year-old girl was referred to our pain clinic 2 days before an operation to remove her right leg above the knee. She had heard about phantom limb pain and was quite frightened about her amputation. We reviewed some basic information about phantom limb pain, including the possible responsible mechanisms and the methods for relieving pain. We emphasized that she would experience some pain after surgery and some phantom sensations, but that phantom pain does not invariably develop. If it did, she would receive adequate analgesic medications. She learned relaxation exercises to assist her to progressively decrease physical tension if she did experience discomfort. Like all other children and adolescents referred to the clinic, she learned about descending pain-inhibitory systems and the internal factors that may activate them. We described the qualities of phantom sensations reported by adults, and asked her to monitor her own experiences so that we could better assist other children by providing them with information from her perspective. We honestly explained that we could not provide accurate estimates of the intensity, quality, or duration of possible phantoms, and encouraged her to describe these dimensions from her own experience as part of her pain control program.

She completed a brief sensation log each day, beginning with the first day after her amputation. The log consisted of a body outline and five questions: (1) Shade the area on the outline where the sensation occurs. (2) What does it feel like? (3) Does this sensation change throughout the day? When? (4) How long does it last? and (5) Is there anything you wish you had known before about these sensations? (This log has been shown previously in Chapter 1; see Figure 1.3.) In addition, she used a VAS to rate the intensity of the sensations.

During the month after surgery, phantom sensations spread gradually from her toes to encompass the whole absent leg, as shown in Figure 7.3. Both the

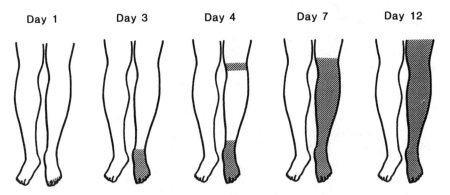

FIGURE 7.3. The template used by a 15-year-old girl to describe how her phantom sensations changed after surgery. She completed the body outline shown for 28 days after surgery. The day postsurgery is shown above each outline.

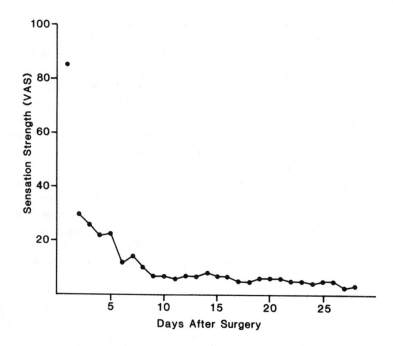

FIGURE 7.4. The intensity of the same 15-year-old girl's phantom sensations (rated on a VAS) is plotted for 28 days after surgery. With the exception of the first day (shown by the high circle on the left)—representing the rating for her postsurgical pain, rather than for phantom limb pain—her sensations were not painful.

intensity and duration of these sensations gradually diminished. The strength of her sensations is plotted as a function of time since surgery in Figure 7.4. As indicated by the first large circle on the graph, she only experienced pain described as "sharp and throbbing" during the first day after surgery. Her phantom sensations were not consistently present throughout the day, but appeared and disappeared at progressively shorter intervals. She felt itching and tingling sensations in her toes for approximately 15 minutes at different times throughout the first day after amputation, whereas she felt a tingling in her leg below the knee for only a few minutes once in a while throughout day 6. On day 7, her sensations moved closer to the stump. She felt as if her "nerves would jump," and the stump would jerk an inch or two for a second. On days 8 through 10, the sensations filled her absent leg. The quality of her sensations remained constant—itching and tingling—but the duration gradually decreased to only a couple of seconds on day 28, and then they occurred only sporadically.

The patient did not require additional analgesic medication while in the hospital. Her only difficult experience with the phantom sensations occurred one day when she had intense itching in her absent right knee. She was so frustrated that she reached down and scratched her left knee in the contralateral location. The phantom itching was relieved within a few minutes. No one had suggested that she use counterstimulation, yet she continued to use this technique when she was irritated by the itching phantoms. A few weeks after hospitalization, the phantom sensations disappeared and had not recurred at a 4-month follow-up.

This case history illustrates how it is possible to combine service and research in a practical and convenient pain control program. This young girl's information provides a framework for preparing other children for amputations and for encouraging them to actively participate in their therapy and to develop their own coping strategies.

Although the peripheral and central mechanisms responsible for phantom sensations and pains are better understood today, many questions remain as to the most effective interventions. It is essential not only to apply what we have learned about the relief of phantom limb pain in adults to children, but also to objectively evaluate a child's phantom sensations and the efficacy of various interventions according to the child, as well as the type of amputation.

Pains Evoked by Repeated Invasive Medical Procedures

All children inevitably experience some acute pain during routine medical or dental treatments, and most children do not become overly apprehensive about these procedures. Children who need frequent invasive procedures, however, may become progressively more anxious and frightened throughout the course of their treatment regimen. The more afraid, anxious, distressed, or tense these children become, the stronger their pain during procedures becomes. Then they become more apprehensive for their next appointment, so that an anxiety–pain–anxiety cycle develops with increasing momentum. These children pose a special pain management problem for medicine and dentistry.

Children with diseases or injuries that require long-term management are at risk for developing excessive anxiety about necessary blood-sampling, injections, dressing changes, LPs, and bone marrow aspirations (BMAs). Children show their anxiety at home prior to scheduled treatment days. They may lose their appetites, develop sleeping difficulties, have nightmares, act aggressively toward peers and siblings, withdraw, or become more dependent on their parents. They may also regress so that they behave as if they were younger. Some parents attempt to minimize children's pretreatment distress by not telling them when treatments are scheduled, but children then become anxious about all clinic appointments, because they never know when they will receive potentially aversive treatments. As their anxiety increases, their overt distress behaviors increase immediately before and during treatments in the clinic. Usually, they require physical restraints despite sedative and analgesic medications. Emotionally distressed children often seem to "fight" sedation until procedures are completed. They report that they are frightened by the drowsiness induced by the drugs, rather than calmed by the medication. Many children complain that they do not want sedation, either because they do not want to sleep for several hours after treatment or because they do not like feeling out of control as a result of the drugs.

Children with cancer, diabetes, growth hormone deficiency, and arthritis are those most frequently referred to our pain clinic for management of acute pain evoked by invasive procedures. Our first step in designing programs for these children is to conduct a thorough assessment to identify the factors contributing to their pain and anxiety. The therapist observes children and parents during routine treatments (including home observations), and then interviews them independently, using the structured format shown in the Appendix. Children and parents complete questionnaires to rate the pains associated with all procedures and to describe the effects of the disease and treatments for them. Their responses (both quantitative and qualitative) are analyzed, so that we can develop normative data bases according to disease, age, sex, number of previous procedures, and so on, and eventually identify those children most at risk for developing these anxiety and pain problems.

As more children with the same diseases who require the same invasive treatments were referred to the clinic, some similar patterns developed, enabling us to design a general multistrategy pain program. The specific interventions within the program are selected according to a child's age, cognitive level, expectations, fears, anxieties, and familial support, as well as in relation to the nature of the disease (life-threatening potential and the extent to which the child is disabled) and the type, number, frequency, and predictabilty of invasive procedures.

Nature of Children's Disease

The diagnosis of a serious illness in a child has a profound emotional impact not only on the child, but also on the parents, the siblings, and the extended family. Sadness, fear, apprehension, uncertainty, anger, frustration, and grief over the loss of health are common reactions. Usually young children are affected more adversely by the immediate effects of the diagnosis, medical tests, treatments, hospitalization, and separation from family than by the future consequences of the disease. Older children are distressed by both the immediate effects and the future implications for a normal, healthy childhood. At diagnosis, parents may be overwhelmed with fear about the disease, particularly the possibility of more severe complications or death. At treatment onset, parents must adjust to a complex course of therapeutic interventions, learn about various drugs and potential side effects, and assist their children to cope with invasive procedures. Parents' and children's emotional reactions to the diagnosis affect the children's attitudes toward all treatments and can influence their pain during treatments.

The emotional adjustment to a chronic disease has long been recognized as a complicated process. Multidisciplinary teams comprised of physicians, nurses, social workers, and psychologists assist families by providing individual and family counseling, financial aid, rehabilitative programs, and acute and chronic pain management. The significance of a disease changes for children both as they mature and as they endure more treatments, so that painful treatments that they may have accepted when they were young may suddenly become difficult. It is necessary to understand how children's perceptions of their diseases evolve throughout their development, so as to understand which features are most important at different ages or at different times in a treatment protocol. The primary physical features of a disease or treatment must be recognized from a child's perspective, as well as from an adult's perspective. Hair loss, bloating or weight gain, dietary restrictions, and the inability to participate fully in family, school, and extracurricular activities severely affect children. They need assistance to cope with how their diseases and treatments have changed their lives. The more difficult their adjustment, the more likely it is that their pain will be exacerbated during routine treatments.

Parents whose children have a potentially life-threatening disease such as cancer, face a more difficult adjustment than parents whose children have non-life-threatening diseases. Despite major advances in the treatment of childhood malignancies, with dramatic improvements in the remission rate, the diagnosis of cancer has a severe emotional impact on parents. Many parents initially equate a diagnosis of cancer with a death sentence for their children. They require informed, realistic support from staff members and other parents whose children have survived. At the same time, they require information about how best to assist their children in coping with repeated blood-sampling procedures, injections, LPs, and BMAs throughout a 2- to 3-year period. These procedures can be quite painful, even when children are sedated prior to treatment.

Finger Pricks, Venous Stabs, and Injections

Many children monitor their own blood glucose levels throughout the day or require regular injections to control their diseases. Usually these procedures cause a brief, stinging pain, which children can easily tolerate when they are administered only occasionally. However, blood-sampling and injections may become very traumatic for children when they must be repeated regularly. After diagnosis, children and their parents learn about the disease and the importance of treatments, and perhaps learn how to perform finger pricks or injections themselves, as shown in the sequence of photographs in Figure 7.5. As a consequence, children can minimize the pain by acquiring a rationale for the treatment, by actively participating, and by developing some personal pain-coping strategies. Yet, in spite of accurate information, adequate preparations, active control, and positive family and peer support, pain problems can still develop.

These problems seem to fall into three categories. First, children under age 5, when first diagnosed and subjected to various invasive procedures, may become extremely distressed by all procedures, even those that should produce minimal

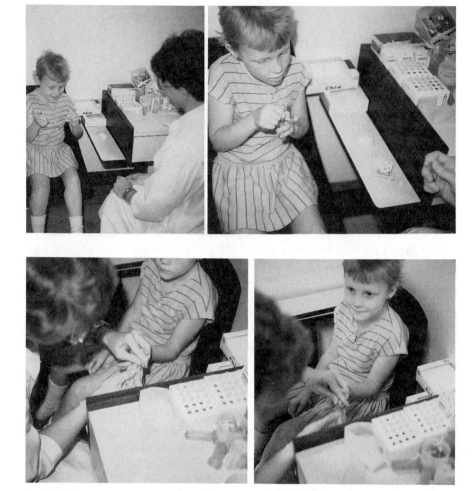

FIGURE 7.5. An 8-year-old girl is shown pricking her own finger and participating in this procedure. She has graduated from the pain program and has learned several strategies to reduce the pain associated with finger pricks, venous stabs, and injections.

tissue damage. Parents are very anxious not only about their children's obvious distress, but also about their own ability to give adequate emotional support to their children and to provide the medical treatments required. Children's distress is exacerbated by their lack of understanding and by parental grief and anxiety. Second, pain problems may develop for children who have coped well with noxious treatments for several months or years, but suddenly and (it appears) inexplicably become so distressed that they are unable to comply with their regimen. Although there seem to be no specific triggers for the dramatic increase in anxiety or for the major difficulty in performing routine finger pricks and injections, children require special assistance to identify and resolve the responsible factors. Third, children who were diagnosed when they were very young, and therefore have grown up on treatment, may develop pain problems as they mature and realize that not all children face the same routines. Similarly, children who are off treatment for several months may have serious difficulties in adjusting to the resumption of treatment, so that they and their families need some brief pain and behavioral interventions.

Although the particular factors contributing to a child's distress and pain depend on the disease, the child, and the family, certain factors have been identified for all children. Inaccurate understanding about their disease, misperceptions of their parents' reactions to the diagnosis, uncertainty of treatment schedules, inconsistency in treatment administration, questions asked by hospital staff about how to conduct procedures (common when new equipment is used, such as portacatheters), lack of control, few coping strategies, and fears about the effects of the disease—all these affect children's pain and must be addressed if their anxiety and pain is to be fully relieved. If parents or staff inadvertently reinforce children's overt distress by delaying treatment or by inconsistent coaching, reassuring, or coercing, then children will become increasingly distressed. Multistrategy pain programs based on the cognitive-behavioral approach described in Chapter 6 are generally necessary for these children, because their problems are caused by a complex interaction of situational, emotional, familial, and behavioral factors.

For example, Jason, a 2-year-old boy recently diagnosed with diabetes, was referred to our pain clinic because he screamed, cried, and required restraints during all invasive treatments; he was beginning to scream when any member of the medical or nursing staff approached him. Although both parents were upset by the diagnosis, his mother was extremely distressed, particularly since she believed that she must assume the full responsibility for his care, including performing injections. She had been very frightened about injections since she was a child.

Jason behaved similarly during finger pricks and injections: He fought and screamed from the moment a staff member approached until several minutes after the procedure. In fact, he was so distressed that he did not seem to react to the actual noxious stimulation any differently than to the cleansing of the site. This observation—that he became distressed prior to the invasive stimulus and remained distressed afterwards, combined with the fact that he reacted the same regardless of the source of noxious stimulation—suggested that he was more upset by the situation than by the tissue damage produced. There was little predictability about what would happen, and little consistency in who was conducting the procedures or where they were conducted.

Consequently, he first required some predictability and consistency. His favorite stuffed animal, a small bear, was used to demonstrate an injection for him, with the bear in the same position as Jason would assume. His parents rubbed the bear's injection site before and after the sham procedure, cuddling it later, all the while explaining to the animal what was happening and why. At the time of the injection, the parents said "Ouch," and as they withdrew the needle they praised the bear. The first time Jason watched, he was very upset; after a few times, however, he calmly observed the procedure, helped to rub the bear, said "Ouch," and cuddled the bear later. At the same time, Jason's own injections were standardized and conducted in the same treatment room. He gradually displayed less distress prior to procedure and cried less during injections.

Jason's mother required assistance from the clinical nurse specialist in endocrinology and from a psychologist to adjust to Jason's diabetes and to realize that the full brunt of the diagnosis was not on her shoulders. We selected two adults who would learn how to inject Jason and who would be available throughout the day when her husband was at work. Some of the immediate pressure she felt about competently injecting and caring for him was partially relieved. She could gradually practice the technique at the same time that she received assistance in overcoming her own fears about needles. Surprisingly, as soon as we established the fall-back system, she immediately felt confident and easily learned how to inject him.

About 2 years later, Jason again began to cry, resist, and refuse injections. He had been preparing the autoinjector, performing his own finger pricks twice daily, and receiving injections, all without any problems. He was now quite angry about the injections, particularly because his 6-year-old sister did not need them. His mother reported that she was having increasing anxiety about his diabetes and obsessive concerns that he would die. She was also becoming increasingly apprehensive about injecting him. Again, a threefold approach was used, consisting of education about treatments (discussion and role play for Jason), behavioral management (a simple program to reduce his overt distress), and simple strategies for pain reduction during injections. At the first session, he participated in a role-play practice for an injection and learned how the more he moved, became upset, or became frightened, the more the injection might hurt. We described how his upset behavior could be reduced gradually by rewarding his nonupset behaviors. He earned a finger puppet for not wiggling, not stalling, rubbing the injection site (before and after), and attending elsewhere during the procedure. He discussed with the therapist and his mother some of the rewards that might help him at home, and suggested that he would like to earn a Mister Freezie popsicle. He helped to draw the calendar on which he and his mother would chart how many popsicles he earned until his next pain appointment.

Within 2 weeks, Jason no longer cried, resisted, or refused during injections. In fact, he did not receive a Mister Freezie for only 3 out of 28 injections. He consistently rubbed his pain site before and after the injections, gathered the equipment, and chose to squeeze his sister's hand, hug a stuffed toy, color, or distract himself during the injection. His mother was more relaxed, since she felt she was no longer causing him severe pain. She wanted to learn more techniques to help him develop a good repertoire of coping strategies, so she learned how to use deep breathing exercises and visual imagery.

A month later at a telephone follow-up, Jason's mother expressed her delight that his pain had decreased and all his distress behaviors were eliminated. She had created a new strategy for him: They cut out strips of colored paper to correspond to the different colors of Mister Freezies available. Before an injection, he selected the color he wanted, held the paper during the injection, and then traded the paper in afterwards for the popsicle.

Jason's successful pain program was essentially the same cognitive-behavioral program that should be used for all acute pain management. His later problems developed primarily as a consequence of his increasing maturity; he became aware that his sister did not need treatments, and that his mother was anxious about his disease and frustrated at having to hurt him during injections. The more difficult his behavior, the more frustrated she became, so that the focus of her interactions with him seemed (to her) more negative than positive. She thus tried different approaches to coerce and coax him into cooperating, inadvertently introducing inconsistency, which increased both their anxieties. The behavioral program provided her with a consistent approach, in which the pain therapist could assume the role of authority figure (or "bad guy," as described by the mother) and mediate the behavioral contract for Mister Freezies that governed the procedures. Jason's mother was able to assume a more positive role in coaching him and in encouraging his sister to share in the treatments. As the immediate crisis passed, she was encouraged to join a support group for parents of diabetic children and to express and resolve her fears about the disease more openly. The education component enabled Jason to develop a better rationale for treatments—a rationale that will be augmented as he matures.

Pain problems from blood-sampling, dressing changes, and injections are quite common for children on lengthy treatment protocols. Often, the external distress signs are similar for all children, regardless of the responsible factors. Health care professionals must conduct thorough assessments and then select the most appropriate interventions. Those interventions may include comprehensive psychosocial care for children, parents, or families; a behavioral management program; or a multistrategy cognitive-behavioral program. Occasionally, even one pain management session, in which parents and children learn some principles of pain modification and simple coping tools, can produce dramatic results, as shown in Figure 7.6. Bill, a 3.9-year-old boy diagnosed with cancer, is pictured on the day he was referred and 2 days later (after one pain session) during insertion of a butterfly needle. Procedures were explained using a puppet; he learned that the butterfly needle actually looked a bit like a butterfly; he was encouraged to choose whether to sit or lie down and to choose a hand; and he was given a few suggestions for distracting himself and squeezing his father's hand. On the observation day, he was extremely distressed when the nurse first held his hand prior to the procedure; he then needed to be restrained throughout the procedure. In the second picture, they had difficulty inserting the needle into his hand, so that they had to start it twice. He showed little distress and reported low pain.

Children who, with their families, have adjusted to their diagnosis may simply require a more versatile repertoire of pain-coping strategies. Adolescents may need to learn self-hypnosis and to share experiences with their peers. Behavioral pro-

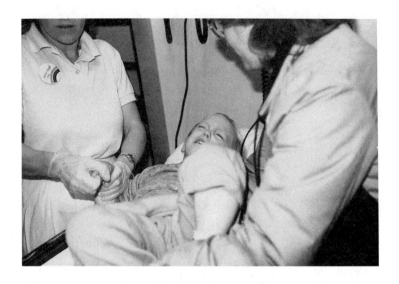

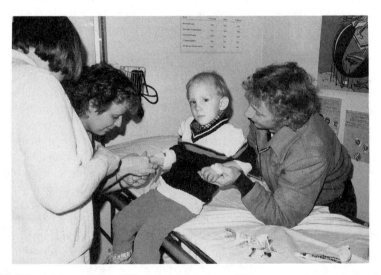

FIGURE 7.6.   A 3.9-year-old boy, Bill, is pictured during an IV insertion on the day of referral to the pain program (upper photograph) and 2 days after his referral (lower photograph).

grams are beneficial for children of all ages, because they provide consistency and motivate children to alleviate behaviors that increase their pain.

Lumbar Punctures and Bone Marrow Aspirations

Children with cancer usually describe LPs and BMAs as the most painful procedures they have experienced (Jay, Elliott, Ozolins, Olson, & Pruitt, 1985). Anticipatory anxiety in children is quite common, sometimes occurring days before procedures are scheduled (Jay, Ozolins, Elliott, & Caldwell, 1983; Katz, Kellerman, & Siegel, 1980; McGrath & deVeber, 1986a). Even though sedatives and cardiac cocktails are administered prior to treatments, children still become anxious. Topical anesthetic creams are often applied with local infiltrations at the puncture site. Although general anesthesia is used in some centers, the frequency of procedures contraindicates its use in most centers. At present, pharmacological approaches are not wholly effective in reducing children's anxiety and pain, so that recent efforts have been directed toward applying cognitive-behavioral approaches to these children.

A variety of multistrategy programs, some similar to our cognitive-behavioral program described in the preceding chapter, have been developed for children requiring repeated LPs and BMAs. The rationale for multistrategy programs to reduce children's acute pain derives from our understanding that pain is a multidimensional experience, and therefore requires a multidimensional approach. The primary components of these programs are hypnosis or hypnotic-like suggestions for analgesia, education about the pain source, management of distress or anxiety behaviors, and improved control in a previously limited-control situation.

Hilgard and LeBaron (1984) provide a comprehensive review of the use of hypnosis to relieve pain and anxiety in children with cancer. Many practical case histories illustrate children's versatility and ingenuity in adapting hypnosis to their unique characteristics, as well as their individual differences in responsivity to hypnosis. Some children can easily learn to reduce their pain with vivid imagery or humor. Hypnotic procedures can be subtly introduced after children and the therapist establish a comfortable rapport, as children's attention is concentrated on a particular event, imagination, or sensory experience. They are thus dissociated from their discomfort. As Hilgard and LeBaron emphasize, children *learn* hypnosis, and, as with all skills learned, some children will require more practice than others. All children will not achieve the same level of mastery through hypnosis.

Hypnotic-like suggestions for analgesia are an integral part of our program for all acute pain management, but particularly for children with cancer or with diseases requiring prolonged care. Suggestions for younger children help them to maintain the necessary body position during treatments, to relax, to pretend they have superhuman powers, and to selectively numb body parts and move their pain. Even very young children can follow suggestions that allow them to keep still with minimal restraints. Ellen, a 4.3-year-old girl with cancer, puts on "magic gloves" before treatment that numb her arms for injections and her back for LPs. Humorous fruit and vegetable analogies (a "fat, round watermelon" for a curled fetal position, a "lean celery stick" for an extended position) and stuffed animals (in the position the child should assume) are very beneficial. Children help the therapist to select the most appropriate model.

Humor can be used to facilitate rapport with young children and to help absorb them in the vivid imagery needed to maintain their position. As cited in an earlier chapter, the image of a big friendly polar bear kissing a child's back during an LP (when the topical anesthetic spray was applied) and of the bear's tooth pricking for a bit (when the local anesthetic was infiltrated at the site) reduced one child's distress. A child's ability to be absorbed by these humorous images, so that the cold sensation and the needle pricks do not hurt as much, is amazing. Often, children respond immediately when these suggestions are presented within a logical context in the first or second pain sessions, but without any formal hypnotic induction.

Older children and adolescents may benefit from more structured hypnosis sessions to acquire the skills to concentrate throughout procedures. Several adolescents imagine trips (each treatment becomes a new holiday in a different country) or vividly describe a past special event. Some place themselves in a drowsy state so that when they receive sedatives before treatment, they can become quite sleepy throughout the aversive stimulation. Few children referred to our clinic for acute pain management have learned only hypnosis, because children's pain complaints usually reflect fear and anxiety about their disease as well as fear and anxiety about their treatments. It is more important to evaluate and manage children's acute pain in relation to how the disease and treatments affect them and their families than it is to evaluate the extent of tissue damage caused by procedures. Even relatively mild noxious stimuli, such as injections through a portacatheter, can be quite painful when children are frightened or lack any coping skills.

The multistrategy cognitive-behavioral program described in Chapter 6 has effectively reduced pain, anxiety, and distress behavior in children of all ages. Histograms of self-reported pain and anxiety from LPs and BMAs are shown for three children in Figure 7.7. The extent of pain reduction varies with children, but as yet there are no clear patterns indicating which children will benefit maximally. This predictive information may be available when more data have been analyzed. However, it is very difficult to establish clear patterns when children vary in terms of age during the program, age at diagnosis, state of disease activity, parental reactions and behaviors, and the type and frequency of invasive procedures, all of which affect children's learning in the program.

Understanding, Predictability, and Control

Understanding, predictability, and control are the most important situational factors that can minimize acute pain evoked by repeated invasive procedures.

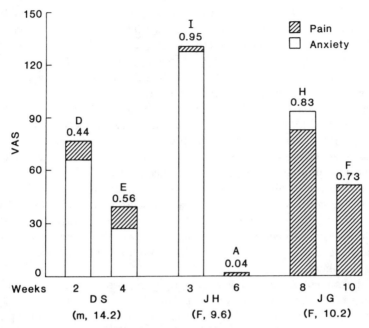

FIGURE 7.7. Ratings of pain (hatched areas) and anxiety (open areas) caused by LPs and BMAs are shown for three children at different points in their pain management programs. Children used visual analog and affective facial scales (described in Chapter 2) to rate the strength and affect associated with their sensations. They also rated anxiety using a VAS.

Children require basic information presented in an age-appropriate format about what is happening to them, why procedures are necessary, and when various treatments are scheduled. The extent of information depends on their interest and their needs. Most children with whom we have worked tell us when they have heard enough, or they ask more in-depth questions as they become accustomed to a treatment regimen. All children require a sense of control, which can be provided by allowing them to have as much choice as possible during invasive treatments, by teaching them some pain-coping strategies, and by motivating them to select and routinely use these strategies.

Naturally, there are some uncertainties about what treatments are scheduled and when they will be conducted, because of children's changing medical conditions. Yet children can understand that their blood and their general health will fluctuate somewhat in the same way that their mood or their energy fluctuates, so that on some days they may require additional treatments. A plan is developed with the child as to how he/she would like to be told about a treatment, how far in advance, and who should be present during that treatment. Even when the opportunities to provide predictability and control seem limited, it is often possible to devise a strategy that assists children.

For example, three children (two girls and a boy, 4.5–5.8 years old) with hemolytic uremic syndrome secondary to an *E. coli* toxin had been hospitalized for 6 weeks, primarily in the pediatric critical care unit (PCCU). They had been on full life-support systems for several days. They received dialysis regularly, varying from hourly to every 4 hours, depending on their conditions. They were referred to the pain program for management of acute pain evoked by invasive procedures. All children had become extremely distressed by even the least noxious procedures, so that they needed to be restrained during blood-sampling, injections, and dressing changes, and they remained upset after treatments. The children were beginning to refuse food and becoming increasingly withdrawn. Since each child received the same noxious procedures, faced the same uncertainties regarding a positive outcome, and exhibited similar distress behaviors, a group cognitive-behavioral program was designed with a special emphasis on alleviating each child's anxieties and promoting his/her unique coping skills. The initial program consisted of 15-minute sessions scheduled daily at nontreatment times. Parents and staff participated by encouraging the children to follow pain management recommendations during treatments.

At assessment, Alice (a 5.8-year-old girl) was no longer able to tolerate blood-sampling from finger pricks or venous swabs. She was very anxious prior to and during noninvasive procedures, such as when nurses monitored her blood pressure. She was extremely agitated and distressed during dialysis. In fact, she had once pulled out her Tenkoff catheter to stop dialysis. Yet she attempted to relax during treatments when her father was present; he encouraged her to relax like a "rag doll." Carla (a 5.2-year-old girl) rated the painfulness of finger pricks as 8 on a scale of 1–10, with 10 the worst possible pain. She rated the pain of venous blood samples as 10. She was extremely distressed during dressing changes and had begun to pretend that she was asleep to avoid all contacts with the medical and nursing staff. She screamed whenever a staff member approached her, reporting that she was frightened because she did not know what would then happen to her. Matt (a 4.5-year-old boy) reported pain even when his bed was touched. He was much angrier than the two girls. He was the most difficult to manage of the three children during all procedures, with the result that he was the last of the three children approached by the intravenous team each morning.

Children were seen individually daily and as a group two or three times weekly, for varying intervals (15–30 minutes) depending on their conditions. A puppet was used to teach them why their treatments (finger pricks, injections, dressing changes) were necessary and how to lessen their fear and pain. Children helped to make posters to illustrate all the materials needed for each treatment (one is shown in Figure 7.8) and posters to remind them what they could do during treatments (one is shown in Figure 7.9). They conducted practice procedures on a special doll and on one another, while the therapist prepared these patients for what they would feel and coached them on how to relax, use visual imagery, or use self-hypnosis. Their pain control repertoire included active participation, hand-squeezing, distraction, rubbing the site, deep breathing, and "magic sparklies" (to

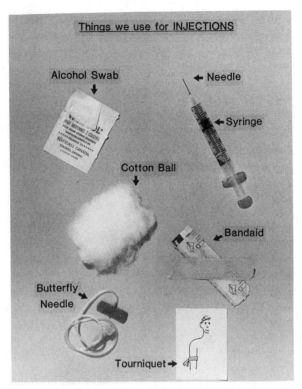

FIGURE 7.8.   Poster illustrating the materials used for injections. Children make posters to illustrate the materials needed for their varied medical treatments.

put their stomachs to sleep). They were allowed as much choice as possible about how to receive treatments and how to assist the staff.

During practice sessions, Alice was able to selectively decrease the sensitivity in one hand. She showed progressive improvements for the next 3 weeks, despite having become so ill that she was again on full life-support systems for several days. She generalized her coping strategies to all procedures and used self-hypnosis routinely. During dressing changes, she pulled off her own tape, rubbed the site, and used deep breathing and hand-squeezing to reduce the discomfort of the cleansing fluids on her stomach. She differentiated the cold sensations from pain, and described her pain as a limited stinging sensation, rather than as a generalized pain throughout the entire procedure. She was able to recognize some of the factors that contributed to her anxiety and pain, her fear of something unexpected, the variety of different sensations produced during dressing changes, differences among staff members, and general lack of control.

Although Carla was even more visibly distressed than Matt, she was able to understand more of her fears than Matt. In her first session, she had explained that

---

Things that I can do to make
finger pricks & needles easier

1. <u>Squeeze someone's hand</u> to tell him/her how much it hurts.
2. <u>Rub the pain site</u> before and after the injection.
3. <u>Keep distracted</u> • talk to someone
                          • count or sing during the injection
                          • do not think about the needle
4. Use "<u>magic sparklies</u>" to relax.
5. Take <u>deep breaths</u> or pant.
6. <u>Stay happy</u> because how I feel influences how much pain I have.

FIGURE 7.9.   Poster displaying the coping strategies for a child. Children help to construct a poster, which can be mounted in the treatment room, to remind them how to reduce their pain during medical procedures.

she was frightened because people did not always tell her what would happen to them. Although she had screamed throughout an intravenous insertion the preceding day, in her second session the therapist helped to prepare her for another insertion. The procedure was divided into two parts: (1) examining and preparing the site, and (2) the actual insertion. She described the first part as "scary" and the second part as painful. Carla was able to remain calm throughout the preparation phase, even watching as the therapist explained what was happening and why. During the actual insertion, she became anxious, her breathing rate increased, and her body began to shake. She squeezed the therapist's hand to communicate pain, while the therapist rubbed her back to help her relax and decrease her breathing rate. She only screamed twice for a few seconds, as opposed to continuously throughout the procedure. She was praised for using some pain-coping methods and later reported that the insertion had not been as scary or painful as usual. She was quite excited about telling her parents what she had learned.

Carla's understanding of most procedures was minimal. She required a consistent approach with clear explanations about what would happen, including seeing the equipment ahead of time. She was the most emotionally distressed of the three children and required shorter sessions twice daily. She was seen individually for a week and participated in two group sessions. For most of the week she preferred to scream during treatments as her main coping strategy, even though she was very interested in watching the other two children use visual imagery and active participation. However, on the last day of the week, she used other techniques. Within another week she actively participated in role-play sessions for all procedures. She was most comfortable rubbing the site and using distraction during treatments.

Matt responded slowly to the therapist's interventions, but was very interested in watching the puppet receive treatments conducted by the other two children. His primary problems were the need to use some coping strategy and the need to control his behavior. When he was not allowed a few minutes to relax before a procedure, he screamed, refused, and fought staff members. Matt benefited most from concrete coping strategies, rubbing, hand-squeezing, and active participation. He required a consistent, firm approach, with procedures paced so that he could relax a few moments between stages. The order of procedures was altered so that Matt was not always last. He was least distressed when his roommates, rather than the therapist, coached him during treatment. He gradually became calm and stopped crying through most, but not all, procedures.

Matt, Carla, and Alice assisted one another tremendously. Their mutual support was always evident, with Alice and Carla supporting and aiding Matt as well as each other. Alice once told Matt, "It's okay to cry and be sad sometimes, but other times you need to work during the dressing change to make it better." They all learned that the nature of their disease meant a certain amount of uncertainty and that some days one or all three might be transferred to the PCCU, but that in general they were improving. The events that could be scheduled with certainty while they were on the ward (blood-samplings, medication, dialysis, dressing changes, pain sessions, school, child life) were emphasized to provide them with a sense of routine.

The components of their pain program were essentially those included in all our acute pain programs: age-appropriate education about the pain source and the disease (or injury); as much predictability as possible in terms of the timing, sequence, and standardization of treatments; improved control by learning some coping strategies; and consistent behavioral management, with staff and parents responding similarly to children and encouraging them to use their skills actively.

Summary

The most common childhood pains are acute pains caused by injuries that produce mild to moderate tissue damage. Many nonpharmacological interventions can immediately reduce pain from mild injuries. Anesthetics and analgesics are usually necessary to control pains from moderate to severe trauma. Although infants and children have been generally undermedicated for all types of pain, serious attention has already been focused on the management of surgical and postsurgical pain, with the result that analgesic prescription and administration are improving in pediatrics.

However, special pain problems continue to exist for many children who receive invasive therapeutic procedures. Despite outstanding contributions from dentistry, health psychology, and behavioral pediatrics toward designing programs to modify children's distress and pain, emphasis has too often been placed more on helping children to cope with painful treatments than on alleviating the pain evoked by treatments. Perhaps health care professionals have accepted too thoroughly the assumption that pain is inevitable during noxious procedures, so that more efforts are directed toward minimizing rather than eradicating children's pain. More ingenuity should be devoted to improving the efficacy of pharmacological and physical interventions for alleviating pain from tissue-damaging procedures, rather than relying almost exclusively on cognitive-behavioral methods.

Multistrategy pain management programs are very effective for reducing children's acute pain, when they have been designed according to the nature of the tissue-damaging stimulus and the needs of a particular child. In this manner, even though the noxious stimulus remains relatively constant, the choice of pain interventions remains flexible and may be adjusted according to the changing needs of children as they adjust to their disease and treatments. Few, if any, children can always achieve the same level of pain relief throughout a lengthy treatment protocol from the same medications or cognitive-behavioral interventions. The emotional, situational, and familial factors that influence their pain are not constant, so pain management that is appropriate in one situation is not necessarily appropriate in all situations.

Pain management for all children's acute pains involves strategic planning based on an assessment of the primary factors that determine pain. The presumed level of tissue damage is a necessary, but insufficient, factor for predicting the level of pain a child experiences from an injury or treatment. Identification of the common factors that modify the different types of acute pain provides a general framework for acute pain management, which can then be adapted to meet the specific needs of all children. Even though children may seem similarly distressed during an invasive procedure, the reasons for their distress are not always similar. Pain assessments enable us to better understand children's unique perspective and choose the interventions most appropriate for them.

8

Recurrent Pain Syndromes

Recurrent pain syndromes may represent a major health problem for children and adolescents. Many otherwise healthy and pain-free children suffer from frequent headaches, abdominal pains, or limb pains. These recurring pains are not symptoms of an underlying disease that requires medical treatment; instead, the pain syndrome *is* the disorder, and the multiple factors responsible for the pains must be identified and managed. Children's pain episodes vary widely in frequency. Some children suffer daily attacks for a few weeks, but then do not have pains for several months. Other children develop pains on a regular weekly or monthly basis. However, there seems to be no predictable temporal pattern for the majority of children. In addition, there are no clear predictors for how long children will have recurrent pains. Some children will be afflicted for a few years, whereas other children will suffer throughout their lives. Pain onset may be coincident with a major source of stress for some children, such as a move to a new city, entry into a new school, parents' separation or divorce, the sickness or death of a family member, or the birth of a new baby. Yet for most children there are no obvious precipitating factors.

Similar variability exists in the onset, intensity, and duration of individual painful episodes. Pain may develop gradually and increase steadily, or may develop suddenly at a strong level. Some episodes are severely incapacitating, but other episodes are mild. Although most episodes last from 2 to 3 hours, pain duration is usually not consistent. Episodes can last only a few minutes or can persist for several days. Generally, there are no predictable patterns for when children will develop painful episodes or for how long they will last. Pains may occur at any time throughout the day and evening, but pains rarely develop at night when children are sleeping.

Parents and children often believe that painful episodes are caused by many external factors, such as weather conditions (extreme heat or cold, humidity, sudden temperature changes), intense sensory stimulation (bright lights, loud noises, prolonged vibrations from riding in cars or school buses), and foods (chocolate, milk, cheese, eggs). Some families recognize that stress resulting from children's anxieties about their performance in school, sports, and social situations can also trigger pains. Children may recognize that their pains can be caused by their emotions, particularly excitement, anger, anxiety, frustration, and sadness. Yet, despite the wide variety of possible pain triggers cited by parents and children, there are usually no specific external or internal factors that always provoke pain. Instead, it seems as if certain combinations of environmental stimuli and emotional factors must be present to trigger pains.

Children can also develop conditioned pain triggers as they and their parents search for the true causes. First, parents usually consider whether any environmental stimuli are responsible. Many parents are so convinced that external stimuli trigger painful episodes that they unduly emphasize the potentially aversive consequences of certain foods, physical activities, and social situations. These external stimuli may have been associated with at least one painful episode, but they did not necessarily trigger the pain. However, children begin to avoid potential triggers and may become excessively concerned about identifying other pain-inducing stimuli. For example, when a young girl is told that she will get a headache from chocolate cake, then she will become nervous and apprehensive in situations where she wants to have cake but knows she should not eat it. Such situations may be coincidentally stressful (e.g., parties with other children where there are noise, excitement, and competitive games), so that she does develop a headache, which she then attributes to the cake. The primary trigger may have been general anxiety about the situation, but not the specific food. Children's increased anxiety about potential pain triggers can cause additional painful episodes. They continue to attribute their pain to external events, not to their anxiety, so that new pain triggers gradually develop and are reinforced. The longer children have endured recurrent pain syndromes, the larger the number of conditioned pain triggers that may be present.

Several features have been noted as common to all recurrent pain syndromes (Apley, MacKeith, & Meadow, 1978; Barr, 1981, 1983a; Chutorian, 1978; Fenichel, 1981; McGrath, 1987b; Schechter, 1984; Shinnar & D'Souza, 1981). Painful episodes occur in the absence of a well-defined organic etiology. Pains are triggered by a variety of external and internal factors, particularly events that provoke stress. Children are healthy and pain-free between episodes. There is generally a history of similar pains for children's parents. Clinical reports describe children as "worriers," "perfectionists," "eager to please," "mature beyond their years," "overachievers," and "little adults."

Parents do not always seek medical assistance for the first painful episode, often believing that the pain represents a common childhood headache, stomachache, or growing pain that will dissipate naturally. After painful episodes recur (particularly if they are severe), parents bring their children to family physicians or pediatricians for evaluation. When routine medical examinations do not reveal any organic disorders, parents may remain apprehensive about the cause for the pains and seek more specialized diagnostic tests. Although some children are diagnosed with a clear pain problem, such as migraine or tension headaches, the majority remain undiagnosed. Few physicians provide concrete information about the features of recurrent pain syndromes, so parents continue to scrutinize their children's lives to identify pain triggers. As a consequence, anxiety increases, and still more emphasis is placed on children's pain complaints and pain behaviors.

The lack of concrete information about how to minimize the painful episodes leads to several management problems, which can paradoxically increase the frequency of episodes or exacerbate the pain. Parents may teach children that many environmental stimuli are pain triggers, even though these stimuli were initially neutral and would not have evoked a painful episode in the absence of a child's anxiety. Parents may respond inconsistently to children's pain complaints, so that children learn to exaggerate their complaints or develop new symptoms to obtain their parents' attention. Their pain may be rewarded inadvertently when they are allowed to stay at home instead of attending school, encouraged to withdraw from potentially stressful sports or social situations, and relieved from routine responsibilities. These secondary gains may prolong pain episodes or contribute to the development of new episodes when children are stressed. Children may cope during painful episodes by relying only on medication and rest, without any attempt to learn some independent coping strategies. They may believe that they will suffer pain throughout their lives, so that they become depressed, anxious, and preoccupied with somatic complaints.

Approximately 400 children and adolescents with recurrent pain syndromes are referred to the Pain Clinic at the Children's Hospital of Western Ontario each year. Their pain assessments have shown that the longer children endure the relatively unpredictable episodes of severe pain, the more likely they are to develop emotional and psychological difficulties. Emotional problems are more common when parents and children have not learned how to control their pain with practical strategies and how to identify factors initiating recurrent episodes. Most previous treatments for recurrent pains have consisted primarily of explicit reassurances that the pains are not related to a disease or disorder, with implicit messages that no further treatments are required. Children who have one type of recurrent pain when they are young often develop another type as they reach adolescence.

Although few prospective studies have been conducted on the prevalence of recurrent headaches, abdominal pains, and limb pains in children, conservative estimates based on clinical referrals indicate that they constitute a major health problem for children and adolescents; approximately 30% of children have experienced recurrent headaches or abdominal pains (Apley, 1975; Barr, 1981; Bille, 1982; Deubner, 1977; Dunn & Jannetta, 1973; Galler, Neustein, & Walker, 1980; Jay & Tomasi, 1981; P. A. McGrath, 1987b; P. J. McGrath, 1983; Rothner, 1979). The incidence of children who continue to experience recurrent pain or who develop new pains has been estimated at 33% for abdominal pain and 40–60% for headaches (Apley et al., 1978; Christensen & Mortensen, 1975; Jay & Tomasi, 1981; Larsson & Melin, 1986; Oster, 1972b). Unless an organic etiology is established, as for certain types of abdominal pain (Barr, 1983b) or headaches (Lai, Ziegler, Lansky, & Torres, 1982), pharmacological methods may reduce the pain during an episode; however, they have not been generally effective at reducing the frequency of painful episodes (Farrell, 1984; Labbe & Williamson, 1983; Michener, 1981). Objective information about the true time course for these pain syndromes and about the efficacy of various methods of pain control is limited, so that many questions remain as to the etiology and control of recurrent pains in childhood. How does the pain syndrome affect children's pain perceptions and coping abilities as adults? Do a subset of children with recurrent pains mature into adults with debilitating chronic pains? If so, would it be possible to reduce the proportion of adults with chronic pain if these syndromes were identified and managed in childhood?

Although further cross-sectional and longitudinal studies are needed to provide definitive answers to these questions, more attention has recently been focused on the special problem of children's recurrent pain syndromes. This chapter reviews the assessment and management of recurrent headaches, abdominal pains, and limb pains, with a special emphasis on the need for a multidisciplinary approach to pain control. (For review on recurrent chest pains, see Coleman, 1984.) The sensory, situational, emotional, and familial factors that contribute to recurrent pains are described. A multistrategy program for the management of recurrent pain syndromes, which was designed to modify relevant contributing factors to reduce frequency and intensity of painful episodes, is also presented.

Headaches

An adult's headache can be classified as acute tension headache, chronic tension headache, classical migraine, common migraine, hemiplegic migraine, migraine accompagnée, basilar migraine, ophthalmoplegic migraine, retinal migraine, carotidynia, posttraumatic headache, cluster headache, or abdominal migraine ("Classification of Chronic Pain," 1986). Although children can experience most of these types of headaches, tension headaches and common migraines represent the major categories of childhood headaches. Tension headaches, caused by muscular contraction, are characterized by a dull, diffuse, and persistent pain that may last for hours, days, months, or years. Migraine headaches, caused by vascular disturbances, are characterized by a throbbing, often unilateral pain and accompanied by nausea, vomiting, and photophobia.

Common and classic migraines are differentiated by the timing of symptoms, by the vasoconstrictive or vasodilation phase, and by the occurrence of auras preceding headaches (generally visual auras, such as blurring, flickering changes in the visual field, and flashing lights). Most young children experience common migraines, which lack early focal neurological symptoms. These common migraines are not always accompanied by nausea and vomiting. Adolescents may suffer from classic migraines, which are preceded by visual auras and accompanied by nausea and vomiting. (For detailed reviews of headache characteristics and differential diagnosis, see Barlow, 1978, 1984; Brown, 1977; Chutorian, 1978; Gascon, 1984; Prensky, 1976; Prensky & Sommer, 1979; Rothner, 1983; Shinnar & D'Souza, 1981.)

Prevalence and Incidence

The current estimates of headache prevalence (number of children with head-aches) and incidence (number of children who develop headaches each year) are derived primarily from past studies in various countries. A large epidemiological survey was conducted in Sweden in 1962 to determine the prevalence of headaches in children from 7 to 15 years old (Bille, 1962). Interviews conducted with the parents of 9,000 school children revealed that 40% of children had experienced headaches by the age of 7. This proportion had increased to 75% by the age of 15. Although these estimates are still cited as relevant nearly 30 years later, the current prevalence and incidence of childhood headaches are not known, despite several surveys and a few epidemiological investigations (Burke & Peters, 1956; Congdon & Forsythe, 1979; Egermark-Eriksson, 1982; Krupp & Friedman, 1953; Michael & Williams, 1952; Sillanpaa, 1976, 1983; Vahlquist & Hackzell, 1949). The majority of these studies used retrospective reviews of children's medical charts and ques-tionnaires completed by parents after children were diagnosed. Few prospective studies have been conducted, so little valid information exists about the age of pain onset for boys and girls, differences in headache type according to sex and age, and the true prognosis for recurrent headaches. Data accrued from retrospective chart reviews may be marred by inconsistent methodology, particularly with respect to the criteria used to diagnose headaches and to assess pain intensity, frequency, and syndrome duration. Also, inferences about the role of developmental, sex, and familial factors in childhood headaches that are drawn from studies conducted in one country may not be applicable to children in other countries.

The failure to recognize that children's headaches are not simply adult headaches on a smaller scale has led to further difficulties. Too little effort has been expended on characterizing the salient features of children's headaches from the children's perspective, to obtain reliable and valid descriptions of their pain and probable causative factors. Although young children may be unable to describe their symptomatology using "adult" terminology, it is possible to obtain accurate information about their pain using their own terminology. A 5½-year-old boy described the quality of his headaches as "elephants running over my head." From his unique analogy, we inferred and subsequently confirmed that his pain had a pounding quality. Important features of their headaches can be overlooked if children are not interviewed thoroughly in a consistent format.

Deubner (1977) emphasized the importance of standardized and reliable diagnostic assessments, including information from both the children and the parents. He evaluated the headache histories of a randomly selected sample of 600 children and adolescents (10–20 years old) in south Wales. Children and their parents were interviewed at home using a standardized approach. Of the 600, 97 children were then examined by a pediatric neurologist, providing a prospective sample to compare with the retrospective data. The demographic survey indicated that only 22% of the sample did not have headaches. Almost half the sample (47.5%) had headaches with at least one of the classic features of migraines (unilateral headache, nausea or vomiting, varied neurological symptoms). Thirty percent of the sample had headaches with no migraine features. Girls were more likely to have headaches than boys (82% and 74%, respectively) and more likely to have symptoms of migraine than boys (22.1% and 15.5%, respectively). The probability of children's experiencing migraines increased when one of their parents had migraines. The probability increased similarly for boys and girls when their mothers had headaches, but was greater for boys than for girls when their fathers had headaches. After diagnoses were confirmed by neurological examination (3.3% were unconfirmed), the revised estimates were that 6.2% and 3.3% of girls and boys suffered from migraines and that 91.8% and 95.4%, respectively, suffered from other types of headaches (presumably tension).

Sillanpaa (1976, 1983) conducted a longitudinal study on headache prevalence; 4,825 children completed questionnaires about their headache experience when they entered school at the age of 7. Sillanpaa was able to survey 2,921 of these children again when they were 14. The latter sample represented 76% of the entire 14-year-old population in two Finnish cities, so that the sample was highly representative of the population. In the second survey, 69% of children had suffered from a headache during the previous year, in contrast to a prevalence rate of 37% when children were 7 years old. Headache frequency also rose between the first and second surveys, with the most pronounced increase in the number of children who had one to four headaches a month. At age 7, the prevalence rate for migraines for boys (2.9%) was greater than that for girls (2.5%), but at age 14 the rate for girls was 14.8%, almost two and a half times greater than that for boys (6.4%). Many children who had migraines at the age of 7 still had migraines at 14 (41%), but headaches disappeared for 22% and lessened for 37%. The prognosis was generally better for boys than for girls, except among children with migraines. The migraine headaches disappeared in one out of three girls, but only one out of five boys.

Although survey studies have yielded varying estimates of the incidence, prevalence, and prognosis for children's headaches, some consistent findings have emerged. First, tension headaches or common migraines are frequent problems for children and adolescents. Second, many children experience headaches before the age of 5; the average age at pain onset determined in most studies is ~ 7 years. Third, headache prevalence differs in some societies (or at some time periods) according to children's age and sex. Headache prevalence increases with age; migraines become more prevalent during the school years. More young boys (under 7) report headaches than girls, whereas the trend seems to reverse as children mature. More adolescent girls suffer from headaches than boys. Fourth, headaches for many children will spontaneously remit as they mature; however, recovery rates estimated from studies vary widely, from 3% to 80%. Children who were very young when they first developed headaches seem to outgrow their headaches more frequently than children who develop headaches in their teens.

These findings are often cited as definitive facts in review articles on the assessment and management of childhood headaches. Yet caution is advocated before such facts are presented to parents and children at diagnosis. It is not known which children will spontaneously recover as they mature or whether differences in recovery rates between boys and girls exist today. As a consequence, children may develop unrealistic expectations about the prognosis for their headaches—expectations that can increase their anxiety and influence their recovery. Health professionals must be informed about published patterns of headaches (the onset, prevalence, and recovery rate), but they must also be aware of the limitations of the studies from which this information is derived. Differences in sample sizes, cultures, study dates, ages of children, headache criteria, interviewing methods, follow-up periods, and criteria for improvement restrict our ability to generalize these findings to all children in all cultures.

The Child with Headaches

Children's descriptions of their headaches naturally differ in relation to their ages, cognitive levels, pain experience, and creativity. Yet it is possible to obtain consistent and accurate information about their headaches, the factors that trigger them, their pain-coping interventions, their understanding of headaches and triggers, and their pain behaviors. Children should be interviewed in a structured format, so that all children answer the same questions in the same order, with the same explanations and prompts provided for difficult questions. As described in Chapter 2, the Children's Comprehensive Pain Questionnaire (CCPQ) was designed to provide objective information about the sensory, situational, emotional, and familial factors associated with recurrent and chronic pains. The final form of this multidimensional pain inventory, administered in a structured interview, evolved after years of use with children who had been referred to our pain clinic. The CCPQ is one of our principal measures for evaluating children with recurrent pain syndromes, enabling us to identify more objectively the factors that initiate or maintain pains, regardless of individual differences in children's vocabularies.

In addition to the CCPQ, children with recurrent headaches complete standardized inventories to assess their anxiety, depression, basic personality characteristics, perception of familial relationships, and general pain perceptions. These measures are listed in Table 8.1. Parents complete a brief questionnaire to describe the pains they have experienced, how they manage these pains, and how they respond to their children when they experience pain. They also complete inventories to assess their anxiety and their perceptions of familial relationships. Approxi-

TABLE 8.1.   Pain Assessment Measures: Recurrent Pain Syndromes

Child	Parent
Calibration task[a]	Headache [or other pain] History and Pain
Children's Comprehensive Pain Questionnaire[a]	Information[a]
State–Trait Anxiety Inventory for Children[b]	State–Trait Anxiety Inventory[b]
Maximum–Minimum Pain Questionnaire[a]	Family Assessment Measure[e]
Children's Pain Inventory—Intensity and Affect[a]	
Children's Depression Scale[c]	
Basic Personality Inventory[d]	
Family Assessment Measure[e]	
Pain diary[a]	

[a]See Appendix to this book.
[b]Spielberger, Edwards, Lushene, Montuori, and Platzek (1973); Spielberger, Gorsuch, and Lushene (1970).
[c]Lang and Tisher (1978).
[d]Jackson (1976).
[e]Skinner, Steinhauer, and Santa-Barbara (1983).

mately 500 children with recurrent migraine or tension headaches have been evaluated in our clinic. A preliminary study of 200 children (McGrath, 1987b; McGrath & Hinton, 1986) yielded interesting data on the common and unique factors associated with children's headaches—data that led to the design of a multistrategy cognitive-behavioral program for reducing the frequency and severity of headaches. (The study results and rationale for this program have been presented in Chapter 6; the specific format for the program is described at the end of this chapter.)

There is much controversy in the research on recurrent headaches with respect to etiology; the most effective interventions; and the roles of stress, anxiety, depression and familial problems in initiating or maintaining the syndrome. Unfortunately, many studies have been marred by small sample sizes, heterogeneous samples of children, and multiple outcome measures. As a consequence, it is often impossible to reach valid conclusions about factors that predispose children to recurrent headaches. For example, a recent study compared psychological functioning in 32 children with migraine with a sample of 32 children without headaches, who were matched for age, sex, and socioeconomic status (Andrasik et al., 1988). Because of the large battery of tests administered (depression, anxiety, and personality inventories; behavior and psychosomatic symptom checklists; social readjustment rating questionnaire; achievement test for reading; and picture vocabulary test) and the small sample size varying within groups by age, sex, and headache characteristics, the power of the study to detect a true difference in psychological functioning between children with headaches and those without headaches was extremely low. The study results, that children with migraines showed higher levels of depression, anxiety, and somatic complaints, are thus questionable rather than conclusive. Although the authors accurately describe some of the study interpretations as speculative, it is hoped that they will extend their research to unequivocally address the psychological aspects of childhood migraine.

Although migraine and tension headaches are distinguished primarily on the basis of their presumed vascular and muscular origins, respectively, the understanding of headache pathophysiology remains unclear. The external triggers responsible for headache onset are not consistently known. Stress is an important factor for both migraine and tension headaches. Consequently, techniques that promote stress management in pain control, such as relaxation techniques, hypnosis, and biofeedback, are considered to reduce both types of headaches.

Migraine may be a lifetime disorder, with different manifestations at different ages. Various food substances seem to play a role in the precipitation of vascular headaches for some children. Tyramine, phenylethylamine, dopamine, histamine, monosodium glutamate, and sodium nitrite have all been implicated. Yet the role of allergies and nutritional triggers is uncertain. Although many foods are believed to trigger migraines, we have not seen any child for whom a particular food was a consistent trigger. Instead, for the majority of children, certain foods seem to represent learned triggers. It is also possible that these foods may trigger headaches only when children are stressed. This may account for why foods trigger headaches occasionally, but not consistently.

In our original study of recurrent headaches, we observed some strikingly similar profiles from the clinical interviews (McGrath, 1987b; McGrath & Hinton, 1987). Some children denied many of the usual emotional reactions that were typical for their age group, particularly any emotions that they judged as negative. These included reactions to common problems at school, with peers, with siblings, or with parents. This denial was quite common and contrasted sharply with the responses of children referred to the pain clinic for other pain problems. Most children had multiple triggers, with some underlying stress. Most children had some maladaptive pain behaviors, but a few children seemed to cope well. Some children presented with serious emotional problems resulting from long-term anxiety, depression, and familial stress. Consequently, a multidimensional pain assessment was necessary to understand children's pain and to adapt the basic pain program to children's needs.

Martin, a 10-year-old boy, had had headaches since he was 8. His headaches lasted a few hours and occurred regularly every 3–4 weeks. They were located bilaterally in the parietal lobes. He described the pain as pounding and throbbing, so that "my head is going in and out a bit." Although there were no other accompanying features (e.g., dizziness or nausea), his eyes were sensitive to light when he had a headache. His headaches often began in the late afternoon before supper and lasted until he went to bed. They were usually gone when he woke. When he developed a headache, he rested and took aspirin. He also had recurrent pains in his stomach every 1–2 weeks. These pains "feel like someone's pulling on my stomach, trying to pull it out, but they are not as bad as a headache."

He identified noise, physical activity, mental concentration, and school tests as pain triggers. Martin limited all activities requiring mental concentration or physical activities during headaches. He also avoided noisy social situations for fear of headaches. He perceived that he had no control over his headaches without medication. Martin was an A student who did not apear to be stressed about school.

Several emotional, situational, and familial factors contributed to his recurrent pains. He was afraid and anxious about the reasons for his headaches and was concerned that he would always have them. He had difficulty expressing his emotions and tried to appear consistently happy and untroubled. He had high expectations for maintaining A grades in school. Martin required some concrete understanding of the factors that affect headaches, some tools for improving his control over the pain, and some assistance in expressing his emotions. Both he and his parents were interested in learning about recurrent headaches, the plasticity and complexity of nociceptive systems, and nonpharmacological methods of pain control. They had positive expectations that our pain program would be effective.

Martin entered the program and used biofeedback to learn about the relationship between his emotions and his body. He learned how to recognize potential stressful situations so that they did not cause headaches. He was happy to share his insights about probable causes (e.g., a headache prior to a test at school) with the therapist. He learned relaxation and distraction techniques to reduce his anxiety. He was encouraged to resume regular activities despite his headaches. Martin helped to teach his family some of the problem-solving skills he learned in the pain program. He had a tendency to avoid problems rather than resolve them; he needed assistance to identify problems, recognize his emotional distress, and manage the problems so that his distress could be genuinely reduced. Once when his mother had a headache, he encouraged her to "relax, take deep breaths, and focus on pleasant thoughts" rather than reach for an aspirin. Within the eight-session program, he learned to identify and modify many headache triggers. His headaches occurred progressively less often and were less strong, so that he was not experiencing any headaches after treatment. At follow-up 1 year later, he had only experienced one headache.

David, a 13-year-old boy, had had one to two headaches every 3 months for 2 years. His headaches lasted approximately 3 days; they were bilaterally located in the frontal and temporal lobes. He described the pain as severe, with sharp, aching, pounding, and hammering qualities. He became nauseated, vomited, and was sensitive to light during headaches. Headache onset was usually sudden. He had tried a variety of medicines to relieve the pain, but was unable to obtain complete relief unless he rested. His headaches mainly started on school days at lunchtime. He had missed 6 days of school during the semester.

There was a strong family history of headaches; David's mother, aunt, and paternal grandparents all had migraines. He could not identify any temporal patterns for his headaches. He believed that changes in barometric pressure and anxiety about school achievement were headache triggers. He had been a straight

A student until 2 years ago, approximately at the time when the headaches began; since then, his grades had fallen to an average range. His mother described him as a mature and quite well-behaved teen. Yet David tended to be socially withdrawn and avoided competitive activities. He worried about his academic performance and others' opinions of him. As an example, he had hidden his last report card for several days before showing it to his mother; he was very disappointed by his grades, even though he had received two excellent marks. His parents were divorced, and David had high goals for himself so that he would please his father. When he was unable to realize these goals, he withdrew and later cried.

Most of his responses on standardized personality measures were within the normal range, but he was extremely preoccupied with somatic concerns and tended to deny problems. He was unable to discuss stressful issues, particularly those related to his family. Several emotional and familial factors contributed to David's headaches. He was a quiet, sensitive child who had extremely high expectations for achievement; he may have developed these expectations in order to receive positive feedback from his father. David was also unable to discuss stressful problems, so that his problems intensified without resolution. He had difficulty coping within the extended family and in social situations with his peers.

David entered a multistrategy pain program. Although his program included a basic cognitive-behavioral focus, the primary emphasis was to teach David to recognize stressful issues, to resolve problems, to set realistic goals, to promote regular relaxed body states (through relaxation techniques, humor, and exercise), and to make decisions in a less anxious manner. The therapist used practical examples from his life (e.g., choosing high school courses) to illustrate the components of problem-solving. During the first few treatment sessions, David's headaches increased in frequency and strength. But by the fourth session, he was no longer developing headaches, and he remained pain-free at the 4-month follow-up.

Shelley, a 16-year-old girl, had had headaches for 1 year. Her headaches occurred daily, each lasting 4–5 hours. They were usually bilateral, spreading around her entire head. Very severe headaches were localized more directly over her eyes. She described the pain as "sometimes sharp, but generally aching, dull, and cutting." Many headaches began at school. She became pale, nauseated, and dizzy. She vomited and occasionally had nosebleeds during severe headaches. She rarely used medication; instead, she tried to distract herself by reading. Shelley reported several headache triggers: some foods (e.g., cheese and French fries), weather changes, anger, anxiety, noise, certain social activities, fatigue, mental concentration, and school. She limited many activities when she had headaches. Shelley also experienced recurrent neck and shoulder pains. These pains had occurred approximately three times a week for 8 months. Unlike Martin and David, who both believed that their headaches would be relieved someday, she had low expectations that she would ever be pain-free and very low expectations that the pain management program she was beginning would benefit her at all.

Shelley had an older brother and younger sister, both of whom were healthy and pain-free. Her mother experienced frequent headaches and back pains. Shelley's mother described her as a very happy and sociable girl, who was active in extracurricular activities and assumed many daily responsibilities at home. Her elder brother had behavioral problems, which created much familial stress. Her father had a chronic and potentially fatal illness. Shelley worried about the family, but she did not openly discuss her anxieties, frustrations, or disappointments.

Her responses on personality testing indicated that she was extremely preoccupied with somatic concerns, was severely depressed, and denied normal stressors. Emotional and familial factors were primarily responsible for Shelley's headaches. The onset of her headaches was coincident with serious conflicts with her older brother and her father. She was unable to express anger and frustration, and generally could not identify or resolve stressful issues. As a consequence, Shelley's pain program emphasizes stress identification and problem-solving skills, in addition to pain reduction strategies. She has just begun her program.

Management of Recurrent Headaches

Many of the pharmacological, physical, cognitive, and behavioral treatments described in Chapters 4 and 5 are available to control recurrent headaches. However, little is known about which treatments benefit which children. In fact, the efficacy of most interventions has not been determined in controlled studies. Interventions have been selected primarily on the basis of headache type (migraine or tension) and pain severity, rather than on the basis of individual contributing factors. Yet, the situational, emotional, familial, and behavioral factors that can trigger recurrent episodes or exacerbate pain are not identical for all children. When selecting an intervention, it is essential to consider not only those factors common for most children, but also the factors unique to each child.

Pharmacological Interventions

Several medications are used to control childhood headaches. Aspirin and acetaminophen are used for symptomatic management, to relieve the mild or moderate pains from common migraines and tension headaches. Abortive treatments are used to prevent classic migraines when a child has some warning that a headache is beginning. These medications are more effective when administered early in the attack. Few children, though, have adequate warning signs (e.g., an aura) for impending headaches. Common abortive medications include ergot derivatives and isometheptene preparations. Ergotamines have a vasoconstrictor action, which interrupts the pathophysiological sequence of vasospasm and dilation. The most widely used preparation is a combination of ergotamine tartrate and caffeine (Cafergot). Some investigators have reported that ergotamine is effective in treating migraines in children (Bille, 1962; Holguin & Fenichel, 1967), but many investigators do not recommend ergotamines for young children (Barlow, 1984; Prensky, 1976; Shinnar & D'Souza, 1981).

Prophylactic or preventive therapy, requiring continuous medications, may be administered when headaches are severe and occur very frequently (e.g., weekly or more often). Propranolol is probably the most commonly prescribed drug for adolescents with severe migraines (Barlow, 1984; Shinnar & D'Souza, 1981). Propranolol effectively reduced migraine headaches in 28 children from 7 to 17 years old (Ludvigsson, 1974), but a later double-blind study on 39 children failed to demonstrate any beneficial effects of propranolol compared to placebo with respect to the frequency, severity, or duration of migraines (Forsythe, Gillies, & Sills, 1984). Sillanpaa (1977) conducted a double-blind treatment evaluation of clonidine and placebo in 57 children with migraine. Both groups of children improved; clonidine was not significantly better than placebo. Other prophylactic drugs include phenobarbital, phenytoin, and amitriptyline. The anticonvulsants phenobarbital and phenytoin were found to be effective in treating childhood migraine in some uncontrolled studies (Buda & Joyce, 1979; Millichap, 1978; Prensky, 1976). Amitriptyline is prescribed commonly for adolescents who experience constant tension headaches and for adolescents who report many somatic complaints in addition to recurrent headaches. Often these adolescents experience some underlying depression. Children who are on long-term prophylactic management for migraines should have their medications discontinued at regular intervals, because of the possibility that their headaches may spontaneously remit. Even if complete remission does not occur, a substantial decrease in headache severity and frequency may occur, which will then preclude the need for continued prophylaxis.

The vast majority of children referred to our pain clinic for recurrent headaches do not routinely use preventive medications, even adolescents who have severe and frequent migraine headaches. Most children and adolescents rely on simple analgesics and rest to control their pain. Many physicians express serious reservations about prescribing medication for children with migraines, because they are concerned about drug habituation, eventual drug dependency, and adverse side effects.

Cognitive and Behavioral Interventions

Few studies have unequivocally demonstrated the efficacy of cognitive and behavioral interventions for controlling childhood headaches, despite their widespread use. Most of the evidence about their efficacy is derived from clinical case reports or uncontrolled treatment evaluations. Hypnosis, stress management, guided imagery, and cognitive coping skills are the cognitive methods most often used; relaxation training, biofeedback, and behavioral management programs are the most common behavioral methods (Andrasik, Blanchard, Edlund, & Rosenblum, 1982; Masek, Russo, & Varni, 1984; Richter et al., 1986; Werder & Sargent, 1984).

However, the majority of treatment programs for children's headaches employ cognitive-behavioral approaches because they include components of each approach.

Diamond (1979) first described the use of behavioral methods for controlling childhood migraine. Of 32 children who used biofeedback and progressive muscle relaxation exercises, 26 experienced reductions in the severity and frequency of their headaches. Since then, recent studies have applied several behavioral approaches. Ramsden, Friedman, and Williamson (1983) described a behavioral management program for a 6-year-old girl with migraines. Her headache complaints decreased as she earned rewards for any days in which she did not report a headache. An exclusively behavioral management program should be effective when headache complaints are due primarily to secondary gains (e.g., school avoidance, reduced expectations for performance) and not due primarily to stress.

Richter et al. (1986) compared the efficacy of relaxation training, cognitive coping, and a placebo intervention for 42 children (9–18 years old) with migraine. The relaxation training consisted of sequential tensing and relaxing of large muscle groups, followed by sequential relaxing without tensing, and then by self-cued relaxation (in which the children gradually learned to relax from a cue, rather than from a lengthy progressive muscle relaxation session). Cognitive coping sessions focused on teaching children to alter their maladaptive thoughts about pain by restructuring, to use simple pain control strategies, and to manage stress more effectively. The children who received relaxation training and those who received cognitive training had significantly fewer headaches than children who received the placebo. But pain severity and headache duration did not decrease after treatment.

In autogenic training, children imagine that their hands are warming as they receive biofeedback of their skin temperature. They gradually learn to warm their hands without the feedback. Autogenic training has been successfully used to reduce migraines in five children, as described in case reports (Andrasik et al., 1982; Labbe & Williamson, 1983, 1984). Autogenic training has frequently been combined with biofeedback to treat childhood headaches. Olness and MacDonald (1981) taught self-hypnosis, with and without thermal autogenic training and thermal biofeedback (skin temperature from their fingers), to 15 children with migraine. All children responded successfully. Houts (1982) taught cue-controlled relaxation and biofeedback to an 11-year-old boy with migraines. His headaches decreased gradually over the 20-week treatment program. At a 1-year follow-up, he had experienced only three headaches during the previous 12 months, in dramatic contrast to three headaches per month prior to treatment. Waranch and Keenan (1985) evaluated the efficacy of a multistrategy program combining relaxation training, biofeedback, and counseling for 15 children (10–17 years old) with recurrent migraine or tension headaches. At the end of treatment (the number of sessions varied from 4 to 11), 13 children had experienced significant reductions in the frequency and intensity of their headaches.

Masek, Russo, and Varni (1984) assessed the efficacy of a multistrategy program of biofeedback, meditative relaxation, and management of pain behavior for

20 children with migraine. Nine 1-hour sessions were conducted over 11 weeks. Children watched a television monitor to obtain feedback of their facial muscle activity from surface electromyograph (EMG) electrodes placed on their foreheads. They received continuous biofeedback as they practiced meditative relaxation. Meditative relaxation consisted of rest and deep breathing while the children concentrated on a single thought or image. The behavioral management component included regular monitoring of headache occurrence, suggestions for behavior change to modify headache onset, and recommendations for parents to encourage children's normal activities and discourage their pain behaviors. Headache occurrence, pain intensity, headache duration, and medication use decreased for all children. This improvement was maintained at a 1-year follow-up.

In 1986, a randomized controlled trial was conducted to compare the efficacy of relaxation training plus biofeedback, relaxation training alone, and a waiting-list control for reducing migraines in 18 children from 8 to 12 years old (Fentress, Masek, Mehegan, & Benson, 1986). Both treatments significantly reduced headaches in comparison to the control condition. Larsson and Melin (1986) evaluated the efficacy of relaxation training, information about headaches (as usually provided in regular health services), and no treatment for 32 children with headaches. Children who received relaxation training had significant reductions in headaches after treatment and at a 6-month follow-up, whereas children who received information or had no treatment experienced only minor improvements.

Biofeedback and relaxation training through mental imagery or progressive muscle relaxation were used by 119 children and adolescents with recurrent headaches (4–20 years old, mean age 12.5) (Womack, Smith, & Chen, 1988). No data were presented as to actual headache frequency and intensity before and after treatment, but the authors reported that most children had fewer and less severe headaches after 2 months of weekly treatment sessions.

Hoelscher and Lichstein's (1984) comprehensive review on the behavioral management of childhood migraine included only 12 studies. At that time, many studies lacked any empirical data; yet there was still convincing evidence that autogenic training, biofeedback, and relaxation reduced the frequency and intensity of migraines. Most studies also included some cognitive coping strategies to teach children how to reduce their muscle activity or skin temperature, although these were not specifically described. These skills were then generalized to stressful situations in which children developed headaches.

Since most clinical studies to date have lacked well-controlled no-treatment groups, the supposed treatment efficacy of some cognitive and behavioral interventions may be confounded by high rates of temporary spontaneous remission. Spontaneous remission rates for recurrent pain syndromes are a special problem. The remission rates for childhood headaches have ranged from 16% to 72% (Bille, 1962, 1981; Congdon & Forsythe, 1979; Sillanpaa, 1976). Such factors as initial headache severity and frequency, length of follow-up, age of subjects, methods of determining remission rates, and type of intervening treatment undoubtedly contribute to this variability and make it difficult to reach a general conclusion about the true remission rates for childhood headache. The controlled treatment evaluations that Hoelscher and Lichstein recommended in 1984 are now beginning. Because few studies have had comparable baseline measures of headache severity, frequency, and duration, so as to ensure that children assigned to different treatment groups are truly similar before treatment and to permit meaningful comparisons among different studies, more attention is now being focused on obtaining accurate and thorough descriptions of the pain syndrome at diagnosis. More emphasis has also been placed on the need for long-term follow-up to estimate treatment efficacy in relation to true spontaneous remission rates.

Multistrategy Pain Control Programs

Multistrategy programs provide a flexible repertoire of physical, cognitive, and behavioral interventions, so that each child can receive the most appropriate treatment based on his/her own needs and preferences. The treatment regimen can also be modified according to a child's progress in the program, so that different interventions may be used at different times, beginning with simple, concrete methods and progressing to more complex, abstract methods.

The multiple causes and factors contributing to recurrent headaches have led to several integrated programs for treating children's pains. Although these programs are quite promising, their efficacy has yet to be determined in randomized controlled trials. Multistrategy programs should begin with a thorough assessment of children's headaches. Interventions are then carefully selected to modify the factors that affect pain. Similar factors may emerge for children of the same age or sex, but some unique factors are present. All children may require information about their pain problem, but not all children will require a strict behavioral component. All children should learn some coping skills, but some children will use hypnosis more effectively than distraction. A basic multistrategy program can provide a rational framework for reducing childhood headaches, as described at the end of this chapter. All programs should be strictly evaluated, so that valid conclusions will be obtained about both their immediate and their long-term efficacy. Headache intensity and frequency should be monitored using daily records completed by the child, as well as recorded in pre- and postassessment interviews. When children have experienced recurrent headaches of variable frequency, it is often difficult to precisely determine headache frequency and pain intensity, unless children complete daily diaries for a specified interval. Although only children complete pain diaries for 1 month in our program, Andrasik, Burke, Attanasio, and Rosenblum (1985) recommend that both children and parents complete pain diaries.

In 1987, we began a randomized controlled trial to evaluate the efficacy of our pain control program for recurrent headaches. The sample sizes for the treatment study (162 children from 5 to 17 years old in each of three treatment groups) were calculated to ensure that treatment evaluation would not be confounded by differences due to age, sex, diagnosis, headache frequency, pain severity, headache duration, and syndrome duration. This large sample will permit us to evaluate the effectiveness of the treatment over a 2-year period; to identify the factors at initial pain assessment that predict the children who will and will not respond to treatment; to determine how situational, emotional, and familial factors change after treatment; and to evaluate the relationships between children's emotions and headache frequency, intensity, and syndrome duration. Such evaluation studies are essential for all multistrategy pain programs.

Abdominal Pain

Recurrent abdominal pain (RAP) is a common problem for children, as can be readily noted in the referral statistics for pediatric clinical practices and for emergency department admissions. Like all recurrent pain syndromes, RAP varies in onset and duration, occurring in unpredictable patterns without clear triggers. Otherwise healthy children report aches and pains diffusely localized over a wide region, often the epigastric or periumbilical areas. Several painful episodes may occur within a short span of time, or pains may occur every few weeks. The pains may last for a few minutes or a few hours. Varied symptoms may accompany pains. Some children feel nauseated and vomit; some are constipated; some have diarrhea; some develop headaches; and some become pale and lethargic.

Apley's (1975) extensive and elegant observations on children with RAP provide a classic description of the syndrome and factors presumably associated with its etiology. He depicts the child with RAP as a child with normal intelligence who has a history of recurrent somatic complaints; who is susceptible to emotional disturbances; and who is timid, anxious, or overconscientious. There is usually a history of recurrent pains or nervous disorder within the child's family. Apley considers RAP as an expression of the child's reaction to emotional stress—a reaction that is often shaped by factors within the family. The differential diagnosis of RAP is complicated by the diverse pathological conditions that can produce similar pains. A thorough medical examination is required for the accurate diagnosis of RAP because similar pain symptoms may be caused by many conditions (Blevens, Buchino, & Fellows, 1984; Buck & Bodensteiner, 1981; Byrne, Arnold, Stannard, & Redman, 1985; Glaser & Engel, 1977; Kirschner, 1988; Marshall, 1967). (For a detailed review of the characteristics and differential diagnosis of RAP, see Apley, 1975; Barr, 1983b; Galler et al., 1980; Levine, 1984; Levine & Rappaport, 1984.)

Prevalence and Incidence

Only a few studies have been conducted on the prevalence and incidence of RAP in children. Most articles on the management of the syndrome are review articles, which cite the same few studies as to prevalence. The most frequently cited study is the prospective field survey on 1,000 school children conducted by Apley and Naish (1958). In addition to conducting detailed clinical examinations, they also collected information for each child about the family history of illnesses and pains, the sensory characteristics of the pain from the child's and mother's perspective, associated symptoms, psychological difficulties, and emotional stressors. Approximately 12% of the girls and 9% of the boys suffered from RAP. Peak incidence occurred at the age when children began school. After school onset, girls had more pain complaints than boys. The families of children with RAP had a higher incidence of abdominal pain and other somatic complaints than control families (randomly selected). Children with RAP often seemed anxious, timid, fussy, or overconscientious. Aply conducted a long-term follow-up of 30 children with RAP, 9–20 years after children had been hospitalized (Apley, 1975; Apley & Hale, 1973). Approximately one-third of the children with RAP continued to have abdominal pain, whereas one-third had developed other somatic complaints (usually headaches). Only one-third of the patients were symptom-free.

Cullen and Macdonald (1963) described the prevalence of recurrent pains, "the periodic syndrome," in 3,440 children of 1,000 families in western Australia. The proportion of children with abdominal pains, headaches, and limb pains were 5.6%, 6.9%, and 4.5%, respectively. Pringle, Butler, and Davie (1966) noted that about 14.5% of 8,000 children aged 7 in a survey in the United Kingdom had a history of periodic abdominal pains.

Oster (1972a, 1972b) conducted an 8-year longitudinal study on recurrent pain syndromes in Denmark. As a school medical officer, he registered the prevalence of abdominal pains, headaches, and limb pains in approximately 2,200 children from 6 to 19 years old. About 14% of all children had RAP (16.7% of the girls and 12.1% of the boys). Peak prevalence for RAP occurred at 9 years of age, approximately 3 years before the corresponding peak for headaches. There were differences in the proportions of children with RAP according to their ages (e.g., a higher percentage of 9-year-olds had RAP than 13-year-olds). However, these estimates may be slightly biased, because the criteria for categorizing children's pains as recurrent pains were not specified and may not have been as stringent as those used by Apley and Naish (1958). About 160 parents of children with recurrent pains (and a comparison group of parents whose children were pain-free) completed questionnaires about their own childhood pain experiences. The parents whose children had recurrent pains reported more pains, both at the time of the questionnaire and when they were children, than the comparison group. Oster suggested that a child's family environment, which may focus unduly on pain expression and somatic complaints, contributes to the development of the recurrent pains.

Christensen and Mortensen (1975) conducted a 28-year follow-up investigation for 34 patients who had been diagnosed with RAP as children. They compared the health problems of these adults to a control group without childhood

RAP. Of the patient group, 53% had gastrointestinal pain consistent with a diagnosis of irritable colon syndrome, peptic ulcer/gastritis, diarrhea, and constipation. Only 29% of the control group reported gastrointestinal pain as adults. The RAP group also reported more nongastrointestinal pains: 32% reported headaches, back pain, and gynecological pains, in contrast to 13% of the controls. There were no differences between the two groups in the incidence of abdominal pain in their children; however, 28% of all the children whose parents reported abdominal pains at the time of follow-up had symptoms of RAP. Only 7% of the children whose parents did not have abdominal pain at follow-up had symptoms of RAP. This finding—that parents of RAP children report similar pain complaints—is supported by other studies (Oster, 1972b; Stone & Barbero, 1970). Stickler and Murphy (1979) conducted a long-term follow-up study for 161 children with RAP. Children completed questionnaires about their pain 5–9 years after intiial diagnosis. Approximately 20% of patients were still experiencing symptoms. The percentage of children who do not recover completely is often estimated at between 10% and 30%. However, an accurate prognosis for children with RAP will remain unknown until more stringent criteria are used to diagnose RAP and long-term follow-up evaluations are conducted regularly.

Although there are no prospective surveys on the incidence of RAP in North America, available research data and clinical anecdotal reports indicate that RAP constitutes a major problem for children and adolescents. Estimated prevalence rates vary from 6% to 30%. As an example, 165 children (75 boys, 90 girls; 2–17 years old, with a mean age of 8.8) with abdominal pain complaints were examined in the emergency department of our hospital during a 5-month period. Retrospective chart review and follow-up with family physicians suggested that 25% of these children were suffering from RAP. The majority of children had been seen previously by several physicians or pediatricians for similar abdominal pain complaints. Also, many children had already been examined in the emergency department, and their parents had received reassurance that there was no organic disease underlying their children's pain.

An estimate that 25% of children had RAP, as derived from those who presented with abdominal pain complaints to the hospital, clearly is not a precise index of prevalence. This percentage does not include children diagnosed and managed by their own physicians. Also, children who arrive at the emergency department may represent a biased sample, with a disproportionately high or low number of RAP children seeking treatment. A comprehensive epidemiological survey is necessary to determine the true regional prevalence. RAP is a common problem for children. Prevalence and incidence may differ according to children's age and sex. Many children with RAP also have recurrent headaches or limb pains. The prognosis is unclear; many children may continue to suffer gastrointestinal pains as adults. Many questions remain unanswered about RAP—the age of onset, the proportion of boys and girls with RAP, the etiology, the optimal treatments, and the prognosis.

The Child with Abdominal Pain

Although children with RAP share some common features, each child may have distinctive factors that maintain the syndrome or exacerbate the pain. Catherine, a 9-year-old girl, had experienced weekly episodes of abdominal pain for 2½ years. She was a shy, sensitive child who was self-conscious about being overweight, but she was active with her peers. Catherine had some difficulty completing her schoolwork in the time allocated, and often worried about schoolwork and test situations. The pains always developed in her lower abdominal area; she described them as aching, pounding, and steady. She also developed headaches when the abdominal pain was severe. Catherine had no coping strategies other than to seek her mother's assistance and receive medication. Her pain responses on the Children's Pain Inventory (CPI) were higher than those for other children her age. Her scores on standardized depression and anxiety inventories were signicantly elevated. She had missed 20 days of school in the first semester because of abdominal pains.

Catherine's parents noted that she had been diagnosed with an ulcer when she was 6 years old. Subsequent medications had proven ineffective, so that parents attempted to reassure her during painful episodes. In fact, during severe episodes she was allowed to sleep in her parents' bed. At the time of assessment she had been sleeping most nights on a mat in her parents' bedroom. They had been unable to encourage her to sleep in her own bed.

The results of the pain assessment indicated that several situational, familial, and behavioral factors contributed to Catherine's recurrent pains, but that emotional factors were primarily responsible. She was a shy, quiet girl who was unable to identify or resolve stressful issues. School difficulties were a consistent source of stress. In fact, the onset of her pain was coincident with her entry into school, and her pain episodes occurred generally before or during school hours. She was anxious and depressed, although neither she nor her parents recognized these emotions. Her parents' inconsistent responses to her pain complaints inadvertently reinforced them. They varied from providing excessive attention, medication, and their bed to simply reassuring her with "Don't worry." In order to earn their attention, her pain symptoms had become increasingly strong. Catherine's lack of independent coping strategies, her lack of understanding about her anxiety, and her parents' anxiety also maintained the recurrent pain episodes.

A multistrategy pain control program was recommended for Catherine to help her and her parents to identify and resolve stressful issues, to teach her some nonpharmacological methods of pain control, and to decrease any exaggerated pain behaviors that had developed. She and her parents participated in an eight-session program conducted biweekly; the cognitive-behavioral program was adapted from our program for recurrent headaches. Her painful episodes decreased over the course of the program, as shown in Figure 8.1, with only one painful episode reported at the 4-month follow-up.

Lani, a 15-year-old girl, had experienced daily episodes of abdominal pain for 5 months. These pains occurred for about 30 minutes five or six times each day in

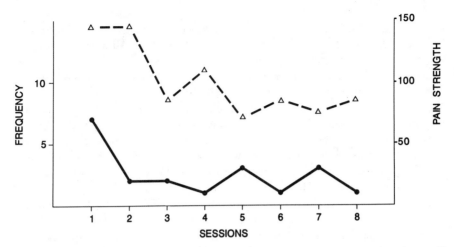

FIGURE 8.1.   The frequency (solid symbols) and intensity (open symbols) of RAP for a 9-year-old girl, Catherine, are plotted throughout the course of her pain management program.

the left upper quadrant. The intensity varied, but was usually quite strong and debilitating. She described the pain as sharp, throbbing, and aching. She felt nauseated and dizzy during some painful episodes. Lani identified stress, anxiety, and several weather conditions as pain triggers. She had missed 9 days from school during the semester because of her pains. The week before her appointment, she began to develop daily headaches.

Lani's scores on standardized measures indicated that she was excessively preoccupied with somatic complaints and had difficulty interacting with her peers. She perceived several problems within her family, such as their inability to communicate effectively, express their emotions, and resolve stressful problems. Her responses on her pain diary showed that Lani was preoccupied with pain complaints. All her pains were listed as "strong, queasy feelings," but she elaborated each response to emphasize such factors as "worse after supper, very hot that day"; "occasional sharp pains, pain in sides when I breathe, pressure in my stomach"; "when I breathe, it hurts my chest, don't get enough air"; "severe pain in chest, strong headache"; and "overheated." She rated all her pains as similarly strong on the visual analog scale (VAS), but she chose faces on the affective scale that were relatively neutral. Most children with strong pain also rate the affective quality as very negative.

Lani's two younger brothers were both healthy. There was no history of recurrent pains within the family. Lani had a positive attitude toward school and achieved average grades. Her mother reported that she had many friends and was outgoing and sociable.

Her pain assessment indicated that emotional and behavioral factors were responsible for the pains. The onset of pain was coincident with the start of ninth grade. Lani was anxious about her peers' opinions of her appearance, popularity, and academic ability. She was gradually withdrawing from organized group activities and sports for fear of failing to achieve adequately. Although her parents assumed that Lani was self-assured, she was quite anxious and unable to express and resolve stressful issues. Her pains were reinforced by her gradual withdrawal from and avoidance of stressful situations with her peers, and by increased support and nurturing from her parents and teachers. A pain management program was recommended to help her to identify and resolve the situations that created anxiety, and to assist her parents so that they responded to her pain complaints in a manner that minimized her maladaptive pain behaviors. She enrolled in the pain program. Her pain increased at the first session, so she was now reporting stronger levels and reporting daily headaches and chest pain in addition to her abdominal pain.

Occasionally a child's pains increase at the beginning of the pain program, especially if his/her pain is the result of emotional distress that they deny. The pain gradually decreases for some of these children, whereas it increases or additional somatic complaints develop for other children. We do not have sufficient data yet to identify at the time of pain assessment which children will respond favorably to treatment. Lani's program is in progress; we do not know whether it will be effective.

Clinical reports suggest that children susceptible to RAP are "good" children, who are eager to please or who worry constantly. Many children with RAP referred to our pain clinic have unusually high levels of anxiety. They are preoccupied with somatic concerns and are extremely worried about how others perceive them. Common sources of stress for children with RAP are familial problems (parental arguments, separation, divorce, illness, pain in another family member, loss of family member, physical move, or major family trauma); peer problems (teasing, loss of friends, peer pressure, inability to socialize in an age-appropriate manner); and school problems (academic pressure, teacher–pupil disharmony, tests, or changes in school situation). Either stress or an illness that would normally produce abdominal pain can be antecedent events for RAP. Much evidence implicates stress either in initiating specific episodes of abdominal pain or in contributing to the maintenance of the recurring pain syndrome, even though there is little substantiated information about the specific relationship between stress and the etiology or maintenance of symptoms. Many children experience familial, peer, and social stress without developing RAP.

Organic etiologies are responsible for abdominal pains in only about 5% of children who have been diagnosed with RAP. The etiology of RAP is generally regarded as "psychophysiological," "nonorganic," or "psychogenic." These terms are often used interchangeably; they imply that the pain is real, but that the causative factors are psychological, presumably anxiety and stress. Barr (1983b) suggested three classifications for children's abdominal pains: (1) "organic pain," or pain that is caused by a well-defined organic disease (e.g., pancreatic insufficiency); (2) "dysfunctional pain," or pain that occurs in the absence of a well-defined organic disease because normal physiological functions are maladjusted, but for which there is no evidence of a psychogenic etiology (e.g., developmental lactose intolerance, chronic stool retention); and (3) "psychogenic pain," or pain that occurs in the absence of a well-defined organic disease and for which there is evidence of a psychological etiology (e.g., conversion reaction syndrome). Barr emphasized the multidimensional nature of the familial, behavioral, and emotional factors that affect children's pains. He described the need for a more broad-based conceptualization of RAP than the traditional and simple "organic versus psychogenic" distinction. Levine and Rappaport (1984) proposed that RAP results from many converging factors for a child—a somatic predisposition, dysfunction, or disorder; lifestyle and habit; environment and critical events; and temperament and learned response patterns.

There is conflicting evidence as to whether RAP children have a differential gastrointestinal response to stress (Feuerstein, Barr, Francoeur, Houle, & Rafman, 1982; Kopel, Kim, & Barbero, 1967). Recently, Gaffney and Gaffney (1987) proposed that RAP may result from a physiological gastrointestinal susceptibility to a normal homeostatic response to stress, such as increases in endorphinergic activity. Endorphinergic stimulation of the gut may cause segmental contractions, colon spasm, and pain. Segmental contractions of the intestine may interfere with sequential peristalsis, increasing transit time and constipation. Increased rectosigmoid motility has been shown in children with RAP (Kopel et al., 1967).

RAP is probably a generic term for a collection of disorders with varying etiologies, rather than a specific problem with a unique etiology. Clinical studies indicate that stress, learning, modeling, emotional factors, familial behaviors, genetic predisposition, autonomic instability, and gut motility may all play a role (Apley, Haslam, & Tulloh, 1971; Bain, 1975; Barr, Levine, Wilkinson, & Mulvihill, 1979; Barr, Watkins, & Perman, 1981; Green, 1967; Levine & Rappoport, 1984; Rubin, Barbero, & Sibinga, 1967; for reviews, see Barr, 1989; McGrath & Feldman, 1986; Levine & Rappoport, 1984; Zeltzer, 1986). Although our research on RAP has not included a large, heterogeneous sample of children, our research findings support this multifactorial nature of abdominal pain. Our pain profiles for children with RAP are strikingly similar to those for children with recurrent headaches. The extent to which each of these factors mediates RAP varies among children.

During the last decade, there has been increasing evidence that the prevalence of depressive symptoms and disorders in children is higher than that previously assumed. Hodges, Kline, Barbero, and Flanery (1985) attempted to assess the presence and severity of depressive symptoms in children with RAP. They used two methods of assessing depression, self-report and semistructured interview, to increase diagnostic accuracy. They also used two comparison groups of children without significant abdominal pain: a healthy control group, and a behavioral-disorders control group with a history of psychiatric illness. They administered the Children's Depression Inventory and the Child Assessment Schedule to all children. In addition, they administered the Beck Depression Inventory to all parents. Children with RAP did not report any more depressive symptoms than did the healthy children, but their mothers reported more depressive symptoms than did the mothers of the healthy children. Twenty-five percent of the mothers indicated the presence of at least a mild level of psychiatric depression, but fathers were not characterized as depressed.

This evidence that children with RAP lacked major depressive symptoms was quite strong, because their results were based on two different depression measures. There was no evidence that children were masking major depressive symptoms or a dysphoric mood during the clinical interview. The high incidence of maternal depression in this study is remarkable. Moreover, the mothers of children with RAP reported symptoms of depression that were comparable to those of the mothers of children with behavioral disorders. Their depressive feelings may have resulted from coping with children who had major problems, or their feelings may have contributed to the development of behavioral or somatic symptoms in children. Factors that underlie mothers' depressive symptoms, such as marital dissatisfaction, may exacerbate their children's pain complaints. Children with RAP are often described as anxious and very sensitive. This sensitivity to maternal affect, regardless of how sensitivity developed, may result in an internalized anxiety state that produces or maintains abdominal symptoms. A young boy referred to our clinic for abdominal pain management developed pains each time his father traveled for business. His mother believed that his father's absence triggered these pains. In reality, his mother's unspoken but evident resentment created the familial anxiety that triggered his pains.

We do not know yet the relationships among familial factors, anxiety, depression, and the development of RAP. The role of familial factors must be examined, since sufficient clinical evidence exists that RAP in some children is maintained by familial dysfunction. In fact, the Hodges, Kline, Barbero, and Flanery (1985) study clearly highlights the importance of treating children within the context of the family. It is necessary to obtain broader empirical data in order to better understand the relationships between family members' affective states and physical symptoms in children.

Hodges, Kline, Barbero, and Woodruff (1985) also investigated anxiety in children with RAP and their parents. Children with RAP reported significantly more stomachaches, vomiting, nausea, headaches, eye problems, and general aches and pains than either a healthy control group or a behaviorally disturbed control group. The RAP and behaviorally disturbed groups had significantly higher anxiety levels than the healthy control group. Both parents of the RAP group scored significantly higher on anxiety than parents of the other children. Although the literature on children with RAP consistently mentions anxiety as prevalent in these children and their parents, few empirical data have been collected about the true incidence of anxiety disorders in these families. Despite the observation that the RAP children were more anxious than healthy children on clinical examination, several RAP children showed no apparent anxiety disorder. The finding that the parents of RAP children were significantly more anxious than other parents is noteworthy. Higher levels of anxiety in the RAP children were comparable to those experienced by children from psychiatric settings who did not complain of abdominal pain.

Autonomic predisposition and family dynamics are frequently suggested as mediating factors for RAP. Abnormalities of rectal mucosa, of abdominal tenderness, of intestinal transit time, of rectal motility, of pupillary reactivity, and of anorectal tonometry have been described for RAP children (Apley et al., 1971; Barr, Levine, & Watkins, 1979; Barr, Levine, Wilkinson, & Mulvihill, 1979; Barr et al., 1981; Black, Welch, & Eraklis, 1986; Dimson, 1971; Hill & Blendis, 1967; Hughes & Zimin, 1978; Hyams, 1982; Janik & Ein, 1979; Lebenthal, Rossi, Nord, & Branski, 1981; MacKeith & O'Neill, 1951; Papatheophilou, Jeavons, & Disney, 1972). These children may have an autonomic dysfunction in which stress or anxiety activates the gastrointestinal tract to produce pain. A physiological predisposition for RAP is consistent with the frequent occurrence of bowel dysfunction. Psychological factors within the family may also contribute to the association between anxiety and somatic symptoms. There may be oversensitivity to other family members and their respective problems, particularly to parental anxiety. Excessive emotional responsiveness among family members, referred to as "enmeshment," has been frequently described as characteristic.

Management of Recurrent Abdominal Pain

The alleviation of RAP requires a comprehensive approach to address all the situational, behavioral, emotional, and familial factors that contribute to the syndrome. Despite the similarity between the causes for recurrent headaches and RAP, many more studies have been conducted to develop and evaluate treatments for childhood headaches than for RAP. Yet the methods that have reduced the frequency, intensity, and duration of headaches may be equally effective for alleviating RAP syndrome.

Pharmacological treatments generally include laxatives, when pains are accompanied by constipation, and simple analgesics to relieve the pain during episodes. These interventions are targeted to control individual pain episodes, not the recurrent pain syndrome as a whole. In two studies, Apley (1975) evaluated the efficacy of an antispasmodic, phenobarbitone, and a placebo for children with RAP. There were no consistent differences between the two drugs. Although some clinicians report the beneficial effects of antidepressants for adolescents, no published studies are available.

The management of RAP by increased fiber intake has been suggested. Feldman, McGrath, Hodgson, Ritter, and Shipman (1985) studied the effects of adding dietary fiber to the diets of children with RAP. They administered high-fiber cookies (5 g of corn fiber per cookie) or a placebo cookie to 52 children in a randomized controlled trial. Children were asked to eat two cookies each day for 6 weeks. Half the children who ate the fiber cookies experienced a 50% reduction in the number of painful episodes. Over one-fourth of the children who ate the placebo cookies experienced a similar reduction in pain episodes. These results are intriguing, since the addition of fiber is a relatively simple and perhaps effective intervention for some children with RAP. It is important to identify the children whose RAP is due primarily to simple dietary factors and those whose RAP is due primarily to emotional factors with lack of dietary fiber as a secondary factor. Both groups of children would be expected to improve somewhat after treatment, but the latter group would not improve completely. Dietary management of RAP is also effective for children whose pain is due to lactose intolerance (Barr, Levine, & Watkins, 1979). Yet children's inability to absorb lactose may still be a secondary cause for RAP.

Behavioral methods have effectively controlled RAP in some case studies. Sank and Biglan (1974) designed a behavioral program for a 10-year-old boy who had suffered from RAP for 2½ years. He constantly experienced a mild level of abdominal pain and had severe pains lasting 5–20 minutes at least once each day. He had been absent from school for 45 of the previous 72 days. There were many secondary gains when he reported pain: His mother stayed home to comfort him, and he was allowed to enjoy any activities with no restrictions. The investigators recorded the frequency, duration, and intensity of all severe pain episodes prior to the behavioral program. During the program, the boy earned points for every half day in which he did not complain about severe pains and had a lower-than-average rating for his constant abdominal pain. As he was able to achieve these goals, the criteria for earning points were increased gradually. He earned a point for every half day he attended school, but he was allowed to attend school only if he did not have any severe pain episodes that day. He exchanged his earned points for nickels to purchase special meals, gifts, or family outings. When he complained about severe pain, he had to stay in bed and could read only school books; all his other pleasurable activities were restricted. His severe pains were eliminated during the program, and his constant pain decreased from a rating of 6 (on a scale of 1–10) to a rating of 3. His school attendance increased, so that he only missed 15 out of 107 school days.

Miller and Kratochwill (1979) used a similar program to reduce abdominal pain complaints for a 10-year-old girl who had suffered from RAP for a year. She had many episodes (an average of 1.5 per day) and frequently missed school. Her behavioral program emphasized time-out procedures, in which she did not receive any positive reinforcements for a specified time period. When she complained about pain, she had to rest for the day in her room with no special privileges. Her pain complaints gradually decreased during treatment, and she remained pain-free at a 1-year follow-up.

Some physicians provide supportive counseling at the time of diagnosis. They reassure the child that there is no underlying disease responsible for the pain, but that stress in the child's life is responsible. Often, their advice includes removing the stress rather than teaching the child to cope with the stress in a more adaptive manner. They are generally unable to integrate other methods that would augment the counseling, such as biofeedback and a behavioral program. Few systematic evaluations of supportive counseling for alleviating RAP are available. Many are needed, particularly to compare the efficacy of psychotherapy conducted by different health professionals. In view of the multiple contributing factors, psychologists and pain therapists may provide the most effective counseling interventions after diagnosis.

Apley and Hale (1973) evaluated "informal psychotherapy," which included reassurance with explanations about the syndrome, encouragement for children and parents to express their emotions more freely, and attention to the role of unrecognized stress in children's lives. Thirty children with RAP received treatment. These patients were assessed 10–14 years later and compared with an untreated group of patients who had been diagnosed in the same clinic. Approximately one-third of adults in both groups had recovered from their pains when they were children. However, the pains did not recur for the treated patients, in contrast to some of the untreated patients. In addition, the treated adults judged that their general well-being had improved, as well as their ability to cope with difficult situations. Berger, Honig, and Liebman (1977) evaluated the efficacy of informal psychotherapy with families and children. Of 19 patients, 17 no longer experienced pain after 18 months of treatment. School attendance and peer relationships also improved over the course of treatment.

The nature of "informal psychotherapy" generally has not been clearly described, so that it is difficult to draw conclusions about which components of the therapy are critical for reducing the painful episodes. Presumably, these include basic information about the syndrome, specific information about causative factors for the child and family, and guidance about how to cope more effectively with stress. Special emphasis should be placed on describing the therapy so that it can be duplicated in other clinics and evaluated for children with RAP according to age, sex, syndrome duration, and salient individual and family characteristics.

Counseling and psychotherapy are the primary cognitive interventions for children with RAP.

Limb Pain

Many children suffer from recurrent bouts of "growing pains"—a generic term that was adopted to describe a variety of limb pains of unknown origin in otherwise healthy children. The specific origin of the term has been lost, but it was used in a study entitled "Maladies de la Croissance" (Duchamp, 1823/1832), indicating that recurrent limb pains were already recognized as a problem in pediatrics. Intermittent limb pains continue to represent a common presenting complaint in childhood more than a century later (Bowyer & Hollister, 1984; Calabro, Wachtel, Holgerson, & Repice, 1976; Conrad, 1980; Illingsworth, 1982; Naish & Apley, 1951; Oster, 1972a; Oster & Nielsen, 1972; Passo, 1982; Peterson, 1977; Schechter, 1984). Recurrent limb pains or growing pains are characterized by the same features described previously for recurrent headaches and RAP. They are variable in frequency, duration, and intensity. Children with recurrent limb pains are quite similar to children with other recurrent pains. In fact, children often develop various combinations of these three types of pain simultaneously or successively.

As with other recurrent pains, the differential diagnosis of limb pain requires a thorough examination, because many organic conditions may produce similar aching pains; these conditions include stress fractures, chondromalacia patellae, juvenile rheumatoid arthritis, osetomyelitis, and leukemia. In addition, pains may be due to psychiatric difficulties, such as conversion reaction syndrome and hysteria. The specific diagnosis of recurrent limb pain should be restricted to children for whom the pain is definitely not a symptom of an organic disorder. Despite frequent episodes of severe extremity pain, many children have no evidence of disease and dysfunction and do not progress to develop serious illness (for a review of differential diagnosis, see Bowyer & Hollister, 1984).

Initially, these pains were assumed to be symptomatic of rheumatic fever. However, children with subacute rheumatic fevers subsequently exhibited other signs of true systemic illness, which differentiated them from children with growing pains (Shapiro, 1939). Oster (1972a) reviews the significance of childhood growing pains and concludes that although these pains are not directly related to children's physiological growth, so that the term is a slight misnomer, they do represent a common affliction that requires objective evaluation and treatment.

Prevalence and Incidence

A few regional surveys have been conducted to determine the prevalence of recurrent limb pains. Hawksley (1938) evaluated growing pains as symptoms of rheumatic disease and reported that 33.6% of 505 children (4-14 years old) had a history of growing pains. In another survey of three geographical (and presumably ethnically distinct) regions, he noted a differential incidence, suggesting different constitutional factors (Hawksley, 1931). Brenning (1960) surveyed two groups of Swedish children: 257 children aged 6-7, and 419 aged 10-11. The incidence of limb pains was approximately 20% for all children in the older group, but was 9.1% and 18.4% for boys and girls, respectively, in the younger group.

Naish and Apley (1951) interviewed 721 schoolchildren in Bristol, England, about their pain experiences and then examined those children who indicated that they had recurrent limb pains. Only 4.2% of these children suffered limb pains, as defined according to their strict criteria: (1) The pains had occurred over a 3-month period; (2) the pains were not specifically located in the joints; and (3) the pains interfered with children's normal activities. Peak incidence occurred between 8 and 12 years of age.

Oster's (1972a) later study showed prevalence of recurrent limb pains in 12.5% of boys and 18.4% of girls. The prevalence was constant for boys until the age of 13, at which it rapidly decreased. The prevalence for girls peaked at age 11 and remained high throughout adolescence. Kaiser (1927) reported that 7.1% of 48,000

Rochester, New York, school children had growing pains; however, this estimate also included children with pains due to rheumatic disease. Seham and Hilbert (1933) estimated that 23% of 208 children aged 7–15 years suffered from recurrent pains as a result of recurrent pain syndrome or rheumatic conditions. At present, there is no valid determination of the proportion of children with growing pains.

Oster and Nielsen (1972) concluded that these pains were common in children and bore no relationship to chronic disease. The pains were interpreted as a manifestation of a specific coping pattern. The current concept of "growing pains" is that of a very specific symptom complex involving deep pain, usually in the lower limbs. There is frequently an emotional component to the pains, but there has been no solid evidence on the actual pathophysiology of this syndrome. It is generally accepted that growing pains do not progress to serious organic disease, and that they often remit over time.

The Child with Limb Pains

Children with recurrent limb pains are strikingly similar to children with other recurrent pains. In fact, most of the children with various growing pains and limb aches who have been referred to our pain clinc have also had frequent abdominal pains and headaches. Laura, a 14-year-old girl, suffered daily from an alternatively sharp and aching pain in her knees, hips, ankles, and wrists. She had experienced various limb and joint aches since she was 2 years old. Throughout the subsequent 12 years, she had been examined by many specialists, but there was no evidence of a disease or disorder that would have accounted for the pains. During the last few years, she had complained about many headaches and stomachaches. She had missed 25 days of school in the past semester.

Laura had experienced much stress since she was 4. Her parents had divorced at about that time, and her sister had died. When she was 10, her mother remarried and had two children within the next 3 years. Her mother described Laura as a very quiet child with others, but a constant complainer and whiner within the family. The results of the pain assessment indicated that Laura had serious emotional problems. Her scores on standardized measures indicated that she was extremely anxious and depressed. Laura would not have benefited from pain management without concurrent psychiatric counseling. The family decided to follow the recommendation for psychiatric consultation. We were unable to contact them for follow-up, so we do not know whether her pains persisted.

Nancy, another 14-year-old girl, had suffered from daily aches in her ankles, knees, wrists, elbows, toes, neck, shoulder, knuckles, and back for the past 5 years. She chose somewhat contradictory terms on the CCPQ to describe the quality of these pains—"sharp," "dull," "aching," "throbbing," "stinging," and "burning." (Few children select all the words provided.) Her pains started in the morning in her foot and spread up her body "like a chain reaction." She believed that most physical activities caused the pain, particularly writing, cycling, and running. She rested on her heated water bed when the pain was too strong to ignore, or she received anti-inflammatory drugs from her mother. Nancy reported 29 pains on her diary in 1 month, with some pains listed in her throat, teeth, and head in addition to her usual sites.

Her scores on standardized testing were atypically high, indicating a strong preoccupation with somatic complaints, severe depression, and high anxiety. She had difficulties with her peers and was unable to make friends. Many aspects of her life were stressful; as a consequence, she tended to avoid events that involved her peers, such as sports and social functions. Although her pains allowed her to escape some stressful situations, they also prevented her from developing appropriate social skills and having any fun with other adolescents. Unfortunately, Nancy's parents did not wish to pursue the recommendations from the assessment after they had been informed by the rheumatologist that there was no evidence of underlying disease.

Michael, an 8-year-old boy, had had a constant pain in his hip and knee for 2 months. At times, the pain was so strong that he was unable to walk. His pain began shortly after he had fallen but had apparently not injured himself. He had tried aspirin, rest, and a vibrator, but none of these interventions relieved his pain. He also experienced frequent stomachaches. At the time of referral Michael was in the hospital for further tests, the results of which were negative. The results of his pain assessment indicated that Michael had some difficulties in relating to his siblings and peers, and that he received many benefits from his pain. His father had taken a leave of absence from his job to care for him. His mother believed that she should encourage Michael to function as normally as possible, but his father adopted a very protective stance and inadvertently encouraged Michael to remain an invalid.

Because behavioral factors were responsible for maintaining his pain complaints, an in-hospital behavioral program was initiated to increase Michael's independence in assuming responsibility for his own care and in completing his physiotherapy. He earned points for completing certain duties; he was only able to see his father evenings instead of throughout the day, and only if he had earned a sufficient number of points. Within 1 week Michael was able to stand, sit, and walk without assistance. However, he continued to complain constantly about pain, and he was very angry. After 2 weeks he reported that his pain was gone. At a 1-month follow-up, he was able to run and play without pain.

These three children were included in a study to characterize the features of recurrent limb pain syndrome. Although the study is in an early stage, the same range of features that have been documented for recurrent headaches seem to be present. The pains have similar variability in onset, duration, and strength, with many situational, emotional, behavioral, and familial factors responsible for initiating new episodes. Salient differences, either between limb pains and recurrent headaches or stomachaches or between the children who suffer from them, are not yet apparent.

Management of Limb Pains

In view of the similarity among the three recurrent pain syndromes, the same interventions that have been applied successfully to control headaches and RAP should be effective for recurrent limb pains. At present, no treatment studies have focused specifically on limb pains, so it is impossible to determine at present which of the wide array of pharmacological, physical, and cognitive-behavioral interventions might be most appropriate for these pains. In my clinical experience, the most effective intervention for reducing limb pains is the multistrategy pain program described in the next section. In spite of the possible wide prevalence of this syndrome, few children with limb pains are referred to our pain clinic. The diagnosis of "growing pains" connotes a normal, benign complaint that will be resolved naturally as a child matures. This diagnosis may not cause the same anxiety and concerns that a diagnosis of headaches and abdominal pains (of presumably unknown etiology, with an unknown prognosis) can create for parents and children. It would be interesting to compare how often physician and hospital referrals for pain complaints are made for children who have been diagnosed with "growing pains" and how often they are made for those diagnosed with other recurrent pains. Although the pains may initially develop as a result of similar factors, the latter group of children may have more complications, simply because of the continuing search for a cause and effective treatment. The label of "growing pains" implies both a cause and a treatment.

Multistrategy Program for Reducing Recurrent Pains

A multistrategy program for children and adolescents with recurrent pain syndromes was designed in our pain clinic. Pain assessments conducted for 200 children with migraine and tension headaches (McGrath, 1987b; McGrath & Hinton, 1987) indicated that there were many common causative factors, so that an integrated approach combining physical, cognitive, and behavioral interventions was necessary. Yet the extent to which these contributing factors represented primary or secondary causes varied among children, so that the program also needed to be flexible to allow different emphases (e.g., behavioral or cognitive) and to provide different strategies (e.g., concrete or abstract), according to the primary factors responsible for the pains and the unique needs of each child and family. Essentially, several methods were selected in order to provide children with accuate information about the syndrome, to teach them a versatile repertoire of pain control techniques during painful episodes, and to teach them how to recognize and resolve stressful issues that could trigger pains. Throughout the program, children learn how to change their behaviors to decrease the frequency of painful episodes. They and their parents also learn about recurrent pain syndromes, endogenous pain-inhibitory systems, and nonpharmacological methods of pain control. As parents understand how their own responses to their children's pain complaints can actually increase the frequency and intensity of the pains, parents modify their own behaviors to minimize any aversive effects.

An eight-session program was developed and gradually refined. Children are seen by the pain therapist for 1 hour every 2 weeks. Their parents are also asked to attend part of each session, but usually only their mothers attend regularly. The program is scheduled over a 4-month period, because children and families require sufficient time to modify factors that contribute to the pains. The handouts children receive and the homework they complete during the program are included in the Appendices to this chapter.

Session 1

The program begins with a thorough pain assessment. Each child's responses on the measures listed in Table 8.1 are scored and interpreted to yield pain profiles comprised of sensory (quality, intensity, location, duration, and frequency of pains), situational (expectations, control, relevance, coping strategies, precipitating events), emotional (anxiety, depression, elevations on personality measures), and familial (parental responses, parent–child perspectives of familial relationships) dimensions.

Although no one pain profile adequately characterizes all children, some typical patterns emerge from the personality inventories. Two common Basic Personality Inventory (BPI) profiles are shown in Figure 8.2. (For information on the BPI, see Jackson, 1976; Jackson et al., 1986.) As shown, many children have significantly elevated scores on the Anxiety scale of the BPI. In addition, many children's scores yield a V-shaped profile, with high scores on Hypochondriasis and Denial combined with a low score on Depression. These children tend to deny many of the usual problems (school, peer, and family) that most children experience. On clinical interview, they present as more mature than their ages and appear as if they are in complete control of their lives. Most children with recurrent pains are not severely depressed, as determined from the clinical interview and their responses on the Children's Depression Scale (CDS; Lang & Tisher, 1978).

The CDS was added to the pain assessment after the first study was completed, when some children and adolescents showed elevated scores on the Depression subscale of the BPI. As yet, we do not have sufficient information to describe the typical CDS profiles for children with recurrent pains. Similarly, sufficient information has not yet been collected about mother–child responses on the Family Assessment Measure (FAM; Skinner, Steinhauer, & Santa-Barbara, 1983). The FAM was added after the first study to provide a quantitative measure for children's perceptions about their families and their roles within the families. Our clinical impressions indicated some common problems concerning children's independence, general problem-solving within the family, and mother–child dynamics. (The children's patterns on the FAM and CDS will be analyzed when we

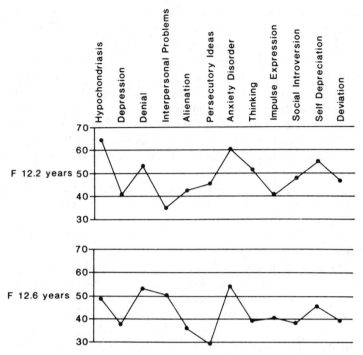

FIGURE 8.2. Profiles on the Basic Personality Inventory are shown for two girls diagnosed with recurrent pain syndrome. Elevations for the Hypochondriasis and Anxiety subscales (see top profile) are common for adolescents who have experienced recurrent headaches for several years. Both profiles show the V shape common for a subset of adolescents with recurrent pain syndrome.

have collected data from ~ 200 children with recurrent pain syndromes, so that we can objectively evaluate differences in profile due to pain intensity, frequency, syndrome duration, sex, and age.)

Session 2

The second session of the pain program is a feedback appointment, in which the results of the assessment are reviewed with parents and information is provided to them about the nature and treatment of recurrent pain syndromes. Parents receive a brief explanation about migraines and tension headaches, abdominal pains, or limb pains (depending on the child's problem), using diagrams to illustrate how pains develop. Common precipitating and maintaining factors are described. Inconsistent parental responses, avoidance of unpleasant situations (social occasions, school), decreased expectations for performance (scholastic achievement, sports, household responsibilities), increased attention or special privileges, and conditioned pain triggers are discussed as the major behavioral factors.

The primary emotional factors affecting children are anxiety and fear related to recurrent pains, an inability to relax, general anxiety about events, depression, an inability to identify and resolve stressful issues, excessively high expectations for achievement, an outward maturity beyond children's chronological age, inability to recognize and express emotions, and somatization of emotional distress. Common familial factors are positive family history of pain, high parental expectations for children's performance, strong dependence on parental reassurance and medication during painful episodes, few or no independent coping strategies, a continuous search for external and environmental causes with little attention to internal factors, overprotective parents, and (in single-parent families) treatment of a child as an adult spouse who is expected to provide emotional support to the parent.

Parents are asked whether any of these factors are relevant for their child, to initiate discussion about the specific results of the assessment. The therapist then describes the primary and secondary contributing factors for the child, without attempting to identify the original factors that began the syndrome. Generally, children's pains cannot be clearly traced to a single traumatic event; therefore, it is more therapeutic to focus on the current maintaining factors than to focus on the probable cause of the first pain episode. The feedback session is based on the present situation. The emphasis is placed on an explanation of the current reasons for the recurrent pains, so that they may be addressed in the subsequent program. Even when the pain syndrome began after the death of a family member or during a marital separation, so that the initial cause is known, the focus continues to be on the factors responsible for maintaining the pains. The multistrategy program is then outlined to the parents and child.

Session 3

Parents

The therapist briefly reviews pain occurrence and any pain interventions used since the feedback session, to determine the number of pains, severity, degree of incapacitation, probable causes, and efficacy of interventions. Parents describe any insights acquired from feedback. The therapist uses this information to provide specific suggestions about how the parents can help the child to reduce pain and any maladaptive pain behaviors, by responding consistently to the child in a manner that promotes independent coping and encourages routine activities, particularly school attendance. The main features (triggers, maintaining factors) from the feedback session are reviewed again, and the plans for the child's session are described.

Child

The child briefly describes any pains and stressful issues that have developed since the feedback session. The therapist leads the conversation so the child can naturally relate what has been happening at home and in school. The child completes the clinic form (a completed form is shown in Figure 8.3) to rate the strength and unpleasantness of any recurrent pains and the efficacy of all interventions. He/she then discusses the possible triggers for these pains, while the therapist emphasizes the triggers and factors identified from the pain assessment. The therapist provides a detailed feedback about why some emotions and situations can lead to recurrent pains, using illustrations from the child's life, and outlines how the various components of the program can reduce the pains.

Homework

Parents are asked to complete a diary of events (Appendix 8.1), not only to monitor potential triggers but also to assist them to evaluate more objectively the relationship between daily events and the child's emotions. The diary enables the parents to note their actual responses to the child's pains. They may believe they respond in a certain manner, and may not recognize how they truly respond. A blank cassette tape is requested for the next session so that the child can make a relaxation tape. The child receives a "pain file" for storing handouts and a few headache logs (see Appendix 8.2; abdominal pain and limb pain logs are also available) to complete for any pains he/she develops until the next session.

Session 4

Parents

The therapist briefly reviews the child's progress and the diary of events to provide suggestions and recommendations about increasing the child's independence during painful episodes. The therapist also explains the biofeedback equipment and presents the rationale for its use. If the parents have responded inconsistently to the child's pain complaints, a behavioral program is designed. The usual goals are to provide parents with a set response (the same verbal reassurances and the same behaviors) whenever the child complains about pain, and to encourage the child to participate in normal activities as much as possible. The parents may need a therapist's support to send the child to school or to refrain from picking the child up whenever he or she has pain away from home. This support seems most effective when a behavioral contract, containing clear information about what should happen throughout the program to eventually reduce pains, is signed with the parents and child.

HEADACHE STUDY - CLINIC FORM

Child's code:...Margaret.D:.............. Date:.....................Session:.3...

Weeks since last session:.....2......... Face sheet color:...blue...............

Have you had any headaches since the last session?   Yes..✓...   No.....

How many pain episodes did you have? ...3....

How long did they last? (Range and average) ....1/2.day......................

How strong was your pain usually, that is, how much did it hurt most of the time?

|————————————————————+——————————————————————————————| 58

How unpleasant was your pain usually, that is, how much did it bother you?

|————————————————————+——————————————————————————————| 59

Which face looked like you felt when your pain was at its usual strength? ...8... .75

SUSPECTED CAUSES	INTERVENTIONS	EFFICACY
? heat	– listening to Sandman tape	– sleep
work		– relaxes
	– no meds	↓ reduces headache

FIGURE 8.3. The clinic form completed by a 16-year-old girl with headaches who was enrolled in the pain program.

The child and parents work together with the therapist to establish reasonable expectations for achievement in all areas of the child's life. The parents may learn that they may be inadvertently placing excessive demands on the child for performance, for emotional support, or for excessively good behavior. If the parents have taught the child not to express emotions openly, they are counseled about the aversive consequences of this and assisted to recognize the need for acceptable emotional outlets. Physical activities and exercise regimens may be modified for a child who has reduced exercise levels to avoid pain, or for a child who is so physically active that sports and exercise have become a source of stress.

Child

The child describes notable events during the preceding 2 weeks and completes the clinic form. The therapist reviews the pain logs and helps the child to identify possible triggers (e.g., stress, school, family, peers, sports). The importance of these triggers for other children is described concretely, with the child encouraged to discuss whether the same situations exist for him/her. The therapist then describes the biofeedback equipment and relaxation training, showing diagrams of the extensor muscles in different states. The purpose of relaxation and self-hypnosis as pain control methods is reviewed, and the child is shown how the machine operates. The child follows standardized relaxation exercises, using deep breathing and guided imagery. The therapist tapes the training session so that the child can practice these exercises at home.

The relevance of relaxation for pain control is emphasized, and the influence of emotional reactions on bodily functions is demonstrated while the surface electrodes are attached. The most convincing demonstration comes when the therapist converses in a regular fashion with the child after the electrodes have been attached. The therapist then introduces stress-inducing topics into their conversation. Although many children do not admit that they are stressed by school events or peer teasing, they often exhibit much higher EMG levels when they talk about these topics. Children quickly learn that their bodies may respond to stress even when they do not acknowledge that they are distressed.

Homework

The child receives the first handout (Appendix 8.3) and a blank calendar sheet on which to record the frequency of relaxation exercises. The child continues to complete pain logs.

Session 5

Parents

The therapist briefly reviews the child's progress. At this session, the child may already have improved, and parents are more willing to discuss the interactions of situational, behavioral, emotional, and familial factors as they relate to the recurrent pains. They have more insight as to the probable triggers and often request specific assistance for responding to the stressful situations that have developed for their child. The therapist checks whether they were able to follow previous recommendations and provides general assistance.

Child

The therapist reviews the child's progress and discusses events as the child completes the clinic form. The pain logs and homework are reviewed, with the therapist assisting and coaching the child to identify triggers and practice relaxation for pain control. The child describes the main points learned in the previous session, so that the therapist can verify that the child remembered the correct information. The therapist describes problem-solving, using the outline shown in Appendix 8.4; the emphasis is on problem identification and emotional reactions. The therapist uses relaxation training with biofeedback.

Homework

A child 9 years old or younger receives Handout #2 (Appendix 8.5) for relaxation exercises and problem-solving, a sheet for matching faces with emotions (Appendix 8.6), and a sheet for "feeling" words (Appendix 8.7). The child also continues to complete pain logs.

A child 10 years old or older receives Handout #2 and the self-awareness activity sheet (Appendix 8.8), and likewise continues to complete pain logs.

Session 6

Parents

The same format as in the preceding session is followed throughout the rest of the program, with an increasing emphasis on parents' assuming the role of facilitating the child's insights about the relationship between pain and emotional distress and promoting the child's use of independent pain strategies.

Child

The same initial format (update, review, and discussion) is used by the therapist to strengthen the child's awareness of potential pain triggers and to teach the child how to modify situations and his/her reactions so as to minimize painful episodes. The problem-solving worksheet is used (Appendix 8.9) to discuss problem ownership and solutions, using both pain-related and non-pain-related examples.

Homework

The child receives Handout #3 (Appendix 8.10) and the crossword puzzle (Appendix 8.11), and continues to complete pain logs.

Session 7

Child

The session begins with the usual review and update. More emphasis is then placed on problem-solving, using further examples selected from the child's own life. The child uses biofeedback and relaxation training, but chooses his/her own methods for pain control (e.g., guided imagery, hypnosis) to use with the therapist. The child also generates a list of relaxing activities that can be used in his/her daily life. The therapist again uses homework from other sessions to demonstrate which coping strategies are most effective for the child.

Homework

The child receives Handout #4 (Appendix 8.12) and continues to use logs.

Session 8

The eighth session constitutes a general summary and review of the child's and parents' progress throughout the preceding 4 months. Emphasis is placed on the parents' and child's applying the principles of pain control, problem resolution, and emotional expression that they have learned to new situations that will naturally arise within the family, the child's peer and social groups, scholastics, and sports.

Program Evaluation

A randomized controlled trial is underway to evaluate the efficacy of this program. The initial success rate in the preliminary study, as defined by a significant decrease in pain and in the number of headaches over a 4-month period, approximated 100%. Improvements were maintained at a 12-month follow-up for about 90% of the children sampled. Only about 20% of the children assessed were randomly sampled for follow-up, because the preliminary study was funded by a small intramural award. The high success rate, however, was compromised because

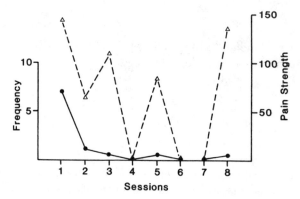

FIGURE 8.4. Headache frequency (solid symbols) and intensity (open symbols) are plotted every 2 weeks throughout a pain management program for a 10-year-old boy.

the pain assessments after children completed the program and at the 12-month follow-up were conducted by a research assistant who knew the children had received this treatment. A current extramural award will enable us to determine the immediate and long-term efficacy of this program more accurately.

Typical changes in headache frequency (solid symbols) and pain intensity (open symbols) are illustrated for two children throughout their programs in Figures 8.4 and 8.5. Headache frequency progressively decreased, whereas pain levels rose and fell more erratically over the 4 months. Figure 8.6 depicts pains for an adolescent whose headaches were primarily related to an underlying depression. Although her responses at the pain assessment indicated that she was depressed, she did not seem severely depressed, and she enrolled in the pain program. As shown, she did not benefit from the program, although other children with similar

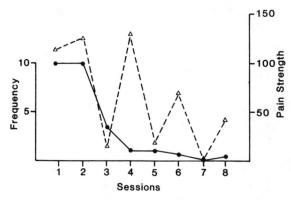

FIGURE 8.5. Headache frequency (solid symbols) and intensity (open symbols) are plotted every 2 weeks throughout a pain management program for an 11-year-old girl.

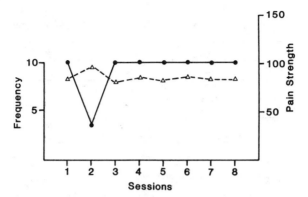

FIGURE 8.6. Headache frequency (solid symbols) and intensity (open symbols) are plotted every 2 weeks throughout a pain management program for a 16-year-old girl whose headaches were due primarily to depression.

pain profiles and some evidence of depression have improved. This program was not designed for children whose pain is due primarily to psychiatric problems and long-standing emotional difficulties. The current study should enable us to identify reliably at pain assessment which children will not respond to this treatment because of their depression and emotional dysfunction and which children will improve.

Summary

Recurrent headaches, abdominal pains, and limb pains share many common features with respect to the pain characteristics (intensity, duration, frequency, and quality) and to the factors that maintain and exacerbate painful episodes. Many children with one type of recurrent pain gradually develop the other types. The common occurrence of all three pains has long been recognized, as when Wyllie and Schlesinger (1933) coined the term "periodic syndrome" to describe this group of disorders. Figure 8.7 displays a pain diary for a young girl referred to our pain clinic for her headaches. As shown, she reported five headaches during a month, but also reported cramps, backaches, and pains in her ankles and legs. She reported more leg/ankle pains from normal activities (wrestling with her dog, dropping a pair of pliers, hitting her ankle) than other children without recurrent pains. She seemed preoccupied with somatic complaints, as evidenced by three pains reported on each of 2 days (April 28 and 29). A preoccupation with somatic sensations is quite common for a subset of children with recurrent pain syndromes. Are these children shaped by the experience of enduring the relatively unpredictable episodes of strong pain, so that they become abnormally sensitive to all sensations? Or are they predisposed genetically or environmentally to develop a variety of aches

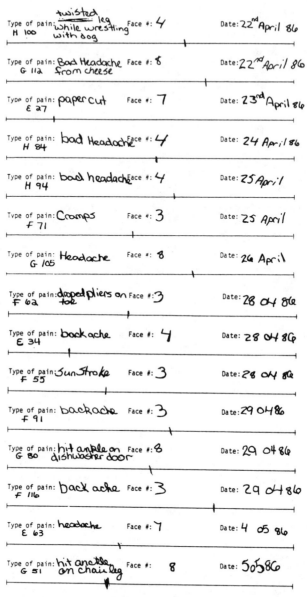

FIGURE 8.7. The pain diary completed by an 11-year-old girl with recurrent headaches. She rated the strength of her pain on a visual analog scale (VAS) and the unpleasantness on an affective facial scale. The actual face values for the nine faces (shown on a card in random order with number codes) are as follows: A, .04; B, .18; C, .32; D, .44; E, .56; F, .73; G, .75; H, .83; I, .95 (0–1 scale, with 1 = maximal negative affect). The faces chosen, along with the VAS pain rating (0–160 mm scale), are shown on the left for each type of pain.

and pains? Can their pains be alleviated? Or are these the children who mature into adults with chronic pain?

"Recurrent pain syndrome" is a generic label that denotes a variable set of common and unique features. However, emphasis must be placed on both adjectives, "common" and "unique." Regardless of the similarity in pains between two children of the same sex and age, there are still unique factors that may be primary causes for one child's pains, but almost negligible as causes for the other child's pains. The same treatment should not be expected to alleviate recurrent pains equally well for all children. Attention must focus on the unique features of the syndrome for each child, as well as on the common features.

There are no accurate estimates of the prevalence and incidence of these syndromes. Since an inability to cope with stress is an important and common feature, the prevalence may be quite high in some societies. Empirical studies and clinical reports indicate that fewer than 10% of these children suffer from undiagnosed organic illness. The vast majority of these otherwise healthy and pain-free children require some treatment, but they require treatment for the syndrome itself and not for an underlying disease. Their treatment begins with a thorough medical examination and pain assessment to obtain an accurate diagnosis. An accurate evaluation is essential—not only to rule out the presence of organic disease, but also to positively diagnose recurrent pain syndrome. The lack of disease should not imply that there is no need for treatment; rather, the confirmation of recurrent pain syndrome indicates a specific treatment regimen for children and their parents. The general framework for the treatment is based on the common factors that contribute to the syndrome, but the specific nature of the treatment depends on the results of the child's pain assessment. The extent to which situational, emotional, behavioral, and familial factors are the primary causes for recurrent pain will determine the unique composition of the treatment.

A pain assessment can be conducted by a physician concurrently with a medical examination. However, a more convenient approach is to schedule a comprehensive pain assessment after the physician has diagnosed the disorder from the medical exam, pain history, and general history of the child's and family's functioning. The information obtained from an independent pain evaluation, with structured interviews and objective measures, should be interpreted by the therapist and summarized in a formal pain assessment reoprt. The report includes specific recommendations to reduce the child's pains by teaching him/her some coping strategies and altering the identified factors that lead to painful episodes.

In general, pharmacological methods alleviate the pain of an episode but do not relieve the syndrome. An integrated, flexible approach combining physical, behavioral, and cognitive methods is more effective for controlling the syndrome. Multistrategy pain programs, designed after a thorough evaluation of the causes of the pains in consideration of a child's sex, age, and cognitive level, are the most practical interventions because they match treatments to the particular needs of each child. The long-term efficacy of these programs, however, needs to be determined in controlled trials.

At present, the specific etiology for recurrent pain syndromes remains obscure. It is probable that there is no single etiology responsible for each of the three syndromes. Family functioning exerts a powerful role for many children. Certain families have been characterized as "psychosomatic families": They are enmeshed (members are overinvolved with one another's lives), overprotective, and rigid (members strive to maintain the status quo), and they immediately suppress any conflicts that may arise, without resolving them (Minuchin et al., 1975). These same family characteristics are important in the development of other somatic complaints and eating disorders. It is still not clear, though, why some children develop pains in response to the same family characteristics and same environmental stresses that lead to different problems or no problems in other children.

The major impediment to deciphering the origins of recurrent pain syndromes is the lack of consistent documentation about children's pain and the situational, emotional, familial, and behavioral characteristics associated with the pain. Unfortunately, relatively little systematic research has been conducted, so that clinicians and researchers must draw broad conclusions from the study of clinical referrals or small-sized regional samples. Their inferences may be biased because of the size or nature of the patient base. Although it is tempting to draw inferences from our own clinical research program, I am reluctant to describe any definite etiological factors. Until the results of our prospective longitudinal studies are completed, I can only describe observed trends and my clinical impressions. Clearly, as indicated throughout this chapter, there are many similarities among children with recurrent pain syndromes and their families. Children seem to develop recurrent pains in response to stressful situations—stress that they fail to recognize and are unable to resolve. The pains remove them temporarily from the source of stress and may lead to some positive benefits through increased parental attention and decreased expectations for achievement. Their bodies' pain responses to stress are gradually reinforced and become aparently involuntary reactions that recur in potentially stressful or aversive situations. Some situations, events, or foods associated with painful episodes become conditioned pain triggers, so that they cause painful episodes in the absence of the original stressor.

The role of stress for initiating or maintaining recurrent pain syndrome is not wholly understood. Many stress factors have been cited, such as parental divorce, serious illness or death of a family member, overprotective or overanxious parents, financial problems, poor peer relationships, and academic difficulties. Yet not all children who encounter these stressors develop pains. It seems more probable that these children are unable to cope adequately with life stresses, perhaps because of parental modeling and their family dynamics. High standards for achievement prevent some children from accepting an average grade or athletic performance, leading to increased stress and pains. There is inconsistent evidence of autonomic dysfunction related to stress, suggesting that some abnormalities develop as a consequence of prolonged stress and then lead to pain. The true role of stress in recurrent pain syndromes will not be elucidated until comprehensive cross-sectional and longitudinal investigations are completed.

The accruing results of our research and clinical program indicate that a multitude of factors can lead to recurrent pains. Since children have had pains for an average of 2 years at assessment, it is impossible to pinpoint with certainty the specific causes of their first pain episodes and the precise etiology. Nevertheless, our focus on the present maintaining causes has led to the unequivocal identification of many factors, which increase and become more complex as children endure the syndrome for longer periods. Yet it is unclear whether the complexity arises from the simple endurance of these pains or from the lack of an explicit diagnosis and treatment, which forces families to continue to search for an explanation and hope for relief. The factors that perpetuate the syndrome may be different from those that initiate the syndrome.

Family characteristics are especially intriguing when one is considering the etiology for recurrent pain syndromes. Some families are particularly frustrating. Although they have searched persistently for a cause and a treatment, some parents refuse to accept the results of the pain assessment and refuse to allow their children to enroll in the multistrategy pain program, even when their children are severely disabled by frequent painful episodes. These parents are often reluctant to discuss family functioning, other than to present an ideal picture of relationships, shared responsibilities, and children's behaviors. Many parents, but not all, show the characteristics described for psychosomatic families. Their responses on the FAM reveal such a high bias toward depicting an ideal family life that the responses are not trustworthy. Yet how many parents whose children do not have recurrent pains respond similarly on the FAM?

Our knowledge of the etiology for recurrent pain syndromes is complicated by our lack of accurate statistics on the familial characteristics for healthy, pain-free children to permit necessary comparisons and enable us to test specific hypotheses. Epidemiological investigations must be conducted for all children's pains to allow us to eventually understand the etiology of recurrent pain syndromes. Until then, we must continue to identify the multiple factors that maintain recurrent pains and recognize that integrated multistrategy programs are required to control the syndrome effectively.

Appendix 8.1. Diary of Events for Parents

The purpose of this diary is to help us identify any patterns and triggers for your child's headaches. Please maintain this diary for two (2) weeks. Use the examples below as a guide. Complete the diary each day, even if your child does not have a headache.

Date	Time	Place	Who present	Activity	Emotional response	Pain complaints	Intervention	Additional notes
Mon 4 March	7:30	Home	Whole family	Getting ready for school—couldn't find his homework	Rushed, snappy, frustrated	No	—	
	12:15	Home	Mom, sisters	Home for lunch—on way out realized he didn't have homework done	Good mood; became mad	No	—	
	3:30	Home	Mom	Home from school—went to lie down and watch TV	Quiet, looked like something was wrong	Yes, "small headache"	Lay down, watched TV	Headache gone by dinner. Got into trouble for not having homework done.

Appendix 8.2. Headache Log

Name: _____ Face sheet color: _____

Please complete the following questions for each headache that you experience.

1. Day _____ Date _____

2. Time started _____ What were you doing when you started to get the headache?
   _____

3. Time ended _____ What did you do then? _____
   _____

4. How strong was your pain? That is, how much did it hurt?

   ├───┤

5. How unpleasant was your pain? That is, how much did it bother you?

   ├───┤

6. Which face looked the way you felt? _____

7. What do you think triggered this headache? _____
   _____
   _____

8. What did you do to relieve the pain? (If you took any medication, write down what and how much.)
   _____
   _____

Appendix 8.3. Handout #1

---

1. Do the exercises you learned today on your own, three times a week. Record when you do these exercises on your calendar sheet.

   Remember: Concentrate on tightening and loosening all muscle groups, then focus on a thought or image that will help you to relax. Block everything else from your mind.

2. What feelings, places, people, or things increase or decrease muscle tension, or make you feel tense or relaxed?

   Relaxed   *Tense*

3. What are the signs for you to show that you are relaxed or that you are tense? That is, how do you know you're relaxed or tense?

   Relaxed   *Tense*

Appendix 8.4. Problem-Solving, Part I

What is a problem?

A problem is a question or situation that makes you feel uncomfortable because you should do something, but it is difficult and you are not sure what to do.

What are some of the feelings that you have when you have a problem?

When people feel upset, it's often because they are having some kind of problem. Problems have some things in common:

- A problem can happen between people, or just with yourself.
- When there is a problem, someone is having strong feelings—uncomfortable or upset feelings.
- Problems that are not solved can sometimes make us not sleep well, lose our appetites, wet our beds, or have headaches or stomachaches.

Some problems . . .	*and feelings*
• Everyone in the playground has someone to play with except me, and that hurts me	• Lonely, left out, not liked
• Someone threw out my artwork and I wanted to keep it	• Angry, upset, hurt
• The teacher asks to see everyone's homework, but I didn't know there was any and now I'll get into trouble	• Anxious, worried, tense, scared

When someone has a problem, how do you know? What are the clues? How does that person look?

Appendix 8.5. Handout #2

---

1. Use your relaxation tape three times a week, especially if you have a headache. Record when you do these exercises on your calendar. (If you have not received your tape yet, do these exercises on your own, as we have done during our session.)

2. During the next 2 weeks, when you feel uncomfortable, think about why. What is the problem? How do you feel? What are the clues to how you feel?

Problem	*Feeling*	*Clues*
a. Teacher yelling at me	Upset, scared, embarrassed	Red face, hot face, butterflies in stomach, frown, heart beats fast

b.

c.

3. What feelings, places, people, or things can make you:

          Relaxed   *Tense*

Appendix 8.6. Matching Faces with Emotions

HOW DO THEY FEEL?

Draw a line from each person to the
word that describes how they feel.

worried

mad

proud

sad

happy

relaxed

frustrated

scared

Appendix 8.7. "Feeling" Words

1. *Charades*

   Play this game with your parents, brothers and sisters, and friends. Cut out the "feeling" words, fold them up, and put them in a box, bag, or jar. Each person picks out a word and acts it out so that everyone else can guess what it is. Can you think of a time when you felt that way?

2. *Fill in the blank*

   Each person picks out a "feeling" word from the jar and thinks of a sentence using that feeling. The person says the sentence out loud, without saying the feeling word. Everyone else must guess what the feeling is. For example, "Sally was really _____ when she came home and found out that her sister broke her favorite toy." (Answer: "angry.")

excited	left out
sad	worried
tense	calm
surprised	proud
happy	scared
angry	puzzled

Appendix 8.8. Self-Awareness Activity Sheet

Finish the sentence:

1. When I'm with my friends I like to _____

_____ .

2. I get frustrated when I _____

_____ .

3. It really makes me mad when _____

_____ .

4. I wish I could _____

_____ .

5. I get excited when _____

_____ .

6. I am disappointed when _____

_____ .

7. My favorite time of the day is when _____

_____ .

8. I feel proud when I _____

_____ .

9. I really get nervous when _____

_____ .

10. I am scared when _____

_____ .

Appendix 8.9. Problem-Solving, Part II

---

1. How do you feel? Last session we learned that we know we have a problem when we feel uncomfortable or _____ .
2. What is the problem? What is making you feel uncomfortable?
3. Whose problem is it? When we are with other people, everything that happens will be either okay or not okay. That is, we may have good feelings or bad feelings. The person who has the bad feelings has a problem.

The problem boxes:

You have a problem

No problem

Another person has a problem

Everything you do with other people can fit into one of these three boxes.

Who owns the following problems? What box do they fit in? What feelings go with the problems?

   a. You and your friends are playing a game.
   b. Your brother/sister is making a lot of noise and you cannot concentrate on your homework.
   c. Your brother/sister takes your toy out of the house without asking you.
   d. Your friend's dog died.

4. What is your goal?

   A goal is the way you want things to end up. If you have a problem, what is your goal? For the problems above, what would your goals be?
5. Before doing anything, *stop and think*! Brainstorm. Solve your problem by thinking of as many solutions as possible. A solution is one way to solve a problem. There are lots of different ways to solve a problem.
6. What are the consequences of these solutions? That is, what do you think will happen if you choose that solution?
7. Decide which ideas are the best. Throw out the bad ideas and keep the good ones.
8. Try one of these good ideas.
9. How well did it work? If it worked well, your problem should be solved. If you still feel bad, you still have a problem—try one of the other good ideas. Remember that only *you* are responsible for the things that you do.

Problem-Solving Example

Sarah has just moved to a new town and a new school. She wants to be friends with other girls and boys, but she is lonely and a little shy.

1. How do you think Sarah feels? What are your clues?

2. What is the problem?

3. Whose problem is it?

4. What is Sarah's goal?

5. What should Sarah do now?

6. Does it work?

Summary: Steps to Solve Problems

1. How do you feel?
2. What is the problem?
3. Whose problem is it?
4. What is your goal?
5. *Stop and think*! Brainstorm solutions.
6. What are the consequences to these solutions?
7. Throw out the bad ideas, keep the good ones.
8. Try one of the good ideas.
9. How well did it work? Is the problem solved? How do you feel?

Appendix 8.10. Handout #3

1. Use relaxation tape three (3) times a week, especially when you have a headache. Record when you use the tape on your calendar sheet.

2. Solve two (2) of your own problems using your problem-solving skills. Use the example given in "Problem-Solving, Part II" as your guide. Write down how you felt and thought and what you did, using the space below.

Appendix 8.11. Crossword Puzzle

WORD LIST

BRAINSTORMING
CANNOT
CHANGED
CONSEQUENCES
CONTROL
GOAL
HEADACHES
MANY
PAIN
RELAXING
SOLVED
WHOSE
WORRIED
WORSE
YOURSELF
PROBLEM

DOWN

1. The amount of pain we experience during a headache can be _____.
2. The first step to problem-solving is to determine how we feel, then we need to determine what is making us feel this way by asking "what is the _____".
3. Problems that are not solved can sometimes make us not sleep well, lose our appetites, bed-wet, or have _____ and other pain problems.
5. It is important for us to learn how to get more _____ over our pain.
6. Being _____ about school, home, or friends can give us headaches.
10. A problem can happen between people or just with _____.
14. A _____ is how we want things to turn out.

ACROSS

2. Solving problems can help make the _____ go away.
4. We have to say or do something to make the problem stop. Problems must be _____.
7. _____ is a good way to reduce pain.
8. It is important for us to determine _____ problem it is.
9. There are _____ different ways to solve a problem.
11. Being upset, sad, or frustrated during a headache will make the pain _____.
12. When deciding on how to solve a problem, we need to think about the _____, that is, what will happen if we choose a certain solution.
13. _____ is thinking of all possible solutions to the problem.
15. Some problems _____ be solved.

Appendix 8.12. Handout #4

Relaxing Activities

Homework

1. Use your relaxation tape.
2. Choose and do one of the relaxing activities above three (3) times a week.
3. Solve two (2) problems using your problem-solving skills.
   Use a separate piece of paper.

9

Chronic Pain

Any pains that persist for a prolonged period or that persist after injuries have apparently healed are classified as chronic pains. Several features, in addition to their persistence, differentiate chronic pains from acute and recurrent pains. Chronic pain generally is caused by multiple sources of noxious stimulation, affecting both peripheral and central mechanisms, rather than by a single source. The cause of pain is usually poorly defined, even when patients are suffering from known diseases. Patients experience prolonged physical and psychological distress as a result of their continuous pain. (The differential classification of pains as acute, chronic, recurrent, and cancer pains is described in Chapter 7.)

Emotional and environmental factors have a prominent role in the etiology of chronic pain for adults. Patients who suffer from prolonged pain inevitably alter some behaviors and activities because the pain prevents them from moving normally. As a consequence, their roles within their families, occupations, and social activities gradually change when they are unable to obtain satisfactory pain relief. Their outlook, their emotional state, and their ability to cope with the pain will be adversely affected. They may become preoccupied with somatic complaints and develop a variety of exaggerated pain behaviors. Patients become less physically active and less interested in the external world, and some adopt a passive sick role in all their relationships. This sick role, which protects patients from the assumption of usual familial and societal responsibilities, reduces personal, familial, and professional expectations for their achievement. The longer patients are protected from the stress of daily living, the more difficult their reintegration into their previous roles becomes. Chronic pain patients are characteristically different from acute pain patients because the persistent pain gradually changes the patients' lives (for reviews, see Bond, 1980; Bonica, 1977; Bradley, Prokop, Gentry, Van der Heide, & Prieto, 1981; Burrows, Elton, & Stanley, 1987; Linton, 1986; Melzack & Wall, 1982; Sternbach, 1978, 1984).

Millions of adults suffer chronic, intractable pain at a cost of billions of dollars annually to the health care system. Chronic pain is not yet recognized as a major health problem for children; however, little objective information exists about the prevalence and incidence of chronic pain associated with different childhood diseases and injuries. Without a precise estimate of how many children suffer relatively constant pains from disease and trauma, it is impossible to know the actual extent to which chronic pain represents a problem for children. Many children do have chronic diseases that cause pain. Presumably, their pain is well controlled, so that they do not suffer the same debilitating, uncontrolled pain that is associated with a diagnosis of chronic pain for adults. Yet, are children's pains from chronic diseases and injuries managed effectively, or have we simply failed to recognize their pains, in the same manner that we have traditionally failed to recognize that neonates feel pain?

In view of the lack of basic research on pain in children and the usual inconsistency in clinical investigations regarding the criteria for assessing pain, the reported incidence of chronic pain in children may be deceptively low. At present, there is insufficient evidence to support the assumption that children experience significantly less chronic pain associated with disease or injury than do adults. Like adults, children do experience chronic pain associated with cancer, arthritis, sickle cell anemia, hemophilia, neuralgia, accidental trauma, and burns. They also develop chronic pain as a result of anxiety, depression, emotional distress related to a chronic illness, and environmental factors that exacerbate acute pain.

Children's perceptions of pain are not simply and directly related to the extent of their physical injuries or to the severity of their diseases. Children perceive a chronic pain, such as arthritic joint pain, in relationship to a certain context. The context is defined by their frame of reference—that is, their age and cognitive level, their previous pain experiences against which they evaluate each new pain, the significance of the disease to their lives, their expectations for obtaining eventual pain relief, and their ability to control the pain by themselves. Children's emotional responses to pain are also determined by the context in which they experience that pain. Children experience different emotions, including anger, fear, frustration, depression, or anxiety, from similar pains when situational and familial factors are different. Certain emotions, such as anxiety about the outcome of an amputation to prevent metastases of a tumor, may subsequently alter a child's perception so that any postsurgical pain after amputation is exacerbated. Phantom sensations in the amputated limb may then be perceived as painful rather than as simple paresthesias. Therefore, it is essential to evaluate contextual factors and emotional reactions for children with chronic pain.

Despite the availability of many pain control drugs, the prescription and administration of analgesics for alleviating children's chronic pains represent perplexing issues. As noted throughout this book, clinical reports indicate that children do not always receive appropriate analgesics in adequate doses to control their pain. The mode of analgesic administration is often inflexible. Until recently, little attention has been focused in pediatrics on the effectiveness of alternate modes of analgesic administration. Yet versatile administration techniques integrated with nonpharmacological interventions are essential for chronic pain management in adults. The management of chronic pediatric pain is further complicated by a lack of objective information about the impact of different diseases and injuries on children and their families. Such information is critical for designing effective multistrategy pain programs for children.

The diverse array of diseases and injuries that can lead to chronic pain precludes a comprehensive description of all children's chronic pains within a single chapter. Consequently, this chapter reviews only a few of the common chronic pains treated in pediatrics. These pain problems have been selected to provide typical examples of each category of childhood chronic pain. Emphasis is placed, first, on the multiple factors relevant for each type of chronic pain, and, second, on the various interventions available for children.

Chronic pain falls into one of four broad categories, according to the primary source of noxious stimulation: pain caused by disease or injury; pain caused by life-threatening disease; pain associated with a primary psychological etiology; and pain of unknown etiology. (Only the first three categories are discussed in detail in this chapter.) Pains in each category share similar physiological, situational, emotional, and behavioral features. However, the strength and unpleasantness of children's chronic pains are also influenced by their ages, cognitive levels, and family support, as well as by the pain source and its life-threatening potential. (Table 9.1 lists the attributes of the various categories of chronic pain.) Therefore, though children with the same type of chronic pains share some common contributing factors, each child's unique circumstances must be recognized.

Chronic Pain Evoked by Disease or Injury

Disease and injuries are the most common causes of chronic pain for children. Arthritis, hemophilia, and sickle cell anemia can produce some prolonged aching pain, with periodic episodes of intense pain. Children who sustain nerve damage may develop painful conditions that persist beyond the apparent healing time of their injuries. Children who have been injured in accidents or developed serious infections may experience persistent pain for several months or intermittent episodes of steady pain throughout their lives. Children who are severely burned will experience constant pain as their skin heals and repeated acute pains during medical treatments.

The management of chronic pains associated with disease or injury begins with an understanding of the source of tissue damage, but must include an understanding of children's perceptions of their illness and the relevant factors that can intensify their pain. These factors will necessarily differ in relation to the type of disease/injury and to a child's and family's reactions to the prognosis. Prolonged pain evoked by disease or injury often results from multiple sources of noxious stimulation, arising in both peripheral and central nociceptive systems. In many instances, the specific source or sources of noxious stimulation are unknown. The

TABLE 9.1. Attributes Associated with Types of Chronic Pain in Children

Attribute	Disease/ injury	Life-threatening disease	Psychological etiology	Unknown etiology
Temporal duration				
Prolonged	A	A	A	A
Source of noxious stimulus				
Single	U	S	S	S
Multiple	S	U	S	S
Well-defined	U	S	S	—
Poorly defined	S	U	S	A
Biological significance				
Adaptive warning	S	S	S	S
No warning	S	S	S	S
Prolonged physical distress				
Fatigue	S	S	S	S
Restricted motion	U	S	S	S
Prolonged emotional distress				
Irritability, anger	U	U	S	U
Anxiety	S	A	U	A
Fear	S	A	S	A
Frustration	U	U	S	A
Depression	S	U	U	U
Hypochondriasis	S	S	U	S
Concern for future health	U	A	S	A
Relevant situational factors				
Limited understanding	U	U	A	A
Poor control	U	A	A	A
Inaccurate expectations	S	S	A	A
Relevance (life-threatening potential)	S	A	S	A

Note. A, always present; U, usually present; S, sometimes present.

pain is usually a correlating symptom of the disease process, rather than an early warning signal for disease onset. As a result of the multitude of internal and environmental factors that modulate nociception, no single treatment may completely alleviate the pain. Typically, several treatments have proven unsuccessful, so that patients are frightened about the possibility that they will have pain for the rest of their lives. Or their pain may only have been reduced to a lower level, so that patients must learn to accept constant, moderate pain.

The impact of chronic pain resulting from disease or injury is profound for children and their families. The responsible disease or injury generally causes some physical disability for a child. The family must adjust to the child's condition and any accompanying physical limitations. Parents are distressed by the condition and its implications—the life-threatening potential (if any), constant pain, and related disability. They tend to emphasize the future consequence of the condition and the pain, whereas children are preoccupied with the immediate consequences. Parents grieve when a child is injured or diagnosed with a chronic disease. Their grief is generally proportional to the severity of the condition, particularly whether it may be fatal, the extent of accompanying symptoms, the number of invasive medical treatments required, the aversive side effects of treatments, the nature of disability, and the intensity of pain.

At the same time, parents must provide information and emotional support to the child, his/her siblings, and the extended family. They may also assume a primary role for the child's daily health care. Often one parent, typically the mother, assumes most of the emotional responsibility for supporting the child and the logistic responsibilities involved for continuing medical care. As a result, unspoken resentments may build gradually between parents. Additional stress is caused if parents feel guilty about a child's condition, as happens when a chronic disease is hereditary or when a child has been injured in an automobile accident. Parents may blame each other for a child's disease or injury.

Parents face a difficult, protracted adjustment when children suffer from chronic pain; the effects are not static for either the parents or the children. Parental stress changes during the course of an illness or injury, as children respond or fail to respond to medical treatments and analgesic interventions. Children place different demands for support on parents throughout a long-term disability because its impact evolves as they mature. Initially, young children are primarily concerned about the interruptions caused in their daily activities and are frightened by their parents' emotional distress. Later, as they become increasingly aware of the future consequences of their condition, they become very distressed; they are frightened that they will not lead full and normal lives.

The dynamics within a family inevitably change as an injury or disease and the resulting pain prevent a child from assuming normal roles. Siblings often perceive that the ill child is receiving special attention, and they resent him/her. There is also less parental time available because of the increased demands involved in care of the ill child, so siblings may feel neglected. They need special assistance to understand their brother/sister's condition. Siblings may fear that they are responsible for the condition or that they may also become afflicted. Like the needs of the child with chronic pain, siblings' needs for information, support, and parental attention will change throughout the course of a long-term disability or illness. Siblings represent a special nucleus, the peers closest to the child, who may be ideally suited to support the child. Their unique needs and strengths should be considered in order to provide a positive family environment for the child with disease- or injury-related chronic pain. The manner in which siblings adjust to the child and to the altered family lifestyle will ultimately affect a child's pain. (Although few articles specifically address the problem of chronic pain in children, for reviews of articles relevant to children's chronic pain, such as children's conceptualizations of disease, the impact of chronic disease on the family, and the need for comprehensive management for chronic disease, see the following: Cadman, Boyle, & Offord, 1988; Campbell, 1975; Cataldo, Russo, Bird, & Varni, 1980; Dunn-Geier, McGrath, Rourke, Latter, & D'Astous, 1986; Herrera, Simmons, & French, 1983; Jordon & O'Grady, 1982; Karoly, Steffen, & O'Grady, 1982; Katz, 1980; Keefe & Bradley, 1984; Kupst et al., 1982; Lacouture, Gaudreault,

& Lovejoy, 1984; Levinson & Shear, 1983; Mattson, 1972; Mennie, 1974; Merskey, 1987; Natapoff, 1978; Neuhauser, Amsterdam, Hines, & Steward, 1978; Newburger & Sallan, 1981; Payne & Norfleet, 1986; Pless, 1983; Potter & Roberts, 1984; Prugh & Kisley, 1982; Simeonsson, Buckley, & Monson, 1979; Wiener, 1970a.)

Although chronic pain resulting from disease or injury causes prolonged physical and emotional distress for all children who suffer from such pain, the nature of their distress has not been well documented. Generally, these children do not sleep as comfortably as pain-free children, with the result that they may become tired, listless, and easily distracted. Children's normal motions are restricted, with the degree of disability related to the extent of tissue damage. Because of physical restrictions, young children may gradually withdraw from much active play with their peers. Since the major focus of social activities in early childhood is active play, the children can become isolated, frustrated, and anxious. They may become increasingly concerned with somatic complaints as other outlets for emotional expression diminish. The children may also feel angry, frightened, and depressed; however, they may suppress feelings of anger and depression in a sincere effort to cope well so that they please their worried parents. Continued emotional suppression can create serious problems as they mature. Older children and adolescents may be more emotionally distressed because they are more aware of the consequences of their condition. They may become extremely depressed and anxious. Some children are so preoccupied with somatic complaints that they are unable to participate fully in any activity. Instead, they are continuously monitoring their bodies for new signs and symptoms of illness/injury or for evidence that any activity is increasing their pain.

Most children and adolescents with chronic pain related to a disease or injury have a limited understanding of the source of noxious stimulation, the internal and external factors that can modulate disease activity, and endogenous pain-inhibitory systems. As a result, they have poor control over the situations that can exacerbate or relieve pain. They usually have few pain-coping strategies that they can incorporate into their daily activities to complement the medical management of their disease and the symptom management of their pain. In addition, children often have inaccurate expectations about obtaining adequate pain relief and about their abilities to lead productive, satisfying lives. As described in Chapter 3, these emotional and situational factors can exacerbate nociceptive responses so that a child's chronic pain increases; consequently, it is essential to begin to understand the nature of these factors for different types of diseases and injuries. Children's pains caused by arthritis, hemophilia, and trauma are reviewed in this section to provide an overall perspective for assessing and managing chronic pains evoked by disease and injury.

Arthritis

Arthritis, which is caused by inflammation of the connective tissues of a joint, may develop in conjunction with many diseases. Diseases of the connective tissue and rheumatic diseases, such as juvenile rheumatoid arthritis (JRA) and systemic lupus erythematosus, are the most frequent causes of arthritis in children and adolescents (for reviews, see Boone, 1983; Boone, Baldwin, & Levine, 1974; Calabro, 1981, 1988; Cassidy, 1982b, 1982c; Hanson, 1983; Jacobs, 1982; Varni & Jay, 1984). Children with JRA may develop pain, swelling, and stiffness in the small joints of the hands and feet, as well as in the wrists, ankles, knees, shoulders, elbows, and cervical spine. Joints may deteriorate progressively, leading to impairment, crippling, and increased pain. Pain arises from multiple sources, including the inflammation of the joints, chronic changes in articular tissues, complications of the arthritis, systemic illness, medication side effects, and affective changes (Hart, 1974).

Approximately 250,000 American children suffer from chronic arthritis, with an estimated incidence of 1.1 cases per 1,000 children each year (Baum, 1977; Calabro, 1981; Gewanter, Roghmann, & Baum, 1983; Petty, 1982). Children may suffer from loss of appetite, fever, lethargy, and depression. Although the specific manifestations of JRA vary widely among children, the common complaints are pain, swelling, and some physical impairment. There is no medical cure for arthritis; thus, the goals of treatment are to control inflammation, preserve joint function, relieve pain, and promote healthy adjustment to a chronic disease.

The diagnosis of arthritis has a profound emotional impact on children and their families. Families may be uncertain about the extent to which children will become crippled, suffer from pain, and not enjoy a normal childhood. The grieving that accompanies the diagnosis of any chronic disorder is exacerbated by these uncertainties. Clinical reports indicate that arthritic children seem quiet, introverted, withdrawn, passive, depressed, and extremely dependent on their mothers, but few empirical studies have evaluated the nature of the emotional distress that these children and their families experience. In fact, many clinical reports contradict one another with respect to the roles of stress, personality, and familial factors in the etiology or exacerbation of arthritis (Anderson, Bradley, Young, McDaniel, & Wise, 1985; Blom & Nicholls, 1954; Heisel, 1972; Ungerer, Hogan, Chaitow, & Champion, 1988; Varni & Jay, 1984). Similarly, reports describing the relationships among disease severity, pain, and psychological adjustment for arthritic children are often contradictory (Ivey, Brewer, & Giannini, 1981; Litt, Cuskey, & Rosenberg, 1982; McAnarney, Pless, Satterwhite, & Friedman, 1974; Varni, Thompson, & Hanson, 1987).

Blom and Nicholls (1954) described 28 children who had JRA as markedly disturbed, with overly involved relationships with their mothers. However, their patient sample was drawn from a group of children receiving psychotherapy, and thus is not representative of all children with JRA. In contrast, Cleveland, Reitman, and Brewer (1965) studied 30 children with JRA, aged 6–16, to determine whether specific personality characteristics were associated with the disease. Their study did not reveal any unique personality type related to arthritis. Heisel (1972) examined life changes in JRA patients for 12 months prior to disease onset. Children's life change scores were twice those of a matched control group. A move to a new school, the birth of a sibling, parental divorce or separation, parental death, and a child's hospitalization were common events that contributed to higher scores. Another study reported comparable evidence that these life stressors precipitated initiation of disease activity (Henoch, Batson, & Baum, 1978). Stress can trigger flares of disease activity, and perhaps can trigger disease onset in susceptible patients. But the relationships among stress, disease activity, and psychological factors cannot be elucidated without further study. Both cross-sectional and longitudinal investigations, which begin before the onset of disease activity, are required to determine any causal relationships among these variables.

Similar ambiguity exists in the relationships among stress, pain, and disease severity. In an initial validity study for the Varni–Thompson Pediatric Pain Questionnaire (described in Chapter 2), 25 children from 5 to 15 years old rated the sensory, evaluative, and affective qualities of their arthritic pain (Varni et al., 1987). The majority of children chose the terms "sore" and "aching" to describe their painful sensations; approximately half the children chose "tiring" as an affective descriptor and "uncomfortable," "miserable," and "horrible" as evaluative descriptors. Children's pain ratings on a visual analog scale (VAS) increased with increases in disease activity.

McAnarney et al. (1974) evaluated the effects of disease severity and existing disability on psychosocial status for children with arthritis. Children were assessed and rated according to the functional classification of the American Rheumatism Association: Class 1, able to carry on all usual duties without handicaps; Class 2, able to engage in normal activity, despite handicap; and Class 3, moderately to severely disabled. These children, like some children with other chronic disorders, had a higher rate of psychosocial disturbance than a comparison group of healthy children. However, children whose disease had produced no significant disability had *more* psychosocial problems than their disabled peers. Almost twice as many of the nondisabled had poor personal adjustment and low achievement scores on school ratings, in comparison to disabled children. In order to understand these surprising findings, the authors examined clinical interview data for children according to their disability status. A clear pattern emerged from children's responses: The less disabled children had higher expectations for personal achievement (education, social activities) than seriously disabled children. The children with fewer disabilities may have had confused perceptions about the extent of their eventual disability; their higher expectations for achievement, perhaps stemming from the comments of parents and doctors, created more difficulty in adjusting to the realities of arthritis. The authors concluded that the attitudes and behaviors of the family are major determinants of a child's adjustment to arthritis, particularly when disabilities are not severe. Wilkinson (1981) also stressed the importance of the family for assisting severely disabled adolescents in coping with their anxieties about self-image, dependency, and social isolation.

The impact of chronic arthritic pain for children is merged inextricably with the impact of the disease and any accompanying disability. As a consequence, a thorough pain assessment must include information about a child's (and family's) adjustment to the disease, pain-coping strategies, and social and emotional factors, as well as information about the sensory dimensions of the pain. Structured interviews with children and parents, quantitative pain scales, and standardized indices of disease severity and disability are the minimum assessment tools for children with arthritis-related pain. When possible, consistent information should be obtained about the emotional impact for a child and for other family members. We have successfully administered all the same pain assessment measures used for recurrent pain syndromes to evaluate children's arthritic pain. (These are described in Chapter 8; the measures are included in the Appendix to this volume.) It is essential to assess chronic pain from the child's perspective. The situational, emotional, and familial factors relevant for childhood arthritic pain are not necessarily equivalent to those identified for adults.

Clinical reports indicate that children with JRA may experience less pain than adult patients. Laaksonen and Laine (1961) compared arthritic pain in 24 children (4–14 years old) with arthritic pain in 30 adults. A total of 95 affected joints were compared for each group. Children reported less pain than adults during palpation, normal joint movement, and weight-bearing; also, children had fewer painful joints than adults. Scott, Ansell, and Huskisson (1977) assessed arthritic pain in 100 children from 2 to 17 years old. Their pain ratings were consistently lower than those for 100 adults. Beales, Keen, and Holt (1983) interviewed 39 children about their arthritic pain. They rated the quality of their pain (e.g., aching, burning), as well as its severity and unpleasantness. All children reported an aching sensation, and approximately half of the children also reported a sharp sensation. Younger children (6–11 years old) reported less severe pain and less unpleasant sensations than older children (12–17 years old). Older children attributed a more negative meaning to the joint inflammation and pain, because they better understood the potential degenerative effects of the disease. The adverse emotional impact presumably increased their pain (Beales, Holt, Keen, & Mellor, 1983).

Interventions that improve children's psychological state and strengthen their ability to cope with a chronic disease should produce reduced pain, because their pain is not directly linked to the extent of their tissue damage. Interventions for arthritic pain should be selected to modify the factors that exacerbate pain, as well as to reduce inflammation. As an example, Sally, a 10-year-old girl with JRA, described dull, aching pains in her ankles, wrists, feet, and shoulder. The pains varied in strength, depending on the time of day and her physical activity. In general, her pains were stronger in the morning. She rated 12 mild pains (average value 15 on the 0–160 VAS) on her diary over a 3-week period. Ten of these pains occurred in the morning when she first awoke; her pain steadily diminished throughout the day as her joints loosened. She took aspirin daily and received physiotherapy twice a week. Her arthritic pain had been generally well controlled, but she now required gold therapy. (Sally completed all of the pain assessment measures described for recurrent pains.)

Sally was referred for acute pain management because she was quite afraid of the scheduled gold injections. Sally was shy and soft-spoken during her pain assessment. She shuffled when she walked, with an exaggerated slouch and stooped shoulders. Sally had few friends and believed that she was unable to participate in most peer activities. She reported that most classmates disliked walking with her in the school corridors because she had to walk so slowly. Her mother provided strong support to Sally, but was very drained by the feeling that she was the sole adult primarily involved with Sally's emotional care and physical treatment. Sally's father seemed to distance himself from her disease and the impact of the treatment regimen. We did not speak with him directly, since he did not accompany Sally to any appointments. Sally had become quite dependent on her mother, even requesting that her mother choose her clothing before school each day.

Sally participated in a multistrategy program for acute pain (described in Chapter 7) and easily learned to cope with the necessary gold injections. Sally asked whether she could use some of the same relaxation techniques and hypnotic suggestions in the mornings to help her arthritis when her feet ached. When she first woke, she breathed deeply and imagined that her joints were warm, comfortable, and loose. She gradually felt more relaxed and seemed less apprehensive about dressing and moving in the morning. Her physiotherapist noticed a general improvement in her mobility and encouraged Sally to use the same techniques in her physiotherapy program. Sally also helped the pain therapist to teach another girl, with whom she attended physiotherapy, to reduce her arthritic pain. Although Sally had learned principles of acute pain management, she easily extended these principles to reduce her chronic arthritic pain and improve her mobility. Her gait and posture also improved noticeably. As she gained confidence, she interacted more comfortably with her peers and increased her participation in organized social activities. In addition, she became less dependent on her mother, with the result that her mother seemed more relaxed and less pressured.

Sally's pain descriptions and interventions are typical of many children with arthritis. Their stiffness and pain are usually worse in the morning and are relieved primarily by physical therapy and anti-inflammatory analgesics. Sally's sense of isolation, lowered self-esteem, and extreme reliance on her mother are also characteristic of some children referred to our pain clinic for growth hormone deficiency, recurrent headaches, and hemophilia, as well as for arthritis. The extent to which these characteristics describe arthritic children in particular is not known, because our referrals for pain management represent a relatively small sample of all children with arthritis.

We do know that children like Sally must adjust to arthritis and to the impact of the disease on themselves and their families. It is essential to recognize the manner in which a child's and family's emotional response to the diagnosis can affect a child's pain perception. These children need reassurance, assistance in relating to their peers as normally as possible, and therapy to control the arthritis and their pain. However, these children also benefit from a cognitive-behavioral program to improve their active pain control and to alter the aversive impact of the disease.

Arthritis should be treated from a multidisciplinary perspective, beginning with a comprehensive assessment of pain (Thompson, Varni, & Hanson, 1987).

Children require physical, pharmacological, and psychological interventions (Calabro, 1988; Cassidy, 1982a, 1982c; Cioppa & Thal, 1975; Sullivan, 1982). Physical treatments include therapy to maintain and improve joint activity through appropriate rest, exercise, and perhaps splints or casts. Aspirin is used widely for its anti-inflammatory and analgesic properties. Intramuscular gold injections are very beneficial for some children whose arthritis does not respond to aspirin (Brewer, Giannini, & Barkley, 1980). Corticosteroids (e.g, prednisone), which have a rapid anti-inflammatory effect to improve joint stiffness and swelling within hours, are used for children with severe active disease. Surgery may be indicated for the management of JRA to improve functional capacity and relieve pain (for reviews of surgical management, see Scott, Sarokhan, & Dalziel, 1984; Scott & Sledge, 1981). Cognitive-behavioral pain programs provide structured interventions that augment standard physical and pharmacological interventions. These programs are designed to inform children and parents about how to cope with the disease, disability, and pain. As children's control and understanding increase, their anxiety and pain decrease.

Hemophilia

Hemophilia, a congenital hereditary disorder of blood coagulation, affects approximately 0.01% of males (Hilgartner, 1976a, 1976b; Lusher, 1987). It is a chronic disorder characterized by recurrent, unpredictable internal hemorrhaging. Patients who have mild hemophilia often lead fairly normal lives; excessive bleeding ordinarily occurs only after significant trauma. By contrast, patients with severe hemophilia have multiple hemorrhages beginning when they are young. Trauma-induced bleeding episodes begin during the toddler stage, when children are learning to walk and fall frequently. Spontaneous bleeding episodes also begin during this period and will continue intermittently throughout their lives. Although uncontrolled bleeding episodes can cause serious complications or even death, hemophilia is not generally regarded as a potentially fatal disease, like cancer.

Bleeding, which can be triggered by physical trauma or emotional factors, may occur in any body part, especially the joints and extremities. Repeated bleeding into the joint areas eventually produces a chronic condition similar to osteoarthritis, marked by articular cartilage destruction, impaired bone function, and chronic pain. This condition affects approximately 75% of hemophilic adolescents and adults, so that chronic arthritic pain is a common problem in the care of adolescent and adult hemophiliacs (Dietrich, 1976). Fortunately, the treatment of children with hemophilia has advanced with the development of clotting factor replacement (Factor VIII). This concentrate enables the blood to clot to reduce bleeding. However, approximately 10% of hemophilic children develop an inhibitor to Factor VIII, which creates a serious problem for the management of bleeding episodes and pain. (For reviews of the management of the disease, see Abildgaard,

1984; Forbes, 1984; Guenthner, Hilgartner, Miller, & Vienne, 1980; Levine & Zeltzer, 1985; Lusher, 1987; Sergis-Davenport & Varni, 1983).

Hemophilia can be diagnosed at birth; in some specialized regional centers, the diagnosis can be made prenatally. The joy of such a child's birth is complicated by the sorrow that he has hemophilia, a genetically transmitted disease. Parents are frightened about the possibility of uncontrolled bleeding episodes that can cause death. They learn that the disease can affect other organ systems and that treatments can produce serious complications. Recently, parents are quite frightened that their children may develop AIDS from infusions. If a son with hemophilia is a first child, the normal parental anxieties about caring for a first-born infant are magnified; parents may be extremely frightened about hurting the newborn during routine physical care. As hemophilic children mature, parents are constantly aware that normal childhood injuries may prove fatal. Children can bleed when they are excited or upset, so that families may approach celebrations with some anxiety as well as joy. The lack of predictable emotional triggers for bleeding episodes further complicates parents' anxieties, as they are unsure about how best to protect their children.

The impact of hemophilia on children and their families has not been well documented. Children grow up with the disease, so during their first few years they do not fully understand how they are different from other children. As they interact more frequently with other children, they begin to realize that they are suffering from a rather mysterious disease. They generally do not understand that bleeding episodes may be triggered apparently spontaneously. They learn that trauma causes some episodes, but other causes (e.g., emotional distress) appear vague. They may begin to avoid certain situations, activities, and people for fear of bleeding episodes. Children's subsequent anxiety when they cannot avoid a particular situation where they had a previous bleeding episode can lead to a variety of learned bleeding triggers. The emotional distress associated with a situation causes bleeding, not the particular situation, in the same manner that anxiety can create learned pain triggers for children with recurrent pain syndromes (see Chapter 8).

Conversely, children may deny the possibility of bleeding episodes and engage in rough physical play against their parents' instructions. These children need to feel that they are like other children. Some children may be so angry and frustrated by their physical limitations that they act out, even if they require hospitalization later. How does the causative relationship between their behaviors and bleeding episodes affect their perceptions of the disease? Parents warn children that certain activities, often normal childhood activities, can be dangerous for them. As children engage in these activities and sometimes develop bleeding episodes, do they begin to feel more responsible for the disease and more guilty? If so, are they more susceptible to depression, anxiety, and lowered self-esteem than children with other chronic diseases? Their emotional responses undoubtedly affect the painfulness of bleeding episodes; children who blame themselves probably experience stronger pain.

Some children may use bleeding episodes to manipulate their parents and families, threatening that they will become upset and bleed if their needs are not met. These children will probably have more frequent bleeding episodes, but remain seemingly less disturbed by them. They may appear relatively unaffected emotionally, because the episodes provide such strong secondary gains. Situational and behavioral factors, rather than trauma and emotional factors, are presumably responsible for these episodes.

Effective control of bleeding episodes requires a thorough evaluation of the context in which children develop the episodes, as well as the responses of significant others. The sensory characteristics of bleeding episodes may be the same for two children, but the contributing factors are often quite different. Children with frequent episodes that are due to emotional factors must be differentiated from children with frequent episodes that are due to reinforced behaviors. Children may complain about chronic pain from hemoarthroses more frequently because of their emotional distress or because of secondary gains. The same situational, familial, and emotional factors that affect the acute pains caused during bleeds can affect chronic pain from degenerative disease.

Browne, Mally, and Kane (1960) described the impact of hemophilia on 28 children and their families. The majority of bleeding episodes were not caused by falls, cuts, and bumps; in fact, several situations were reported in which severe trauma did not cause bleeding. A boy fell from his porch and struck his head on a concrete walk, but he did not bleed. A few days later, however, he bled spontaneously into his knee joint when he became excited about a proposed fishing trip. This association between excitement and spontaneous bleeding episodes was a prevalent theme among families. Many common triggers were cited, including the start of school, holidays, Christmas, and family outings. These children were outwardly quiet and docile; yet the authors noted some rebellion, aggression, and anxiety. They concluded that the children's major psychological problem was a conflict about physical activity. All of the boys were concerned about their internal organs and the threat of harm resulting from their activity. They were also very concerned that they were always watched and spied upon because of their parents' constant concern.

The boys' mothers reported that they had felt guilty when they were informed that they were carriers of the disease. The authors described these mothers as depressed and anxious. Many expressed resentment and questioned whether they had been punished. Most mothers encouraged the children to pursue only passive activities and to develop younger, smaller friends. Only one mother encouraged her son to be physically independent—to climb, ride bikes, and swim. The reactions of the fathers were more varied than those of the mothers. Many remained aloof, attempting to deny the disease. They were generally active men who wished that their sons could be active and masculine. Some were apprehensive about playing with their sons because they might be injured. Many fathers belittled the manner in which their wives protected their sons. In fact, the authors described a common interwoven theme of mothers' guilt, fathers' ambivalence, and children's conflict about activity. The children's disease, both frequency and severity of bleeding episodes, appeared to be exacerbated by this family context.

The current impact of hemophilia on children and their families is not known. Advances in education, medical management, and psychological support should have contributed to less adverse consequences for children and their families than those documented by Browne et al. in 1960. We do know, however, that the factors they described are factors that can intensify a child's pain. In order to control hemophilia-induced pain effectively, it is essential to modify these factors.

The management of chronic bleeding-induced degenerative joint pain is similar to the management of any arthritic pain, except for the use of medication that may reduce blood coagulation. Anti-inflammatory drugs can relieve tissue damage and pain, but nonpharmacological interventions should be included for comprehensive pain management. Varni, Katz, and Dash (1982) described case reports to illustrate the efficacy of behavioral management approaches for reducing arthritic pain. Varni (1981a) taught two adult hemophiliacs progressive muscle relaxation exercises, meditative breathing, and guided imagery techniques. The therapist assisted patients to visualize blood flowing gently from the forehead down through all the body parts to reach their targeted arthritic joints, their ankles. They imagined themselves in a warm and pain-free setting, surrounded by warm red and orange colors, with warm sensations from sand and sun on their ankles. As the joints became progressively warmer, the pain lessened. Later, three patients followed this program using thermal biofeedback to regulate the temperature of the most severely affected joints (Varni, 1981b). The surface skin temperature over joints showed an average increase of $4.1°F$. Patients' pain decreased from 5.1 during baseline to 2.2 at follow-up (scored on a 1–10 scale).

Varni et al. (1981) reported a case study of a 9-year-old child with Factor VIII inhibitor. The child required narcotics to tolerate the pain of each new hemorrhage, as well as to reduce daily arthritic pain in his extremities. He followed the self-regulation program described for adult hemophiliacs. His pain lessened, and he required fewer analgesics; his mobility also improved, so that he was able to attend school more regularly and socialize with his peers. These case studies must now be complemented by controlled studies to ensure that the promising results are due to the treatments and not to random circumstances. Both the pain relief and the general health benefits of cognitive-behavioral programs should be objectively evaluated for children with hemophilia, so that the most effective aspects can be identified.

Hemophilia, like any chronic disease, requires a multidisciplinary approach including pharmacological and nonpharmacological interventions for optimal pain management. Pain management begins with a thorough assessment of the pain in relation to the child and parents. A therapist must learn how the family responds to the child and how they are coping with the disease. The structured interviews and standardized measures described in Chapter 8 provide a framework for distinguishing between learned and natural bleeding triggers. The assessment allows the therapist to interpret the extent to which a child's pain is exacerbated by situational, emotional, and familial factors, so that an appropriate treatment program can be designed. Children derive enormous benefits when cognitive-behavioral programs complement analgesic administration. They seem especially adept at using simple pain control strategies to reduce their pain. Their enthusiasm motivates them to actively seek new methods for reducing pain that they can adapt for their own lives. The more they understand about the causes for bleeding episodes, the less anxious they become during social situations. Children should receive guidance to enable them to distinguish between learned bleeding triggers and natural triggers. A therapist can help them to develop appropriate coping strategies in situations that may cause bleeding, and can teach them to gradually relax in situations that will not cause bleeding for nonanxious children.

More research must be conducted to identify the factors associated with hemophilia, in order to ensure that adequate pain programs are developed to meet the unique needs of these children and their families. At the present time, the probable factors that exacerbate their chronic pain and that can lead to repeated bleeding episodes can only be inferred from clinical reports. Children's anxiety, depression, guilt, lack of independent pain control methods, family support, beliefs about presumed bleeding triggers, and inaccurate expectations about functioning normally all undoubtedly influence their pain. Analgesic administration alone cannot control the pain-increasing effects of these factors.

Trauma

Trauma resulting from accidental injuries (including burns, lesions, and fractures) and surgery can lead to chronic pain for children. Either the tissue damage is so severe that healing requires many months (as with serious burns and multiple injuries resulting from automobile accidents), or the acute pain triggered by the original injury persists beyond the apparent healing time. The nature of the injury, the aversive impact, the potential for disfigurement and continued disability, responses of family and peers, expectations for recovery, and perceived control are all important determinants of how children cope throughout the healing period. The management of chronic trauma-induced pain begins with the recognition of the multiple factors that affect children's adjustment, and subsequently their pain. Pain interventions are naturally selected according to the primary source of nociceptive activity, as defined by the nature of the injury and extent of tissue damage (peripheral vs. central; need for anti-inflammatory action as well as analgesic action), but interventions must also be selected according to the unique factors that affect each child's pain. Optimal management of trauma-related pain, like that of disease-related pain, requires a comprehensive approach encompassing pharmacological, physical, and cognitive-behavioral interventions. Phantom limb pains and reflex sympathetic dystrophy are reviewed briefly here to illustrate why children require multidimensional assessment and management for the relief of chronic trauma-induced pains. (Burn pains have already been described in Chapter 7.)

Phantom Limb Pain

When a child loses an arm or a leg in an accident or surgical amputation, the child may feel as if the lost limb is still present. The sensations arising from the "phantom," the term used to denote the amputated limb, are quite vivid, so that the child may not believe that a limb was removed until he/she looks for it. Although approximately one-third of adults suffer from chronic phantom limb pain after amputation, children do not seem to suffer from persistent phantom pain. In fact, they have primarily acute pain from the surgery combined with some varying phantom sensations, as illustrated in Chapter 7 by the case history of a girl with phantom limb sensations.

Simmel (1962) investigated the incidence of phantom limb pains in children and in adults who had experienced amputations as children. Only a small proportion of children who had amputations before they were 4 years old reported phantom sensations and pains. However, after 4 years of age, the incidence of phantom sensations increased rapidly, until phantoms occurred predictably on amputation for children at or above 8 years of age. Phantoms occurred only when there had been some sensory and/or motor function before the loss of a misshapen limb for children who had undergone amputation for congenitally malformed extremities. Phantoms were not present for congenitally missing extremities (Simmel, 1962).

Browder and Gallagher (1948) interviewed 28 children and adolescents who had amputations. Phantom limb sensations developed after amputation for half of the children, whereas all adolescents experienced typical phantom limb pains. Although it had been generally believed that phantom limb sensations did not occur when limbs were congenitally absent, Weinstein and Sirsen (1961) reported that 5 of 30 children with congenitally absent limbs experienced phantom sensations. The authors presented a convincing argument that the reports of phantom sensations in these children did not simply represent the responses of suggestible children. The reports were elicited only after detailed questioning. Children's responses were consistent; they did not vary when estimating the lengths of their intact limbs or their phantom limbs.

The specific peripheral and central mechanisms responsible for phantom limb pain have not been precisely detailed (for reviews, see Bonica, 1953; Jensen, Krebs, Neilsen, & Rasmussen, 1984; Postone, 1987; Shukla, Sahu, Tripathi, & Gupta, 1982). The quality and intensity of phantom limb pains vary considerably in adults. Pains may develop in one site within the phantom or throughout the stump; pains may be sharp or dull; pains may be consistently present or recur in discrete episodes.

Many environmental and emotional factors can trigger or intensify pain, including cutaneous stimulation, other pains, weather changes, attention, and emotional distress. Similarly, a variety of methods can relieve pain, such as rest, distraction, heat or cold, and movement or massage of the stump. Pharmacological, physical, and psychological interventions are used for pain management in adults. However, since children do not have the same persistent pains as adults, they seem to benefit most from accurate educational programs as preparation for surgery, with appropriate supportive counseling after amputation. Children require reassurance that they will not have uncontrolled pain after surgery; some have been told about phantom limb pains and are quite frightened. They should be told that they will feel phantom sensations and should be encouraged to use rating scales to describe the quality and intensity of their sensations. They should also learn some acute pain control strategies to assist them with any pain after surgery. Many of the children who receive amputations in our hospital are quite active after surgery, receiving prostheses as soon as possible. Usually, these children experience vivid phantom sensations that dissipate over time, but they do not suffer from chronic phantom pains.

The psychological impact of amputation is related to many of the same situational and familial factors that affect children's ability to cope with a chronic disease. The extent of the amputation, the limb involved, the life-threatening potential of the disease that necessitated amputation, children's ages and cognitive levels, their coping strategies, their expectations about participating actively in their lives, and their families' responses to the amputation all play a role. Children require honest information and consistent emotional support to minimize the psychological distress of an amputation. They may require such support intermittently throughout the first 2 years after amputation, because the impact of their missing limbs will inevitably change as they mature. Children who initially cope very well may encounter a difficult period later as they face the reality of living with a prosthesis. Their emotional distress may lead to heightened stump pain or the development of phantom pains.

Reflex Sympathetic Dystrophy

Reflex sympathetic dystrophy (RSD) was first described by Mitchell (1871/1965). This syndrome is characterized by burning pain involving the peripheral portions of an extremity. The pain and dysthesias are not restricted to the area supplied by the nerve that is injured. Pains may be so intense that patients cannot tolerate the slightest pressure upon the extremity. Pain is almost always accompanied by mild to severe vasomotor dysfunction, either vasodilation or constriction. Frequently, the syndrome duration is prolonged, with functional recovery delayed out of proportion to any nerve deficit (for a review, see Ruggeri, Athreya, Doughty, Gregg, & Das, 1982).

The pain develops after some trauma (usually a mild injury) and is not correlated with significant nerve injury. Patients describe their pain as a constant burning sensation, which is exacerbated by movement, stress, and cutaneous stimulation. This pain develops weeks after the original injury and often persists indefinitely. The pain occasionally spreads to the contralateral limb. The specific mechanisms responsible for RSD have not been precisely detailed. Sympathetic blocks, physical therapy, sympathectomy, and corticosteroids have been used to relieve pain for adults.

Clinical studies indicate that several features of childhood RSD are different from those described for adults. Although pain, tenderness, and swelling are the predominant features, the syndrome seems milder for children. Many children do not exhibit trophic changes or vasomotor instability (mottling and temperature changes on skin), and seem to respond better to conservative treatments than adults do. In fact, RSD often appears to remit spontaneously for many children.

The relationship between emotional factors and childhood RSD is intriguing. Bernstein et al. (1978) described 24 cases of RSD in 23 children. The major complaints were pain, swelling, and vasomotor instability; however, certain personality traits were common. Children were entering into adolescence, but there was a notable lack of rebellion or overt resistance to parental expectations and authority. The authors concluded that the illness offered children a safe means of frustrating their parents' demands for performance without having to assume responsibility for their behavior. It also offered them a respite from home responsibilities, and perhaps from anxiety about coping with the broader freedoms of adolescence. A case from our clinic supports these observations.

Ellen, a 15-year-old girl, had sustained a minor injury on her left arm during a basketball game. Approximately 2 months later she reported a burning pain in her arm, spreading over the area she had injured. She was diagnosed with RSD and received physiotherapy. Her pain gradually increased and spread to a larger area on her arm. She began to lose some of her grip strength and adopted a protective arm position, preferring to wear a sling during the day. At the time of referral to our pain clinic, Ellen was barely able to use her arm and complained about constant pain throughout her arm and shoulder; she also reported a localized pain in her right arm. She was hospitalized for further neurological evaluation and intensive physiotherapy.

The neurological examination proved negative. Her physiotherapist described an unpredictable performance pattern: Ellen would have almost normal grip strength one day, but would be unable to grasp even a light object the next day. Ellen requested her medication (Tylenol plus codeine) at regular intervals, waiting at the nursing station at the specific dosing times. The nursing staff did not believe the extent of her pain, because she seemed quite happy and occasionally moved her arm when no one was looking at her. She was hospitalized Mondays through Fridays for treatment and was allowed weekend leaves to return home.

Ellen was the eldest of five children and assumed many family responsibilities. She was an A student who excelled in sports as well as in her studies. She cotaught a religious class for her church's preschool each Sunday. She denied any of the usual adolescent concerns regarding independence, peer versus family values, and sex. Assessment showed that there were strong secondary gains asssociated with her pain complaints, which may have prolonged the duration of her RSD. In addition, the nursing staff was inadvertently teaching Ellen to develop maladaptive pain behaviors to demonstrate more convincingly that she had pain. A treatment plan was designed to reduce maladaptive pain behaviors, increase independent pain control strategies, and eliminate secondary gains from the pain. Nurses rewarded Ellen (verbal praise) when she inadvertently used her arm; she was also told that some days her strength would improve and she could do more—the more normal arm movements did not indicate that she did not have any pain. Ellen learned some hypnosis and relaxation techniques to reduce her pain; she also relied less on analgesic medication. The nurses praised her independence. Her grip strength and flexibilty improved.

However, the therapist was quite concerned about her affect, particularly the fact that Ellen denied any normal adolescent feelings. This concern was discussed candidly with Ellen's mother during the feedback session from the pain assessment. Special attention was devoted to the issue that her pain was removing much stress, and that as the pain decreased Ellen might not be able to resume her previous activities without appropriate psychological counseling. Throughout the session Ellen's mother concentrated on her 2-year-old son, who, she insisted, could not be separated from her. She listened to the therapist's concerns, but responded that her daughter was unlike other daughters, that her family was unusually strong, and that they did not need any further assistance. About 3 months after discharge, Ellen developed a strange paralysis beginning in her left arm and spreading to her legs. She was readmitted with a diagnosis of conversion reaction syndrome and required intensive psychotherapy.

Ellen's case is typical of the features of RSD and the problems that can arise when pain behaviors are inadvertently reinforced. Fortunately, most children do not follow such a difficult course; however, more research should be conducted to evaluate the psychological status of children and their families to identify which children may be most at risk for RSD. In all cases, comprehensive pain management programs are required. Physical therapy is essential for the management of RSD and should be individualized according to the severity and duration of the symptoms. Patients benefit from both active and passive range-of-motion exercises. Pharmacological therapy is often indicated. More studies are needed to evaluate the efficacy of conventional interventions, as well as nonconventional interventions such as the use of electrical stimulation at acupuncture points described by Leo (1983). The psychogenic components of this syndrome are particularly important. These children are not malingering. Some children are responding to familial stress, which prolongs or perhaps initiated the syndrome. Children can also be manipulative so that they receive secondary gains at home; these children are better managed in a controlled environment, so that the pain–disability–pain cycle can be broken. Supportive counseling and long-term psychotherapy should be provided.

Chronic Pain Evoked by Life-Threatening Disease

Cancer, cystic fibrosis, and sickle cell anemia are potentially fatal diseases that can cause chronic pain for children. The quality, extent, and intensity of pain vary in relation to tissue damage and in relation to the individual child. Pains may recur intermittently in different sites and at different strengths, predictably reflecting disease progression, or pains may recur in an unpredictable manner with no clear relationship to advancing disease. In some conditions little pain arises from the disease, but invasive treatments cause intense pain seemingly out of proportion to the extent of tissue damage. In other cases pain may increase steadily throughout an illness, so that children experience severe pain in the terminal phase. Additional chronic pains can arise during the course of an illness when children suppress their emotional reactions to the disease and treatment.

The diagnosis of a potentially fatal disease has a profound impact on a child, parents, siblings, and extended family. As the initial shock subsides, parents attempt to understand a variety of new information presented in sophisticated terminology. They must learn about the features of the disease, treatment protocols, and adverse treatment effects. Most importantly, they must cope with the possibility that their child may die. Some uncertainty about a child's prognosis is inevitable; continual advances in medicine constantly improve a child's chance for recovery. However, this uncertainty can heighten parents' anxieties. Parents may question the probable benefits of treatments, particularly painful treatments. Some parents assume that certain diseases, notably cancer, will definitely cause their children's death. In contrast, other parents regard some potentially life-threatening diseases such as diabetes and hemophilia as nonfatal, despite the possibility of serious medical complications. These extreme assumptions, which underlie exaggerated fears and unfounded hopes, hinder parents' ability to support their children. Such unrealistic expectations can intensify children's distress and pain.

As listed in Table 9.1, the physical, emotional, and situational factors associated with chronic pain are magnified when children may die. The onset of chronic pain does not always provide an early warning sign for life-threatening disease. Even when pain initially prompts parents to seek medical treatment, later prolonged pain serves no adaptive function. Multiple sources of noxious stimulation are usually responsible for chronic pain, as the disease progressively affects many systems. Increased disability, toxic side effects of medication, and loss of normal social outlets can lead to further pains as a result of increased activity in nociceptive afferents and decreased activity in non-nociceptive afferents.

Children usually experience periods of extreme fatigue. They are restless and unable to participate normally in physical activities. Medications may cause adverse effects, including aches, nausea, bloating, disfigurement, and loss of hair. Changes in their physical appearance can lead children to become overly self-conscious and ill at ease with their peers. They may begin to withdraw from activities because they fear the reactions of their friends. Increased withdrawal and isolation can exacerbate their pain, or they may begin to complain about pain to avoid social situations. Children may become overly dependent on their parents to support and entertain them; at the same time, they miss their friends, so they become increasingly sad. When their prognosis is uncertain, they may become excessively concerned about all body sensations in a search to discover whether the disease is spreading. Children may be extremely frightened about dying.

Some children become increasingly irritable, as evidenced by an inability to concentrate on schoolwork or to enjoy social activities and family interactions. They act out in various manners—by provoking arguments with siblings, by disobeying parents, and by regressing so that many of their behaviors resemble those when they were younger. Children's anxiety may also be manifested in eating and sleeping difficulties. Their anxiety is heightened when they do not understand why their families are upset, why they require different treatments, and why they are sick. Some children openly resent their healthy friends and siblings, particularly if they require painful treatments and are becoming progressively disabled. Older children and adolescents will grieve for the loss of a normal future.

As with other types of chronic pain, children may outwardly cope with the diagnosis, the treatments, and their reduced ability to participate in their typical activities. However, they may actually suppress their true emotional reactions—anger, anxiety, and depression. These children may develop new pains and somatic complaints because their emotions have no other outlet. Children do not have any control over the course of their illness, and they generally have little control over their pain. Their lack of control has been exacerbated by our past failure to recognize when they are in pain and to provide adequate pain relief. They frequently have inaccurate expectations about their illness and treatments. Parents may prefer to withhold information from children, assuming that the children will be less distressed by few specific facts. Or parents may be so distressed when they discuss the illness that children refrain from seeking additional information so as not to upset them.

The impact of chronic life-threatening disease on children and their families has been well documented in regard to the physical, situational, behavioral, and emotional consequences. (For more comprehensive reviews, see Aronson, 1980; Burton, 1974; Drotar, 1981; Friedrich, 1977; Kellerman, 1980a; Lavigne, Schulein, & Hahn, 1986a, 1986b; Magni, Carli, deLeo, Tshilolo, & Zanesco, 1986; Morrow, Carpenter, & Hoagland, 1984; Pless, 1983; Pless & Roghmann, 1971; Pless, Roghmann, & Haggerty, 1972; Slavin, 1981; Sourkes, 1980a, 1980b; Wood et al., 1988; Zeltzer, 1980; Zeltzer, Kellerman, Ellenberg, Dash, & Rigler, 1980.) However, there has been little documentation of the specific impact of these factors on children's chronic pain. A child's chronic pain is undoubtedly affected by the same physical, situational, emotional, and familial factors associated with his/her disease. The pains evoked by two potentially fatal diseases are described here to illustrate how different factors affect children's pain and why comprehensive pain management requires recognition of their powerful mediating role.

Cancer Pain

Prevalence and Nature

Cancer is a relatively rare disease in children, with an approximate incidence of 2 per 1,000 (Altman & Schwartz, 1983; Diamond & Matthay, 1988; Sutow, Vietti, & Fernbach, 1977). However, cancer ranks second to accidents as the leading cause of death in children from 1 to 14 years old. Fortunately, the life expectancy for children with cancer is continually increasing because of advances in surgical, pharmacological, and radiation therapies. Many children with leukemia will remain free from disease after completing their treatment regimens. Thirty years ago the median survival time for a child with acute lymphoblastic leukemia, the most common form of childhood cancer, was only 3–6 months. Today, over 60% of these children will survive for 5 years, with increasing numbers becoming long-term survivors (Kalwinsky, Mirro, & Dahl, 1988; Katz & Jay, 1984; Siegel, 1980; Willoughby & Siegel, 1982). The prognosis is also improving for children with Hodgkin's disease, Ewing's sarcoma, and osteogenic sarcoma. The presumption that a diagnosis of cancer is synonymous with death is no longer valid. (For reviews, see Li & Bader, 1987; Sallan & Weinstein, 1987; Steinherz, 1987; Steinhorn & Myers, 1981.)

But the presumption that cancer is synonymous with pain is still valid. All children with cancer will undoubtedly experience some pain during the course of their treatment. Cancer pains are classified according to the primary source of noxious stimulation as disease-related, therapy-related, and coincidental with but unrelated to the disease (Foley, 1979). Children can experience chronic pain when the disease process generates nociceptive activity by invading bone, compressing nerves, infiltrating blood vessels, and injuring healthy tissue. Both acute and chronic pains arise from the tissue damage produced by blood-sampling procedures, lumbar punctures, bone marrow aspirations, intramuscular and intravenous injections, surgery, chemotherapy, and radiation therapy. The quality of these pains varies in relation to the nature of tissue damage. However, pain strength varies widely in relation to the individual child, as well as to the nature of tissue damage. In addition, children with cancer can develop pain as a result of the psychological stress of living with a potentially fatal disease. (For reviews of the nociceptive mechanisms associated with different types of cancer, see Bond, 1985; Bonica, 1953, 1979a, 1984, 1985; Foley, 1979, 1985; Janig, 1984; Wall, 1985.)

Children with cancer generally do not experience the same chronic debilitating pain as adults with cancer, presumably because of the different types of cancer that they experience (Altman & Schwartz, 1983; Jay, Elliott, & Varni, 1986; Kellerman & Varni, 1982; Schechter, 1985). Leukemia is the primary type of cancer that afflicts children, in contrast to the lung, breast, gastrointestinal, and skin cancers common in adults. Leukemias and lymphomas are not extremely painful diseases for children, even though they can produce joint aches during periods of active disease. Nevertheless, children with cancer do suffer pains caused by the disease, pain during and after treatments, and pains resulting from their psychological distress. Pain is often a presenting symptom for childhood cancers (DeSousa, Kalsbeck, Mealey, Campbell, & Hockey, 1979; Haft, Ransohoff, & Carter, 1959; Rogalsky, Black, & Reed, 1986). But there are no accurate estimates of the magnitude of different cancer pains in children. It is only recently that investigators have begun to specifically document the prevalence of childhood cancer pain within their own treatment centers (Cornaglia et al., 1984; Miser, Dothage, Wesley, & Miser, 1987).

Hahn and McLone (1984) reviewed the prevalence of "verbal" and "nonverbal" pain descriptions in the charts of 54 children with spinal cord tumors. The children ranged in age from 5.5 months to 15 years. There was a similar number of recorded pain notes for all children, but children under 3 years old expressed pain more through their behaviors, whereas older children voiced their pain complaints.

Miser, Dothage, Wesley, and Miser (1987) surveyed the prevalence and nature of pain in all patients (139 patients from 7 to 25 years old; median age 16) treated by the pediatric branch of the National Cancer Institute over a 6-month period. Approximately half of the hospitalized patients and a fourth of the outpatients had some pain at the time of assessment; the majority of pains were mild as assessed by VAS ratings (the median VAS score was 26, on a scale of 0–100 mm). Only seven patients had chronic pain for over 1 year after the eradication of all known tumors from the site of pain. Only one patient received massive doses of narcotics, which may have been high in relation to his underlying pain.

Miser, McCalla, Dothage, Wesley, and Miser (1987) surveyed the incidence and nature of pain in 92 children and young adults (ages ranged from 6 months to 24 years; median age 16 years) with newly diagnosed malignancy. At the time of assessment, 72 of the patients had been experiencing pain for a median period of 74 days. Pain had been an initial symptom of the cancer for almost two-thirds of the patients. Although each patient had been recently evaluated by a physician, many patients with pain were not receiving any analgesics. Patients were followed longitudinally from the initiation of cancer therapy until they became pain-free, until they died, or until their pain persisted continuously for 9 months. The median duration of pain after therapy started was 10 days. One patient died 5 months later without obtaining adequate pain relief. Four other patients experienced persistent pain for more than 9 months despite achieving tumor remission.

The two studies by Miser and colleagues evaluated a special group of children who had been referred to a treatment center; such a center selects patients whose malignancy generally has a poor prognosis if treated by standard therapy. Although the results of these studies may not be wholly representative of all children with cancer, the majority of children with cancer do experience pain at some time during their course of treatment and follow-up. Outpatient referrals to our pain clinic confirm the prevalence of acute therapy-related pains. In our hospital, increased anxiety during invasive procedures has been the predominant pain problem for children with cancer. Children are referred less often for the management of disease-related pain. Some children have been referred for pain assessment when they complain about pain in sites distal to identified areas of tissue damage or when their pain suddenly intensifies. Usually, their pain complaints have preceded detectable metastases. In a few children, however, the pain arises from emotional distress related to a relapse in disease remission, especially when the children have relapsed previously. Children who relapse are anxious, apprehensive, and frightened as they wait for the results of tests to define the extent of their relapse (e.g., central nervous system involvement). Their anxiety leads to additional aches and to increased pain during procedures. The children who realize that they may die are severely upset. Their anxiety is also manifest in muscle aches, headaches, and stomachaches.

Children's and Families' Attitudes toward Death and Cancer

The cumulative effects of some robust cancer therapies can lead to chronic pain. Children receive varied treatments over many years. Some children develop chronic back pain from disc deterioration; other children may develop chronic pain from irreversible damage to their gastrointestinal tracts. These pains augment any disease-induced pain. Children who are dying may be more susceptible to increased pain because of the emotional impact of the situation. Some children have been referred to the pain clinic because they complain about pain, despite seemingly appropriate palliative management. Some children require more potent analgesics, whereas others require counseling about their deaths. These latter children need to discuss their fears with an objective adult outside their immediate families. They often ask, "Will I be alone? Will I miss my family? What will happen?" Children should receive accurate information, consistent with their religious beliefs, presented in a calm reassuring manner. They may need concrete reassurance that they will not suffer when they die, that they will not be alone, and that their families will remember them. Children often know when they are dying, even though no one has discussed the possibility of death explicitly. Some children would like their brothers and sisters to know that they will die, particularly when their deaths are near.

Little clinical information about children's concepts of death was available until Nagy (1959) explored the attitude of a group of healthy children in postwar Hungary. Children's concepts of death varied with age. Children under 6 regarded death as a reversible condition, like sleep. Children aged 6–10 envisioned death as a person, like a witch or devil, who would take them away. At about the age of 10, children began to realize that death is an irreversible biological process. Children with acute leukemia on a special research ward were allowed to talk spontaneously about their own and their friends' disease. They were acutely aware when a child had died, despite some evasion by the staff. The children appeared to be helped by expressing their own fears about death and their feelings of their illness. Behavior problems often disappeared as more honest communication increased.

Much has been written about helping children and families cope with the children's illness and death from cancer (Armstrong & Martinson, 1980; Spinetta &

Deasy-Spinetta, 1981a). Children's understanding varies with their developmental level. Similarly, their need for information and support will change with maturity. Even preschool children can be sensitive to the cues of their families when death is near. Children and adolescents choose when and with whom to discuss their impending deaths. Useful discussions of guidelines, practical considerations, and how-to approaches grounded in clinical research have been compiled (Spinetta, 1980; Spinetta & Deasy-Spinetta, 1981a). First, one must understand each family's philosophy of life and views on death in order to discuss issues with the child within the proper context. Second, one must understand the family's emotional reactions and experiences with death. Families express their fears and their grief in different ways, and the therapist must understand each child's view of illness and death in relation to the family pattern. Third, one must understand how age, experience, and developmental factors affect children with cancer. Children of different ages conceptualize death differently, and their experiences with illness and death may advance their comprehension beyond what would be expected of normal, healthy children of similar age. Fourth, it is necessary to understand each family's usual manner of dealing with a crisis, so that one can support the family members themselves. Fifth, one must understand that children are more attuned to process than to content in communication. What one says to children may be less important than how one says it. Children require assurance that it is okay not to want to talk about death and that when they are ready to talk, someone will be there. They need to know that they will not be alone at death or afterwards, and that it will not hurt. Communication about death or illness must be geared to each child's needs and desire for information. An open and honest approach does not mean that children should be confronted with information that they may not want to hear or may not be ready to hear. Rather, it entails assessing children's communication needs and styles and learning how to respond sensitively and carefully to their questions and to their nonverbal cues.

How children face death depends on their developmental capacity to understand its meaning and on the environmental climate provided by their caretakers (Schowalter, 1970). It is very difficult to obtain direct information on death from dying children. Because of intellectual immaturity or emotional defenses, some children do not realize they are dying. Other children do not talk about the possibility of death because those around them overtly or covertly deny it. Schowalter (1970) reviews children's responses to terminal illness according to their developmental phases, from the infant and toddler periods to the preadolescent and adolescent periods. The younger the child, the more his/her affective responses to dying are influenced by those around him/her. During the first few years, the mother is the child's whole life. She not only emotionally cares for the child, but also literally keeps him/her alive. The toddler does not yet know death, only absence. It is important that a parent be as close to a child as possible, since the separation is perceived as something extraordinarily frightening. Continuity of the parent's presence and the character of this presence are critical in determining the child's response to dying.

The young child requires special nurture, care, and support from parents. Between the ages of 3 and 5, most children first understand that death is something that happens to others. Their concepts of death are relatively unstable, but they are better able to understand short separations. Children in this age group respond more spontaneously and with less anxiety to questions about death than do other children. Some children may fear that their illness is a retribution for bad thoughts or actions. Children will become passive and withdrawn if they assume guilt for their deaths; they become angry and rebellious if they project this guilt. Children from 6 to 11 years of age attribute death to an external agent that causes the organism to die. Children at this age may believe that they are themselves responsible for their illness. Once parents have been told about a child's fatal prognosis, it is impossible for them not to change their attitudes toward the child. It is also impossible for the child not to recognize the change. He/she may not recognize overt signs, but the child senses that the parents are distressed and that his/her relationship with them is somehow different. There may be subtle intensifications of feelings, which anticipate the process of mourning. During preadolescence and adolescence, children realize that death is permanent. Their responses to terminal illness become more like those of adults. They grieve more for the loss of a future than do younger children, who are more focused on the moment and the present. Shame, guilt, anticipatory mourning for themselves, and depression are not unusual for adolescents. Dunton (1970) describes how informing a child about his/her impending death must be based on each child individually. (A comprehensive review of children's concepts of death, the reactions of family members, and the manner in which information should be presented is beyond the scope of this chapter. The reader is referred to Armstrong & Martinson 1980; Craig, 1974; Drotar, 1977; Dunton, 1970; Feifel, 1959; Furman, 1970; Kalnins, 1977; Kellerman, 1979, 1980a, 1980b, 1980c, 1980d; Nagy, 1959; Reilly, Hasazi, & Bond, 1983; Schowalter, 1970; Spinetta, 1980, 1981a, 1981b; Spinetta & Deasy-Spinetta, 1981a, 1981b; Spinetta & Maloney, 1975; Spinetta, Rigler, & Karon, 1973; Wiener, 1970a, 1970b.)

Problems of Pain Control and Living with Cancer

Special problems in pain control may arise when children die at home, unless parents and medical/nursing teams communicate openly about the availability of potent analgesics and the flexibility of dosing routes and regimens. Parents may be unduly anxious because even small children, like adults with cancer, require larger opioid doses at frequent intervals. Parents' fears can lead them to deny the extent to which their children are in pain. Or children may fail to report pain because they do not want to distress parents further or because they fear injections. As yet, we do not know how many children have uncontrolled cancer pains before they die.

Beales (1979a) noted critical differences between adults and children in their perceptions of pain, especially cancer pain. Children's cancer pain seemed even less positively correlated with pathology than adults' cancer pain. Beales suggested that some of the psychological mechanisms involved in pain perception may be manipulated more easily in children than in adults. Many of our clinical and research findings support Beales's interpretation. Children's cancer pain may be more plastic than adults' pain. Children have an ability to absorb themselves completely in a task, game, or imagined event; thus, they may be more able than adults to trigger endogenous pain-inhibitory mechanisms, which may require total concentration for activation. Children seem able to perceive more control over a noxious stimulus than adults, and as a result they may feel less pain from the same stimulus. In contrast, when children have little control, they may experience even stronger pain than adults in a similar situation. Children lack the normal coping abilities that adults acquire throughout life.

The model for children's pain perception shown in Chapter 1 (see Figure 1.7) illustrates how emotional and situational factors can attenuate or enhance pain. It is essential to consider the role of these factors when designing programs to alleviate children's cancer pain. Children's ages, cognitive levels, family responses, general coping strategies, expectations about treatments, beliefs about probable recovery, and perceived control shape their understanding of cancer. Since their emotional responses arise from their understanding and abilities to cope, we need to understand how each child views his/her cancer. In general, younger children are affected primarily by the immediate impact of the disease, the necessary treatments, the constant interruptions of their routine activities, separations from family and friends, and their parents' sadness. Because of their limited concept of death, an ominous prognosis is generally not the major source of distress for young children. Restrictions in play, in contact with family and friends, and in their ability to take part in favorite activities may be more distressing to them. Older children are affected by the future impact of the disease as well as by the present situation. Since older children have an increased awareness of the grave potential of cancer, even minor noxious stimuli may be augmented by their emotional reactions. Their emotional responses naturally differ more from those of young children as their view of death more closely approximates an adult perspective. They grieve when they are diagnosed and worry that they may die. As a consequence, their pains may differ, even though the peripheral source of tissue damage is not different. Children and adolescents may worry that all pains and unusual body sensations are related to the disease. Acute pains unrelated to cancer should be concretely identified so that children are reassured. It should also be borne in mind that children with cancer are still subject to all the normal aches and pains experienced by other children.

An extensive array of research has been conducted to learn about the adverse effects of living with cancer for a child, parents, and siblings. (For reviews, see Beales, 1979a; Binger et al., 1969; Brunnquell & Hall, 1982; Frydman, 1980; Gogan, Koocher, Foster, & O'Malley, 1977; Hilgard & LeBaron, 1984; Jay, Elliott, & Varni, 1986; Katz & Jay, 1984; Katz, Kellerman, Rigler, Williams, & Siegel, 1977; Kellerman, 1980a; Koch, Hermann, & Donaldson, 1974; Koocher, 1980; Koocher &

Berman, 1983; Koocher & O'Malley, 1981; Kupst et al., 1982; Lascari & Stehbens, 1973; Lavigne & Ryan, 1979; Lewis et al., 1988; McKeever, 1983; Michael & Copeland, 1987; Morrow et al., 1984; Moss & Nannis, 1980; Schuler et al., 1981; Spinetta & Deasy-Spinetta, 1981a; Susman et al., 1982; Tritt & Esses, 1988.) Many of the psychosocial issues identified in these studies seem particularly relevant to children's cancer pain. Children are distressed by separation from parents and friends, loss of health, inability to participate fully in regular activities, loss of control and independence, increased reliance on parents, altered social and school relationships, possible disfigurement, and the uncertain outcome. They can become frightened, depressed, and anxious. When children are first diagnosed, parental reactions vary from a loss of control to outward calm and resignation. Many studies report that parents suffer an initial period of physical distress, depression, inability to function, anger, hostility, and self-blame. These symptoms persist for some parents or recur intermittently throughout a child's treatment. However, most parents say that they gradually accept the diagnosis and are able to focus on the day-to-day aspects of living with cancer. Siblings also experience profound distress at the diagnosis and at varied intervals throughout treatment. Siblings react to the general emotional distress within the family, as well as to their brother/sister's specific distress.

Binger et al. (1969) interviewed 20 parents whose children had died from leukemia about the families' reactions to the children's illness. Parents had manifest anticipatory grief reactions when the prognosis was poor. Some worried about the exact circumstances in which their children would die. Many fathers tended to absent themselves as a method of coping, causing even more distress for mothers, who assumed the primary responsibility of caring for children. Siblings often showed distress through enuresis, headaches, school difficulties, depression, separation anxieties, and abdominal pains. They feared that they might also develop a fatal illness, and resented the special attention the sick children received. Later, Cairns, Clark, Smith, and Lansky (1979) reported that siblings from 71 families in which a child had cancer tended to be anxious, to fear for their own health, and to feel isolated. However, recent prospective research on parents' and siblings' reactions to a child's cancer has shown that most families cope quite well during the course of the illness and treatment, despite periods of extreme stress. Not all siblings exhibit prolonged anxiety, excessive fears, or feelings of isolation. Instead, siblings, like their parents, react and then adjust to a profound alteration in the family environment caused by the diagnosis of childhood cancer. Some siblings, like some parents, are more at risk for developing emotional problems from the prolonged stress of the illness and treatment.

Accurate information about the illness, combined with consistent parental support and discipline, provides a reassuring family environment for the siblings of children with cancer. Many outpatient clinics have play areas where siblings can interact with children waiting for treatment, as well as with other siblings. A sibling may ask to observe the ill brother/sister's treatment. The direct observation allows the sibling to understand more concretely what is happening and why. In our program, siblings are encouraged to participate in pain management programs according to their level of interest. Their involvement must be individually tailored to their cognitive level and emotional strength. Clearly, all siblings should not watch invasive medical treatments, particularly if the ill children themselves are distressed. Some siblings should not even accompany their families to the clinic. A few parents advocate overincluding siblings, which only heightens their fear and anxiety. Even though there are no specific guidelines as to which siblings (e.g., by age, sex, cognitive level, or birth order) should participate in cancer treatment programs, the best approach seems to be the simplest approach: Ask the child. A health professional must ascertain a sibling's need for involvement. Parents often unintentionally bias siblings in regard to how they should cope, subtly encouraging them to share in treatments. Some parents may bring younger siblings to the hospital, in an unconscious effort to minimize their own anxiety. The need to maintain the siblings' attention serves as an important diversion for parents. Other parents may block siblings' attempts to understand why the ill children require repeated trips to the hospital, regular days off from school, and other apparently "special" benefits.

The new multidisciplinary approach for assisting children with chronic disease enables children with cancer, their parents, and their siblings to receive the individual assistance each requires. Various team members are specially trained to evaluate each family member's needs for knowledge and support. They recognize that the family constitutes a child's primary environment, so that the reactions of parents, siblings, and relevant members of the extended family are critical to the child's own adjustment. The family's response to the ill child modifies the psychosocial effects of cancer for a child and provides the framework for the situational and emotional factors shown in the model of children's pain (see Figure 1.7). Thus, the family environment shapes the factors that can alter nociceptive processing to increase or decrease a child's disease-related and treatment-related pain. Comprehensive pain control requires changing the psychosocial effects of cancer so that they do not exacerbate nociceptive activity. Predictability, control, and independence should be increased by adopting practical strategies to help children cope with the tangible effects of cancer on their daily lives. The aversive significance of the disease should be minimized by enabling children to realize that they are normal with respect to all the other children in treatment, rather than abnormal with respect to their healthy siblings and peers. Consistent emotional support is required to enable children to express, confront, and lessen their fears and anxieties. Several practical approaches can be used to alter the psychosocial impact of cancer for children and thereby to minimize their cancer pain.

Children with cancer should return to school as soon as their condition permits it and resume as many activities as possible. A normal, predictable routine provides them with a sense of reassurance and enhances their feelings of control. Children derive additional positive benefits because they enjoy these activities.

Physical exercise facilitates periods of natural stress reduction to help them cope with their illness. Parents should discipline children in the same manner as before they were diagnosed; rules should not be altered because they are sick. Parents should attempt to maintain the same expectations for children with respect to their family responsibilities, even if some responsibilities must now be shared with siblings. No matter how much the children are reassured verbally that they will be fine, major changes in parental expectations and discipline convey a stronger message. Children will believe that they are very different, presumably very ill. The aversive significance of cancer can be reduced when children are treated normally, interact with their friends, and maintain regular schedules. Children should meet and play with other children who are receiving similar cancer treatments. Children in our oncology program derive enormous benefits from an opportunity to swap favorite pain control strategies with one another (strategies for invasive treatments are described in Chapter 7). They enjoy playing in the ambulatory clinic before treatments, coaching one another during blood-sampling and injections, and motivating one another to earn stickers for using a pain control tool during treatments. They learn how to respond to teasing comments about the hair loss and periodic bloating that may result from treatments, as described by Ross and Ross (1984b).

Clearly, children require special support from parents and staff to cope with cancer throughout varied and lengthy treatment protocols. But this support should be extended in a manner that promotes the children's understanding, provides accurate expectations, improves control, increases independence, reduces fear, and lessens anxiety. Children have more control when they know what treatments are required, when procedures are scheduled within the protocol, and why some treatments seem unpredictable (e.g., when the blood lab must first contact the clinic with the results of an earlier finger prick). Children are not distressed by the unknown when they are prepared for the exact sights, sounds, and smells of each treatment. Most health professionals can recall a child who was unduly distressed by an unexpected change in protocol, so that he/she reported more pain than usual during treatment. In our clinic, a 3-year-old boy was quite upset by overhearing a relief nurse ask how to clean his portacatheter. His pain rating was extremely high, even though the actual cleansing procedure was consistent with previous procedures, when he had reported no pain. An 8-year-old girl was very distressed when a new resident requested that she lie in a different position during a bone marrow aspiration. She rated the aspiration as more painful than previous procedures. A change in the texture of topical anesthetics, the smell of antiseptic or anesthetic creams, or the number of test tubes that are used can profoundly alter a child's ability to cope. These seemingly simple changes to an adult represent major modifications to most children. Such changes reinforce children's sense that they have no control and that treatment variations are not predictable. In addition, they may distrust some staff members because they assume that only certain "regulars" can conduct procedures in a painless manner.

Management of Cancer Pain

Studies on childhood cancer conclude that comprehensive psychosocial support is essential to assist children and families in living with cancer. Multidisciplinary teams consisting of art therapists, child life specialists, psychologists, and social workers share the total care of the child with nurses, hematologists, and oncologists. However, few teams include members who are specially trained in the management of childhood pain. The emphasis is often placed on the pharmacological approach to disease-related pain, with very little awareness of how psychosocial factors affect a child's pain. As a consequence, children may not receive optimal pain relief during treatments, because the factors that exacerbate their pain remain unidentified. Each parent, child, and sibling reacts to a fatal illness individually, in a manner consistent with his/her own personality structure, past experience, current crises, and the particular meaning or special circumstances associated with the threatened loss. To help children live with cancer, one must know the children and their relations to their families, their beliefs about life and death, and their current sources of support.

Similarly, to help control children's pain, one must know the relevant situational, emotional, and familial factors that affect their pain. The optimal relief of a child's cancer pain begins with an assessment from a dual perspective—an objective appraisal of the sources of nociceptive stimulation, and a thorough evaluation of the factors that modify nociceptive processing for that child. The characteristics of the pain, the chronology of the disease, previous therapy, and the child must be carefully considered. Many interventions are available to relieve cancer pain. The difficulty in pediatrics arises more from a failure to employ an integrated therapeutic approach than from the lack of available interventions. As emphasized by Bonica (1979a) for adults, "Consideration of the numerous mechanisms of chronic pain in general and cancer pain in particular and of the various modalities currently available for its therapy makes it obvious that no one individual has the knowledge, expertise, and skill to provide optimal relief to each and every patient" (p. 129).

Several misconceptions impede the control of childhood cancer pain. First, many of the individuals who treat children's cancer lack information about the plasticity and complexity of the nociceptive system. They manage pain from the perspective that tissue damage is synonymous with pain, rather than from a multidimensional perspective. Second, the source of pain is not properly evaluated with respect to the origin of nociceptive stimulation and with respect to the psychosocial factors that affect nociceptive processing. Third, children are not taught simple pain-reducing strategies. Fourth, parents are not taught the importance of modifying situational, emotional, familial, and behavioral factors to lessen children's pain. Fifth, some clinicians and patients believe that opioid analgesics should only be administered as a last resort, in order to prevent drug addiction. And, sixth, analgesics are not always administered in adequate doses, at frequent time intervals, or via effective routes. It is disappointing that nonpharmacological interventions are not usually included to supplement or complement analgesics.

Cancer pain management requires education about the plasticity and complexity of the nociceptive systems, the diversity of interventions, and the advantages of different modes of administration. Regardless of the type of cancer pain, children's pain can be controlled if basic principles of pain management are followed. First, the pain source must be accurately identified. Various pharmacological and nonpharmacological interventions will effectively alleviate different types of pain, depending on the source of nociceptive activity—single or multiple sites, peripheral, central, or both. The general principles of analgesic administration must be followed, particularly the progression from weak to strong analgesics and the upward titration of the dose until analgesia occurs (as reviewed in Chapter 4). The progression of disease may dictate an increase in dose. Nonpharmacological interventions can reduce both acute and chronic cancer pains for children, when they are selected carefully to modify the factors that exacerbate pain according to the unique needs of children. Overviews of adult cancer pain syndromes and their management have been presented in a monograph (Health and Welfare Canada, 1984) and in a special issue of the *Journal of Pain and Symptom Management* (Brescia, 1987a, 1987b; Cleeland, 1987; Foley, 1987; Kanner, 1987). The control of pain resulting from advanced cancer consists of three main approaches: anticancer modalities to decrease or eliminate the neoplasm and therefore eliminate the source of pain (through chemotherapy, endocrine therapy, radiation therapy, radioisotope therapy, palliative therapy); interventions to control the pain without affecting the neoplasm (through systemic drugs, therapeutic nerve blocks, neurosurgical operations, and psychological methods); and a combination of the two approaches (Bonica, 1979a, 1984, 1985).

Pharmacological Interventions. Continuous infusion should be considered when children require prolonged administration of parenteral narcotics. Continuous infusion has several advantages over intermittent subcutaneous, intramuscular, or intravenous routes. This method circumvents repetitive injections, prevents delays in analgesic drug administration, and provides continuous levels of pain control without side effects at peak level and pain breakthroughs at trough level (Coyle, Mauskop, Maggard, & Foley, 1986; Miser, Davis, Hughes, Mulne, & Miser, 1983; Ventafridda, Spoldi, Caraceni, Tamburini, & DeConno, 1986). Miser et al. (1983) controlled severe pain resulting from malignant neoplasm in 17 patients (ranging in age from 22 months to 22 years) with a subcutaneous infusion of morphine sulfate using a syringe pump. The pump was attached to the patient, the bed, or a vertical free-standing pole, whichever was most convenient. Adequate pain control was defined as freedom from pain and the absence of pain complaints more than 95% of the time. All patients achieved adequate pain control, regardless of the cause of pain, without any adverse side effects. These investigators stated that continuous infusion should be considered when patients have severe pain for which oral and intermittent parenteral narcotics do not provide satisfactory pain control, when intractable vomiting prevents oral medications, when intravenous lines are not desirable, and when children would like to remain at home despite severe pain.

Patient-controlled analgesia (PCA) is a relatively new mode of administration that has been used to treat chronic cancer pain (for a review, see Barkas & Duafala, 1988). This technique enables patients to administer predetermined analgesic doses in accord with their pain levels. Few reports have been published as to the efficacy of PCA for controlling children's pain. (Research on PCA is reviewed in Chapter 4.) Yet adolescents have assumed responsibility for adminstering their own doses at some hospitals. The criteria defining which children would be appropriate for PCA should be determined. The first step is to carefully document the cases in which it was used, noting the advantages and disadvantages. It would be inappropriate simply to use age as the primary criterion. Some younger children (e.g., above 7 years of age), particularly those who have endured much medical treatment and many pains, may be able to understand the concept and use the devices appropriately. Clearly, PCA offers special advantages to children who have little control and who are extremely frightened about uncontrolled pain. More efforts should be expended to evaluate the efficacy of this mode of administration for children.

Analgesic potency, dose, dosing interval, and mode of administration must be carefully considered for managing a child's cancer pain, as illustrated by the following two case histories. Wiley and Rhein (1977) described how severe bone pain was controlled for a terminally ill adolescent with end-stage metastatic rhabdomyosarcoma. He suffered "great" pain at many sites along his back and in long bone areas. Any movement exacerbated his pain. As the disease progressed, oral opioids were no longer effective in relieving his pian. Radiographic examination revealed diffuse metastases of both femurs, the pelvis, and the spine, with compression of multiple thoracic and lumbar vertebrae. He required opioids administered intravenously at larger doses and at frequent intervals to control his pain adequately (e.g., 15 mg of morphine every half hour on the day he died), but he did not experience any adverse side effects. In addition, analgesic medication was provided in a positive environment, in which he was actively involved in decisions regarding his care and participated with nursing and medical staff, a social worker, and his family and friends.

Rogers (1986a) described pain management for a 3-year-old girl with neuroblastoma. She had been receiving morphine (5–10 mg intravenous push), but the morphine provided inadequate pain relief and caused too much sedation and irritability. The analgesic was changed to hydromorphone (Dilaudid) administered through a continuous intravenous infusion (1.5 mg per hour). This analgesic was selected because of its shorter-duration effect; the continuous infusion prevented the seesaw analgesic effect of intraveneous pushes. The patient reported no pain on this regimen, and she remained alert and active.

Nonpharmacological Interventions. The control of acute pain evoked by repeated invasive treatments has been recognized as a special problem for children with cancer (Hilgard & LeBaron, 1984; Jay, Ozolins, Elliott, & Caldwell, 1983; Katz,

Kellerman, & Siegel, 1980; Kellerman & Varni, 1982; Kuttner, Bowman, & Teasdale, 1988; Linn, Beardslee, & Patenaude, 1986; McGrath & deVeber, 1986a, 1986b; Schechter, 1985). Children experience lumbar punctures, bone marrow aspirations, intravenous and intramuscular injections, blood transfusions, and radiotherapy. Many children experience anticipatory nausea and vomiting before their treatments (Dolgin & Katz, 1988; Dolgin, Katz, McGinty, & Siegel, 1985; Hilgard & LeBaron, 1984). Consequently, most attention in pediatrics has focused on the assessment and management of acute therapy-related cancer pain. This focus has been extremely valuable, yielding effective interventions to minimize treatment-related pain. In the future, more attention must be devoted to the management of other types of childhood cancer pains, particularly neuropathic pains, mucositis pain, and postoperative pains.

Nonpharmacological interventions, including relaxation training, operant conditioning, desensitization, and hypnosis, have been used to reduce anticipatory anxiety, nausea, emesis, pain, and behavioral distress for children undergoing cancer therapy (Dash, 1980; Ellenberg, Kellerman, Dash, Higgins, & Zeltzer, 1980; Hartman, 1981; Hilgard & LeBaron, 1984; Hillier & McGrath, 1987; Hockenberry & Bologna-Vaughan, 1985; Kellerman, 1979; Kellerman, Zeltzer, Ellenberg, & Dash, 1983; LaBaw, Holton, Tewell, & Eccles, 1975; McGrath & deVeber, 1986a, 1986b; Olness, 1981a, 1981b; Zeltzer & LeBaron, 1982). Hypnosis has been the most widely used intervention for controlling children's therapy-related cancer pain (for reviews, see Hilgard & LeBaron, 1984; Spinetta & Deasy-Spinetta, 1981a). Several case reports show that children can easily learn self-hypnotic techniques to reduce pain during medical treatments (Crasilneck & Hall, 1975; Elkins & Carter, 1981; Ellenberg et al., 1980; Gardner, 1976; Gardner & Olness, 1981). A few investigators have used hypnosis to supplement analgesics for the control of disease-related pain. Crasilneck and Hall (1973) described the multiple benefits of hypnosis for a 4-year-old boy with inoperable brain cancer who was suffering continual pain. He was hypnotized and given suggestions for reduced pain, better appetite, better sleeping, and increased enjoyment of television. He had daily hypnosis sessions for a month and then three sessions each week. During this time, his pain lessened so that he gradually required fewer opioid injections. Also, his appetite increased, he slept more comfortably, and he enjoyed television and picture books more. Gardner (1976) described how David, an 11-year-old boy, used self-hypnosis to lessen his nausea and vomiting during cancer treatments. David then worked with his therapist to reduce his cancer pain and lessen his anxiety about dying. He was able to derive more positive experiences each day, despite his fatal illness.

Ellenberg et al. (1980) used hypnosis with a 16-year-old girl suffering from leukemia. She experienced severe pain during bone marrow aspirations, as well as severe headaches and backaches, which began after the first course of her chemotherapy. She was hypnotized before bone marrow aspirations, with specific suggestions that she would be aware of sensations during the procedure but that these sensations would not lead to discomfort. Hypnotic suggestions also included time distortion, so she could perceive that the procedure was completed more quickly, and glove anesthesia, so she could transfer a numb sensation to her back. Her pain ratings decreased after hypnosis for both her acute treatment-related pain and her persistent headaches and backache. As her illness progressed, she required the assistance of the therapist to use hypnosis effectively. She was unable to use hypnosis a few weeks before her death, because she felt that she could not relax. At this time she showed signs of central nervous system dysfunction, including periods of hallucination, cloudy consciousness, motor tremors, and agitation. She was very distressed about the severity of her illness. The investigators questioned whether her inability to use hypnosis during this terminal phase reflected an unwillingness to relinquish consciousness because she was afraid that she would die.

LaBaw et al. (1975) described the general efficacy of self-hypnosis for 27 cancer patients (4–20 years old). Progressive muscle relaxation and positive visual imagery were used to induce relaxed hypnotic states. Children then received suggestions to improve their appetites, to increase fluid intake, to rest more comfortably, and to feel less pain during treatments. Although children's ability to use self-hypnosis varied from poor to excellent, the investigators concluded that hypnotic trance therapy is an important adjunctive treatment for most children with cancer. Olness (1981b) described her clinical experience teaching 21 children with cancer how to use self-hypnosis and imagery. She preferred the term "imagery exercises" because it more appropriately summarized the nature of children's training. Children practiced using various images—a "pain switch" to turn pain off during treatments, a pleasant activity or sensation that was incompatible with pain, and specific numb areas along their bodies. Children worked with the therapist to choose the most effective images for them. Only two children did not experience substantial reductions in overt distress, pain, and anxiety; one child died on the day of referral, and the other child was 3 years old and participated in only one session. Children between 5 and 11 years old were able to control their pain more rapidly than adolescents—usually within two training sessions, in contrast to four sessions for older children. Six children also used positive imagery to visualize their powerful immune systems fighting the cancer cells.

Kellerman et al. (1983) evaluated the efficacy of hypnosis (progressive muscle relaxation, deep breathing, visual imagery) to reduce adolescents' anxiety and pain during bone marrow aspirations, lumbar punctures, and chemotherapeutic injections. Once patients were observably relaxed (slow and regular breathing, immobility, focused attention), they were given specific suggestions for reduced discomfort and increased mastery. They were taught self-hypnosis and encouraged to practice before procedures. For 89% of the patients, anxiety and discomfort were significantly reduced. Hilgard and LeBaron (1982) also investigated the efficacy of hypnosis for reducing treatment-related cancer pain. They collected baseline measures of anxiety, overt distress, and pain from 63 children during bone marrow aspirations. Twenty-four children volunteered to learn hypnosis. They completed the Stanford Hypnotic Clinical Scale for Children, which provided a rating of their hypnotizability. Children were hypnotized individually before their next scheduled bone marrow aspiration; the therapist coached each child during the procedure. Fifteen children successfully used hypnosis. The average pain rating for procedures decreased from 7 (on a 10-point rating scale) to 5. Children's behavioral distress also decreased noticeably. Children who had higher hypnotizability scores generally had greater pain reductions than children with lower scores.

Zeltzer and LeBaron (1982) conducted the first randomized treatment evaluation of hypnotic analgesia for children with cancer. They compared the efficacy of hypnosis and nonhypnotic distraction techniques for 33 cancer patients (from 6 to 17 years old). The nonhypnotic techniques included deep breathing, distraction, and practice sessions to help control children's fears. Children in the hypnosis group were encouraged to become increasingly involved in pleasant and interesting imaginings. Images were selected specifically for each child's interests so that children could focus intensely during treatments. Pain and anxiety ratings for bone marrow aspirations decreased significantly from 4.42 and 3.97 (on a 5-point scale), respectively, to 2.92 and 2.85 after hypnosis. Children in the nonhypnosis group reported lowered pain and anxiety, but the reductions were not as large as for children in the hypnosis group. Although the intense imaginative involvement was the main distinguishing feature between the two treatments, it is not clear whether the distraction might have been equally effective if children had been distracted by activities or conversations that were truly interesting to them. In fact, the investigators suggested that the active component of the intervention was the successful diversion of children's attention away from the noxious stimuli.

Recently, Katz, Kellerman, and Ellenberg (1987) compared the efficacy of hypnosis and nondirected play for reducing distress and pain in 36 children (6–11 years old) with cancer. Children in the hypnosis group received specific suggestions to reduce pain sensations, increase control, relax, and use distraction. The other group of children participated in nondirected play for the same amount of time with a sympathetic hospital professional. Children in both conditions experienced significant reductions in pain. There were no significant reductions in children's observed behavioral distress. The comparable efficacy of the hypnosis and play conditions may have been due to the powerful therapeutic role of the therapist who conducted both treatments. The positive rapport between children and the therapist, coupled with the therapist's presence during the bone marrow aspiration, may have led children to feel reassured so that they were less fearful, anxious, and therefore felt less pain. The novelty of the therapist in the room may have proved an ideal distractor for children in the play group. It is also possible that hypnosis is not optimally effective unless children receive active coaching during painful procedures.

Much more research is needed to determine the comparative efficacy of hypnosis, hypnotic-like suggestions for analgesia, distraction, relaxation, and visual imagery for reducing children's cancer pain. Too few controlled studies have been conducted to enable us to identify the critical components of the hypnotic process or to identify confidently the children who would most benefit from such interventions. Many of the clinical reports and research studies on hypnosis in children with cancer are quite valuable for our understanding of how to minimize children's treatment-related pain. Yet caution must be advised when interpreting the results of these studies. There is enormous variability in clinical research on childhood cancer, even for children on the same treatment protocols. Children are usually at very different stages in the protocol; they have generally received different types of analgesic and sedative preparations; they have different coping strategies; they have different expectations; they have different imaginings that will attract their full attention; they have different parents; they have different numbers of and types of people present during procedures; and there may be slight (from an adult perspective) procedural modifications that differentially increase their anxiety. As a consequence of the huge number of variables that could confound the pain-reducing effects of hypnosis, it is quite possible that no study has yet included a sufficient sample of children to permit a valid determination of treatment effects. It may be that controlled studies on the efficacy of nonpharmacological interventions for children can only be conducted at multiple sites with large numbers of children, so that clinically meaningful and statistically valid conclusions can be drawn.

Several cognitive-behavioral interventions have been used to reduce children's therapy-related pain, as reviewed in Chapter 6. The interventions used for cancer pain generally include many of the same components used for hypnotic analgesia, such as progressive muscle relaxation, deep breathing, guided visual imagery, and cognitive restructuring. Dahlquist, Gil, Armstrong, Ginsberg, and Jones (1985) taught three children (aged 11–14) to use cue-controlled muscle relaxation, deep breathing, pleasant imagery, and positive self-talk during chemotherapy venipunctures. Children's overt behavioral distress decreased substantially. Jay, Elliott, Ozolins, Olson, and Pruitt (1985) designed a multistrategy intervention package that included filmed modeling, positive reinforcement, breathing exercises, imagery and distraction, and behavioral rehearsal. This intervention reduced behavioral distress in five children (aged 3.5 to 7 years) during lumbar punctures and bone marrow aspirations. Recently, Jay, Elliott, Katz, and Siegel (1987) demonstrated the efficacy of this intervention in comparison with Valium and a minimal-treatment/attention control. Fifty-six children (3–13 years old) participated in the study; they had significantly less pain and overt distress during bone marrow aspirations when they received the cognitive-behavioral multistrategy intervention.

A similar multistrategy program was designed in our clinic to reduce procedure-related pain for children with cancer (McGrath & deVeber, 1986a, 1986b). This program combined several nonpharmacological approaches in pain management, whose common focus was that they altered situational factors identified as important modifiers of pain. The approaches included relaxation training, hypnotic-like suggestions for analgesia, behavioral management, cognitive restructuring, guided imagery, desensitization, and (most importantly) education about the plasticity and complexity of nociceptive processing. (The program is described in detail in Chapter 6.) The principal objectives of the program were to provide children with accurate information about the source of noxious stimulation, to improve children's control, and to alter the relevance of the aversive situation to minimize fear and anxiety.

Pre-Lumbar Puncture

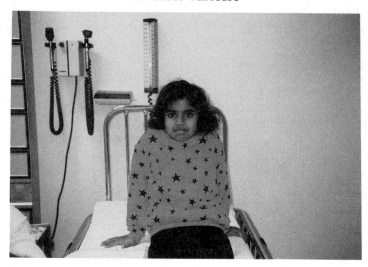

Are you now afraid (or anxious) about this procedure? Yes ✓ No____

|——————————————————————————|————————————————————————————|
Not at all   Most afraid possible

Which face looks like you will feel deep down inside when you have this procedure today?

FIGURE 9.1.   Carol, an 8.10-year-old girl with leukemia, is shown before receiving a lumbar puncture. She rated her anxiety, affect, and anticipated pain using the scales listed below the photograph.

A child enrolled in this program is shown in Figures 9.1 and 9.2, before and
after a lumbar puncture. Her anxiety and pain ratings are listed below her picture.
This program was initially designed for acute pain during lumbar puncture
procedures and bone marrow aspirations. However, the program has now been
extended to encompass all the invasive procedures scheduled for children with
cancer and is now routinely offered to all children as part of our pain clinic. There

Post-Lumbar Puncture

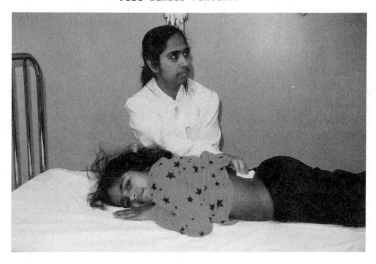

How much did it hurt during the procedure?

Not at all   Very much

(With all you have learned), how much do you think you made the
procedure easier for you today?

Not at all   Very easy

Which face looks like you felt deep down inside when you had the
procedure?

FIGURE 9.2.   Carol is shown immediately after her lumbar puncture; she rated her pain, affect, and
improved control during the procedure.

have been significant reductions in pain, anxiety, and distress during blood-sampling, injections, and dressing changes, as well as for lumbar punctures and bone marrow aspirations. The emphasis on specific program components (e.g., deep breathing or hypnosis) varies to meet the needs and skills of each child, as reviewed in earlier chapters. Consequently, the particular tools that lead to pain reduction vary among children, but the critical components are the same—that is, the modification of relevant situational and emotional factors. An unanticipated benefit of this program has been the enthusiastic interest shown by children as they generalize their new knowledge of pain control to other painful situations. They have used the same strategies they learned for acute pain control when they have disease-related pain or suffer routine childhood injuries.

Cancer pain provides a special model for the management of both disease-related and therapy-related pain caused by a chronic disease. A judicious blend of pharmacological and nonpharmacological interventions can effectively alleviate childhood cancer pain. However, these interventions must be administered after assessment of the unique situational, behavioral, emotional, and familial factors that affect a child's pain.

Sickle Cell Anemia Pain

Sickle cell anemia, which only affects blacks, is a significant cause of mortality and morbidity in children. This disease has an approximate incidence of 1% for American blacks (Lanzkowsky, 1980). Sickle cell anemia is a painful inherited blood disorder in which the red blood cells are distorted into elongated sickle shapes. Although these cell distortions occur continuously, painful sickling crises occur when the rate of sickling increases, so that many more cells are temporarily or irreversibly sickled. The sickle-shaped cells then obstruct oxygen flow into capillaries, causing local hypoxia with deoxygenation of more red blood cells, which leads to more sickling.

The location and number of occluded capillaries determine the extent and severity of noxious stimulation. The severe pain generally has a sudden onset (within 1–4 hours) and can last from 1 to 10 days. Sickling crises develop in the extremities, lower back, chest, abdomen, and bones. The frequency of painful episodes is extremely variable, with some patients experiencing only one episode each year and other patients experiencing episodes every few weeks. Several physical factors can precipitate painful episodes, including events that cause dehydration or change the oxygen balance (e.g., infections, overexertion, and ingestion of alcohol). Emotional factors, particularly stress and depression, may also initiate painful crises. (For reviews, see Davis, Vichinsky, & Lubin, 1980; Platt & Nathan, 1987; Rozzell, Hijazi, & Pack, 1983; Scott, 1982; Thomas & Holbrook, 1987; Vichinsky & Lubin, 1987; Whitten & Fischhoff, 1974.)

The impact of painful sickling crises on children and their families has not been well documented. Presumably, the unpredictability of crises leads to emotional problems similar to those encountered by children with hemophilia, whose bleeding episodes are likewise unpredictable. These problems are often confounded by the socioeconomic status of many black children, who generally do not have the same opportunities as children with hemophilia. The extent to which children with sickle cell anemia are anxious and depressed is not known. Clinical reports indicate that adolescents with the disease are depressed, hostile, and apprehensive. Their feelings result from a long-term lack of control over the disease and pain. Although children and adolescents with sickle cell anemia supposedly have lower self-esteem than their peers, few studies provide support for this claim. Similarly, it is not known what situational, familial, and behavioral factors may contribute to their pain. More research is needed to document the special needs of these children for pain management. It may be inappropriate to assume that the factors that affect their pain are identical to those detailed for children with other chronic diseases in different social and family environments.

Many acute and chronic complications may arise from this disease (Charache, 1981; Platt & Nathan, 1987). There is no cure, so the treatment includes controlling the pain and identifying the factors that can trigger sickling crises. Analgesic administration, hydration, and oxygen therapy are the primary interventions used. Many painful crises can be successfully treated at home with increased fluid intake and oral analgesics. Severe crises require hydration and potent analgesia. Morphine effectively controls the pain when it is administered in adequate doses; however, it is not clear to what extent children with sickle cell anemia are receiving adequate analgesics in appropriate doses. There is still a reluctance to prescribe narcotics to children and adolescents in some areas (Schechter, Berrien, & Katz, 1988). More pain management problems may arise for adolescents, particularly in large cities, where there are specific concerns that they are at risk for drug abuse and addiction.

Few clinical studies have been conducted to evaluate the efficacy of different analgesics, modes of administration, and combined pharmacological and non-pharmacological interventions in the management of sickle cell anemia pain. A double-blind crossover study compared low doses of aspirin and placebo for controlling painful crises in 49 children (Greenberg, Ohene-Frempong, Halus, Way, & Schwartz, 1983). Aspirin did not significantly reduce the frequency and severity of painful crises. Opioid analgesics are necessary to control severe pain. Cole, Sprinkle, Smith, and Buchanan (1986) reviewed the records for 38 children who received continuous opioid infusions (morphine or meperidine) to control their sickling pain. Pain was adequately relieved for all children. Since most hospitalized patients receive intravenous infusions for hydration, children already have ready access for intravenous analgesics. There were no discernible differences between equianalgesic doses of morphine and meperidine with regard to clinical efficacy and most side effects. Narcotic withdrawal and addiction were not noted. The authors stress that caution should be used in administering opioid analgesics in combination with hydration and vigorous blood transfusion therapy in children with chest syndrome (defined as signs or symptoms of pulmonary disease and an abnormal chest roentgenogram).

More recently, a pilot study was conducted to evaluate the use of PCA by three adolescents with sickle cell anemia (Schechter et al., 1988). The patients, who were 11, 12, and 17 years old, all understood the system and were able to responsibly administer opioid doses to control their pain. They used fewer analgesics each day (with the exception of one patient on the second day) as their pain crises subsided. Some patients required higher doses of medication than have been traditionally assumed necessary for pain control. The typical regimen (approximately 10 mg every 4 hours) was inadequate to control the pain initially for two of the patients. A larger first dose may be necessary, as well as larger supplemental doses for some adolescents.

One study has evaluated the efficacy of transcutaneous electrical nerve stimulation (TENS) for the treatment of painful sickling crises (Wang et al., 1985). Twenty-two patients (12–27 years old) participated in a randomized, double-blind crossover study. Approximately three-fourths of the patients believed that the treatment was helpful, but there was no significant difference in pain ratings between the TENS and placebo groups. TENS may prove a valuable physical intervention for sickling pain, but its efficacy has not yet been established.

Cognitive-behavioral methods can enhance the pain relief provided by analgesic medications. Zeltzer, Dash, and Holland (1979) taught self-hypnosis techniques to two young adults (20 years old) with sickle cell anemia. When they were in very relaxed states, patients received suggestions to feel increasingly warm and comfortable sensations and to visualize their blood vessels dilating, allowing the sickle cells to pass through along with the healthy blood cells. Patients practiced these visualizations at the onset of any sickling crises. The frequency and severity of their sickling crises decreased over an 8-month period, along with their analgesic needs. In addition, the visualizations increased their peripheral skin temperature.

Programs that integrate education, psychological support, and medical disease management offer optimal health care and pain management to children. Vichinsky and Lubin (1987) described an effective multidisciplinary program of comprehensive care for children with sickle cell anemia. Their program includes social support, regular medical monitoring, nutritional support, counseling for school and social activities, and physical therapy. Children require assistance to understand sickle cell anemia and to cope with the relatively unpredictable crises that disrupt their lives. Each of the components in the multistrategy treatment program gives children better understanding of and better control over the adverse effects of the disease. Yet children would also benefit from learning some simple strategies to reduce pain during crisis episodes and to promote relaxation during stressful periods.

Relaxation, hypnosis, and behavioral approaches provide children with more control to reduce feelings of helplessness, stress, anxiety, and frustration. The knowledge that they can actively participate in their own pain management should alleviate some of the distress of the disease for them and for their families. Consequently, a flexible repertoire of cognitive-behavioral interventions should be included for the management of children's sickling pains. These programs should be designed after careful identification of the relevant factors that contribute to a child's pain.

Chronic Pain Associated with a Primary Psychological Etiology

As described in the preceding sections, the optimal relief of any childhood chronic pain requires consideration of a child's and family's psychological states. Since children's emotional reactions affect their pain, psychological factors must be recognized as powerful contributing factors for all chronic pains. However, occasionally, psychological factors are the primary rather than the secondary source of a child's pain. Although attention has been focused on understanding the relationships among chronic pain, anxiety, depression, and anger for adults, less attention has been paid to these relationships for children and adolescents.

Children can develop chronic pain as a result of excessive anxiety and depression. In essence, pain represents the somatic expression of their emotional distress. Usually, such children who are referred to our pain clinic are unable to identify their true stressful reactions to situations. They attempt to accept teasing, disappointments, and frustrations without allowing themselves to feel hurt and frustrated. They keep their emotions controlled while they present an apparently calm disposition to the world. A subset of the adolescents who are referred for management of recurrent headaches suffer from masked depression. They tend to suffer more frequent headaches than other children (several headaches each week or a constant daily headache), while appearing less bothered by the headaches than other children. Testing on the Basic Personality Inventory (profiles shown in Chapter 8) reveals that they have exaggerated somatic concerns, low scores on the Depression subscale, and high scores on the Denial subscale. Their responses on standardized depression inventories are often extremely high, indicating serious affective problems.

Children's emotions may surface in the form of pain complaints, as more stress affects them and they are unable to cope with it. Often children's failure to recognize true stress-inducing situations (school, peers, family) means that it is not possible for them to respond appropriately in these situations to reduce the stress. Their attempts to deny the stress associated with common childhood situations prevents them from learning how to resolve conflicts and solve problems effectively, so that each new conflict or problem adds progressively to their underlying anxiety. The headaches or stomachaches that they develop as a result of their anxiety are real, not imagined, and help to remove them from the situation or source of anxiety. The pain can eventually become an unconscious method for coping with stress, because it temporarily removes children from an aversive situation and perhaps provides emotional support through the attention of parents, teachers, and friends.

Children can develop additional chronic pain from their anxiety about a disease. Some children referred to our pain clinic have experienced various pains that were seemingly unrelated to their illness. For example, a 6-year-old girl who required regular growth hormone injections complained about a persistent ache throughout her body. Pain assessment indicated that her ache was related to her concerns about being small, despite the injections she regularly received, rather than directly related to her medical condition. Her ache disappeared after a brief period of counseling to provide her with more accurate expectations about the results of treatment. Children with chronic pain associated with a disease can also experience increases in their pain because of fears about the possibility of dying, anxiety about necessary treatments, or frustrations about living their lives differently than other children. In addition, the anxiety that children may perceive in their parents' reactions to their disorder can cause them to feel guilty, upset, and frustrated, so that the pain increases or becomes more unpleasant for them.

The prevalence and incidence of childhood chronic pains with a primary psychological etiology are unknown. The specific sensory characteristics of most of these pains have not been well described. Unlike other types of chronic pain, these pains do not always lead to prolonged emotional distress; instead, they evolve from prolonged emotional distress and seem to serve a temporary protective function by removing stress. Unfortunately, no controlled studies have been conducted to identify the specific situational, behavioral, emotional, and familial factors associated with the development of these pains in childhood. Similarly, few controlled studies have evaluated the efficacy of pharmacological, cognitive-behavioral, and physical interventions for alleviating these pains.

Retrospective studies with adults reveal that the onset for certain mental disorders in which pain is the predominant complaint is adolescence. "Somatoform disorders" are conditions in which patients experience physical symptoms that suggest underlying physical disorders, but for which there are no demonstrable organic mechanisms. However, there is positive evidence that their symptoms are linked to psychological factors (American Psychiatric Association, 1980). In general, the location, distribution, quality, and intensity of their pains are not consistent with physiological patterns. There may be a marked discrepancy between a patient's rating of pain severity and his/her behaviors. It is not uncommon for adults to grimace and writhe during a pain assessment, but to participate in strenuous leisure activities outside the clinic. Often, their pain episodes are associated with obvious periods of stress.

"Somatization disorder" is a common somatoform disorder in adults, which usually begins during adolescence. Patients suffer from recurrent and multiple physical complaints, among them pains, for which they continually seek medical attention. Retrospective data indicates that they commonly complained about headaches, abdominal pain, and varied diffuse aches and pains when they were adolescents. However, no prospective research has been conducted from an adolescent's perspective to determine the actual prevalence of somatization disorders in children with recurrent pain syndromes. Ernst, Routh, and Harper (1984) retrospectively reviewed the medical records of children with recurrent abdominal pain. Children whose pain was not related to a clear organic etiology had more symptoms of somatization disorder than children whose pain had an organic etiology. The frequency of somatization symptoms increased with pain chronicity; the longer children had had abdominal pains, the more symptoms were present. Such findings are compatible with our research on recurrent headaches. Future research should be directed at identifying which of these children are at risk for psychiatric disorders.

"Psychogenic pain disorders" are somatoform disorders characterized by pain complaints without clear indices of tissue damage and nociceptive activity. Again, there is evidence of responsible psychological factors, as noted by stress triggers for individual pain episodes and by the presence of significant secondary gains. Often adult patients are unwilling to consider even a contributing role for psychological factors in the etiology of their pain; instead, they continually search for a different medical diagnosis and treatment. This disorder can develop at any age, but seems to begin most frequently in adolescence or early adulthood. There are no prospective studies of childhood psychogenic pain. But even clinical anecdotes do not authenticate the same features of this disorder in children that are characterized for adults.

However, a different perspective emerges when one considers the child in relation to his/her family. Then many of the features of adult psychogenic pain are present; only it is the parents, not the child, who are unwilling to accept the role of psychological factors. The major reason why parents refuse to allow their children to participate in our treatment program for recurrent pains is that the parents refuse to accept that their children's pain has no organic etiology. Children may readily understand that how they feel mentally can affect how they feel physically, but parents are reluctant to believe that emotions can lead to real pain. It is quite frustrating when children express interest in the program, but parents refuse the treatment. Some older children and adolescents do fit the profile of the adult psychogenic pain patient. Because these adolescents who refuse participation in pain programs share their parents' beliefs about pain causes and have generally had pains longer than other adolescents, it is probable that their families' attitudes have shaped their perspective.

The management of chronic pain with a primary psychological etiology requires a comprehensive program integrating individual and family therapy with appropriate analgesic interventions and psychotropic medications. Cognitive-behavioral therapies, physical rehabilitation programs, and long-term counseling are needed to achieve complete pain relief.

Summary and Recommendations

Children can experience many types of chronic pain caused by disease, injury, and emotional distress. Like that of adults, children's chronic pain affects the entire

family and must be viewed within a broader context. Pain management is complicated by the multiple sources of noxious stimulation, affecting peripheral and
central nociceptive mechanisms; by prolonged emotional suffering; by impaired
physical functioning; by decreased independence; and often by an uncertain
prognosis. Nevertheless, effective pain control is possible if one treats chronic pain
in relation to the child experiencing it. A judicious balance of pharmacological
and nonpharmacological interventions is required; these interventions should be
selected according to the source of pain and the relevant situational, emotional,
behavioral, and familial factors that affect pain.

It is impossible to relieve chronic pain adequately from a unidimensional
perspective, in which pain is considered as synonymous with the nature and extent
of tissue damage. Childhood chronic pain must be viewed from a multidimensional perspective because multiple sensory, environmental, and emotional factors
are responsible for the pain, no matter how seemingly clear-cut an etiology may be.
Treatment begins with a thorough assessment of these multiple factors, using
structured interviews and standardized measures. Pharmacological, physical, and
psychological strategies must be incorporated into a flexible intervention program
for children, in which parents and siblings form an essential component of
treatment. No single discipline has the expertise to assess and manage chronic pain
independently, because the multiple causes transcend the knowledge of any one
discipline. Multi- and interdisciplinary teams are required to identify causes and to
select the best treatments available for those causes.

In general, children require accurate, honest information about the cause of
their pain, presented in a calm, reassuring manner. This information must be
presented according to their developmental level and their desire to know what is
happening. Children should learn some simple strategies for reducing pain, consistent with their pain source. They should be encouraged to live as fully and
normally as possible. Parents and siblings require special assistance in coping with
chronic illness, but they should be encouraged to share in the children's treatment.

10

Children's Pain: Current Status and Future Directions

Interest in the assessment and alleviation of children's pain has increased dramatically during the last decade. Special attention has been focused on the unique pain problems of premature infants, children requiring repeated invasive procedures, adolescents with recurrent pain syndromes, and children with chronic diseases. Clinicians and scientists are enthusiastically addressing a myriad of issues to improve children's pain control. These include the refinement of age-appropriate pain measures; an objective evaluation of various drugs, dosing regimens, and administration routes for controlling postsurgical pain; an assessment of the multiple factors that affect chronic pain; and the routine integration of nonpharmacological interventions for pain management within children's hospitals.

The unprecedented attention on children's pain is evidenced by numerous clinical reports and research articles published in a broad spectrum of medical, nursing, psychology, and health journals. Three books on childhood pain have been published in the past 2 years. The first International Conference on Pediatric Pain convened in July 1988, and the first European Conference was convened in June 1989. The journal *Pain* has formed an editorial panel on pediatrics; the *Journal of Pain and Symptom Management* is hosting a special series of review articles on childhood pain; and both the *Pediatrician* (Vol. 16, 1989) and the *Pediatric Clinics of North America* (Vol. 36, No. 4, 1989) have published issues devoted exclusively to pain management in children. Although documented concerns about the adequacy of pain relief for children can be traced to the nursing profession, many disciplines are now sharing pediatric pain as a primary clinical specialty or research interest. Several pediatric pain clinics have been created recently in Canada and the United States. Although these clinics vary with respect to administration, funding sources, and composition, they share a common goal: to provide a multidisciplinary approach for children's pain management.

As a consequence of this dynamic interest in children's pain, incredible breakthroughs have occurred in our ability to assess and alleviate a child's pain. Although many questions remain to be answered, much is now known about how children perceive pain and how their pain can be modified. Many of the myths that have guided the manner in which we treat children's pain have been refuted. We recognize that infants perceive pain at birth and that the failure to alleviate their pain has adverse physiological consequences in addition to the suffering that they experience. We recognize that children understand the physical and emotional dimensions of pain at an early age. Children can describe their pain qualitatively, using langauge that reflects their own experiences, and can rate their pain quantitatively on a variety of standardized scales. But we must interpret their use of pain measures in accord with their developmental level and their frame of reference.

One of the most exciting breakthroughs has been the increasing realization that children's pain is plastic and complex. The traditional assumption—that a child's pain is simply and directly proportional to the nature and extent of tissue damage—is no longer credible. A child's pain can be modified by many internal and environmental factors. In fact, children's pain seems even more plastic than adults' pain. Children may possess a natural ability to reduce their pain with a variety of deceptively simple, practical nonpharmacological techniques. Relaxation, distraction, guided imagery, and hypnotic-like suggestions for analgesia may be more effective for children than for adults, because children do not share the common adult bias that only potent pharmacological interventions can truly reduce pain. The gradual acceptance that children's pain is plastic has initiated more ingenious approaches for managing their pain. Methods that have been generally restricted to adults, such as biofeedback, transcutaneous electrical nerve stimulation (TENS), acupuncture, and multistrategy cognitive-behavioral programs, are now adapted for children's pain problems. Traditional therapies for reducing children's anxiety, such as play, art therapy, entertaining films, and music, are now also used to reduce their pain. As a result, we are becoming increasingly sophisticated in our ability to alleviate pain in infants, children, and adolescents.

Yet much effort must still be expended to achieve a comprehensive understanding of children's unique pain problems. Like adults, children experience many different types of pain throughout their lives. Acute pains caused by tissue damage are the most common type, as children sustain mild to moderate injuries during their daily activities. Pain subsides as injuries heal. Children also experience varied muscular, skeletal, and vascular acute pains associated with stress, trauma, and disease. Most acute pains do not produce a constellation of emotional, situational, and behavioral factors that intensify a child's suffering. But acute pain caused by repeated invasive medical procedures can create a unique situation characterized by lack of control, inaccurate expectations, fear, anxiety, and overt distress behaviors—all of which adversely affect a child's pain experience. Children with cancer, diabetes, sickle cell anemia, and growth hormone deficiency, who require repeated blood-samplings, intramuscular and intravenous administrations, lumbar punctures, and bone marrow aspirations, are at risk for experiencing stronger pains from these procedures because of the context in which they are experienced. These children require special assistance. Age-appropriate guidelines must be developed in all treatment protocols to achieve the optimal balance of sedation, anxiety reduction, and pain control during invasive procedures.

Although children suffer prolonged chronic pain caused by disease, trauma, and psychological factors, chronic debilitating pain is not currently recognized as a major health problem for children, as it is for adults. Yet the assumption that children's chronic pain is adequately controlled must be confirmed with epidemiological data on the prevalence of chronic pain related to different childhood diseases. For example, chronic cancer pain has only recently been documented as a problem for some children in the terminal stage of the disease. Increased attention is now being focused on the source of persistent bone pain for some children with cancer. Questions have also arisen as to the extent to which children may be suffering from persistent pain as a result of the disease process or of the potent treatments they receive on certain cancer protocols. In contrast to the availability of many pain control drugs, the prescription and administration of analgesics are probably still inadequate for alleviating children's chronic pains. Clinical reports that children do not always receive appropriate analgesics in adequate doses to control their pain persist, despite advances in our understanding of pharmacology and opioid systems. The mode of analgesic administration is often inflexible, even though versatile administration techniques integrated with nonpharmacological interventions are essential for chronic pain management in adults. A more concerted effort is required to document all types of chronic pediatric pain and the efficacy of conventional pain control interventions. Guidelines for pain management, analogous to those developed for disease and injury management, should be developed and applied consistently for all children with chronic pain.

Recurrent pain syndromes, which afflict otherwise healthy and pain-free children, may pose a more critical health problem for children than chronic pain. Many children do not receive adequate pain relief because their headaches, abdominal pains, and limb pains are not correlating symptoms of active disease. Since disease treatment with symptom (i.e., pain) management has been the traditional approach for children's pain problems, the customary treatment for children with recurrent pain syndromes has been reassurance about the benign nature of their pain and recommendations for analgesic use as necessary during painful episodes. The internal and environmental factors responsible for initiating recurrent pains have received short shrift, so that children's pains continue and often intensify. The benign nature of these childhood pains is questionable, in light of the sequelae of continued pains throughout adolescence and adulthood. Particularly troubling are the recent studies indicating that adolescents who have endured recurrent pains for several years develop numerous emotional problems—

perhaps arising from the years of unpredictable pain episodes. As for acute and chronic pains, descriptive studies on the incidence and prevalence of recurrent pains are mandatory. Furthermore, longitudinal studies must be conducted to evaluate the effects of uncontrolled recurrent pains on children as they mature. The origins of some adult chronic pain conditions may exist in childhood recurrent pain syndromes.

Despite enormous advances in our knowledge about children's pain, serious challenges remain. We do not know the true incidence and prevalence of acute, recurrent, and chronic pains for children. We do not know the extent to which children receive inadequate pain relief. We do not know which interventions are maximally effective for reducing different types of pain in infants, children, and adolescents. And we do not know whether some types of chronic pain for adults originate as recurrent pains in childhood. Clinical and research emphasis must continue to be placed on pediatric pain, so that we can develop definitive guidelines for pain assessment and management. Our future aspirations for alleviating acute, chronic, and recurrent pain in children will only be achieved by a conscientious effort to integrate education, research, and clinical service.

An inevitable lag exists between the scientific accumulation of knowledge about the plasticity of nociceptive mechanisms and the application of that knowledge to clinical practice. The dissemination of information relevant for controlling children's pain is further complicated because few university curricula (medicine, nursing, dentistry, rehabilitative medicine, and psychology) include up-to-date details about nociceptive mechanisms, endogenous pain-inhibitory systems, and nonpharmacological methods of pain control for adults. Fewer still provide any pertinent information about unique pain problems in infants and children. Moreover, most hospital and many university libraries do not subscribe to any of the three major pain journals, so that health professionals lack the opportunity to learn about new advances in pain management unless they are specializing in this area themselves.

All health professionals should be educated about the plasticity and complexity of pain perception. Courses on the physiology, anatomy, and neurochemistry of nociceptive systems should be included in the general curricula of nursing and medical schools. Within these schools, more attention should be focused on the most appropriate pharmacological and nonpharmacological interventions for reducing pain in infants, children, and adolescents. Hospitals should subscribe to the primary pain journals to facilitate communication about nociceptive mechanisms and new techniques for pain control. Hospitals should adopt guidelines for pain management from a multidisciplinary perspective, to ensure that pain control is regarded as a priority within the health care system. Pediatric pain management is not the sole responsibility of any one discipline within hospitals, nor should it be. Instead, each discipline should assume a critical role and share a common responsibility, in order to provide the most appropriate interventions in an environment where a child will obtain optimal pain relief.

Research is a critical component for the provision of adequate pain control in pediatrics, because many questions exist that can only be answered by reputable studies. Unfortunately, the term "research" has an objectionable connotation within many hospitals. The term has become synonymous with large, expensive, controlled investigations; unwieldy data bases; biostatistics; and a core of full-time scientists and research personnel. Although some questions about children's pain must be answered by scientists who have the expertise necessary to design multi-center studies and who can obtain funding to support research costs, much valuable research can be conducted practically through the ongoing care of children with pain problems.

In fact, even though the management of children's pain has been hampered by a general lack of scientific study, a more serious obstacle has been our failure to routinely document the nature of children's pain complaints and the effectiveness of therapeutic interventions. Hospital chart notations may include "voiced pain complaints," "crying and fussing," or "irritable," along with appropriate documen-tation for prescribed and administered drugs, but pain notations are not ordinarily standardized as to terminology, recording frequency, and criteria for evaluating pain. Consequently, wide variation in pain documentation is common within a single ward. It is almost impossible to obtain any retrospective information on the prevalence of pain complaints for hospitalized children. Documentation on spe-cific analgesic effectiveness is extremely rare, apart from "comfortable," "resting," or "no pain complaints." Little prospective information about either the extent of pain reduction or the quality of pain relief (e.g., analgesia vs. sedation) can be obtained from our current charting systems, so that critical data that could improve pain management in pediatrics are ignored. We have seemingly, albeit unintentionally, dismissed pain as irrelevant for clinical care.

The adoption of consistent pain documentation throughout hospitals would do a great deal to remedy our previous neglect of children's pain. Critical attention would then be focused on objectively assessing the presence and level of pain, as well as on evaluating the efficacy of conventional treatments. Most clinical intake forms already include questions as to whether the child has pain, and, if so, the location, duration, and quality of the pain. Such information is essential for the differential diagnosis of any child's health problem. The manner in which this information is obtained from children could be standardized so as to allow comparisons among children and among hospitals. A simple rating scale could be incorporated into intake procedures to enable children to directly assess the strength of their pain. Age-appropriate questions about the location, duration, strength, and quality of a child's pain should be included as part of a clinical interview. Pain should be systematically assessed in hospitals when charting chil-dren's vital signs. Consistent documentation would provide not only accurate data about the presence and strength of childhood pain associated with different diseases, injuries, and surgeries, but also an objective gauge of how well various interventions lessen their pain.

Research is often regarded as contrasting sharply with conventional clinical practice. Yet ordinary clinical care can be regarded as research, because a clinician is determining the cause for pain, selecting an intervention from various alternatives, evaluating the effectiveness of the intervention and any side effects, adjusting the treatment as required to maintain a proper balance between effectiveness and side effects, and integrating the results of the treatment into his/her mental data base for future decisions about patient care. All health professionals constantly evaluate the effectiveness of their treatments, even if they do not detail their evaluations in a consistent manner for all children. Simple documentation of the clinical decision matrix would provide very valuable information about children's pain, while not adding excessive time to the management of a child's health problem.

The failure to document each child's pain has broad implications for pain management in all children. As an example, variations of the statement "Children with cancer do not have chronic pain in the terminal stages of the disease" are commonplace, even though many oncologists who treat dying children with leukemia or solid tumors dispute this statement. Furthermore, some acknowledge that they administer potent opioid analgesics to these children in higher doses and at more frequent dosing intervals than normally recommended, without fear of excessive sedation, respiratory depression, or addiction. But there has been a failure to document such clinical practice in informal presentations, case reports, published abstracts, letters to the editor, or review articles published in medical journals. The unfortunate result is that factual information about relieving pain in terminally ill children with cancer is suppressed, while the misleading statements as to the lack of pain in these children are perpetuated. These latter statements, therefore, convey an implicit message that children dying from cancer do not require potent analgesics.

Careful documentation provides a more objective basis for evaluating the efficacy of any treatment and for guiding decisions about patient care. The nature of the documentation will vary, depending on the clinical setting and the type of pain. Pain from chronic disease should be routinely assessed, coincident with medical evaluations of disease state. Postsurgical pain should be monitored regularly from the postoperative recovery room until children are discharged. Consistent monitoring might prevent the common pain problems encountered when medication is switched abruptly from intravenous opioid analgesics to oral nonopioid analgesics, with the assumption that the weaker oral administrations are equally effective for controlling pain. Acute pain caused by invasive procedures should be assessed routinely for most children, especially children who require repeated medical treatments over a long time period. These children are at risk for developing high anxiety, fear, and depression that will increase their pain. Children with cancer must be assessed at regular intervals throughout their treatment protocol, to evaluate any pain caused by the disease or by the cumulative effects of the potent chemotherapy regimens.

Consistent pain documentation promotes optimal health care. For example, children treated in the emergency department for lacerations may be asked to rate the pain caused by the infiltrations as well as pain caused by the suturing procedure. The location of the injury, nature of the infiltration (number of needles, anesthetic solution), and delay time from infiltration to suturing are probably already recorded. The addition of pain ratings to these statistics provides a salient component for quality assurance. The director of the emergency department can examine differences in pain according to site, extent of injury, type of anesthetic, variables in anesthetic administration, nature of child's preparation, and presence of significant others (parent, child life worker, pain therapist). In this manner, the situational factors that enhance pain relief can be identified and incorporated as part of the standard procedures. Similar benefits in patient care will accrue throughout hospitals and pediatric clinics when pain documentation is implemented. Routine documentation will yield a comprehensive data base that will enable clinical investigators and epidemiologists to determine more accurately the nature and scope of pain problems for children according to their age, sex, and health status. Such information will provide a major resource for health planning and will permit resources to be allocated in a more cost-effective manner. The enormous wealth of information that could be achieved by relatively minor revisions in patient documentation would provide a major resource for improving pain management for children in the clinic and for addressing many research questions about their pain perception, pain expression, and pain behavior.

Despite significant advances in our ability to control pain, the clinical management of children's pain is still deficient. Guidelines for analgesia must be developed and adopted in pediatrics. Recommendations should be based on the source of noxious stimulation (e.g., peripheral or central, duration, extent of trauma), pertinent health factors, age of the child, and modifying situational factors. Analgesic drugs must be selected according to their potency and site of action. Opioid analgesics are indicated when children experience severe pain; children should not suffer because of unfounded fears of addiction. Unfortunately, clinical surveys indicate that opioids have often not been prescribed even when children are dying. All analgesics should be administered in the most effective manner (e.g., oral, intravenous, intramuscular, continuous infusion). Novel administration routes, such as lollipops, should be evaluated for young children. Dosing intervals should be frequent enough to control pain adequately, so that children do not experience an alternating cycle of pain, drowsy analgesia, pain, and so on. Children who require injections should also receive some simple training so that they can reduce the acute pain caused by the needle. Topical anesthetic creams should be used more widely to complement local infiltrations. The use of patient-controlled analgesia should be considered for some children hospitalized with acute postsurgical pain or chronic pain. Although the expertise is available to permit us to develop principles of analgesic administration for controlling different types of pain in infants, children, and adolescents, continued clinical emphasis is required to ensure that this objective is realized.

A diverse array of nonpharmacological interventions may be used to relieve children's pain. Physical, behavioral, and cognitive methods should be integrated more fully into clinical practice in pediatrics. The choice for pain control is not merely "drug" versus "nondrug" therapy; rather, a therapy that mitigates both the causative and the contributing factors in pain should be implemented. Because pain is a multidimensional perception, a multidimensional approach is essential. The most appropriate pharmacological and nonpharmacological interventions should be carefully selected after a comprehensive pain assessment to identify the source of noxious stimulation and the relevant contributing factors.

In fact, multistrategy programs in which pharmacological and varied cognitive, behavioral, and physical interventions are combined (as in the program for recurrent pain outlined in Chapter 8) are beneficial for many types of childhood pain. Because of their continuous physical and cognitive development, children require a consistent, but flexible and versatile, approach to pain management. The wide variety of nonpharmacological interventions enables health professionals to choose the age-appropriate interventions most effective for a particular child. Multistrategy programs can provide a sensible solution for certain acute, recurrent, and chronic pains when they are designed after a thorough evaluation of the pain problem in relation to the specific context (situational, emotional, familial, and behavioral factors) in which children experience pain. The assessment provides a basic framework for identifying the factors that must be changed to alleviate pain. A flexible program can then be designed, with various treatment components selected to address the primary factors common for children. However, the specific interventions may vary, depending on the age of a child and any unique factors affecting his/her pain.

The gradual recognition that children's pain is plastic has enormous implications in clinical service. Practical nonpharmacological interventions can be incorporated in hospitals, such as deep rubbing prior to heel pricks in newborn infants; deep rubbing of fingertips after blood-sampling in all children; the use of TENS for reducing postsurgical pain in critically ill infants for whom opioid analgesics pose a serious risk; and the routine incorporation of distraction, imagery techniques, and simple coping tools into emergency and outpatient ambulatory procedures. The benefits of allowing children more choice, improved control, increased participation, and a better understanding of invasive treatments are revealed dramatically by reductions in overt distress, anxiety, and pain. Most children can easily understand the concept of "closing their pain gates" and eagerly learn new methods to shut the gates to lessen pain. Although some children require special programs from an experienced pain therapist, all children benefit from a general cognitive-behavioral approach (as described in Chapter 6) in which the primary focus is to modify the contextual factors that exacerbate the neuronal activity initiated by a noxious stimulus. Naturally, the specific methods effective for modifying these factors depend on the child as well as on the type of pain.

Few nonpharmacological interventions are used consistently for children. This is unfortunate, because many represent practical, versatile, inexpensive, and effective pain-reducing techniques that can be adopted for all children. A concerted effort should be expended on integrating these interventions into routine hospital practice. Special consideration should be given to whether other nonpharmacological interventions, such as TENS, hypnosis, biofeedback, and acupuncture, have wider utility in pediatric pain control. Standard hospital preparatory programs for children should include some information on pain and pain control. The focus should include information about how to close the pain gates, with an emphasis on the fact that any pain can be adequately controlled so that children (and parents) do not become unduly anxious about necessary treatments. Films, modeling, and direct instructions should incorporate information about the sensory aspects of a procedure, rather than the label "hurt."

Pain management programs should be designed for children with different pain problems (e.g., diabetes, recurrent abdominal pain, arthritis, sickle cell anemia, cancer) from a multidisciplinary perspective. Parents should be an integral part of the program. They become coaches, assisting children to use pain-reducing strategies and encouraging them to be independent and assume control. Children learn techniques that are adaptable to all situations in which they experience pain. The success of the technique does not depend on the therapist who has trained them, but rather on their own ability to use the methods they have learned. Group and individual programs should be developed so that children have an opportunity to learn from one another. The group dynamics can tremendously accelerate children's progress through the pain program. A tangible symbol should be provided as recognition of a child's successful completion of the program and mastery of pain management principles. Colorful buttons reading "Pain Program Grad" (shown in Figure 10.1) have been appreciated by our children.

In summary, despite much progress over the last few years, there is still a reluctance to develop a consistent approach for pediatric pain management. Often, few programs are available within hospitals to facilitate a multidimensional approach to the assessment and management of children's pain problems. Although

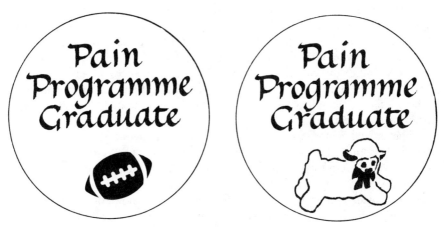

FIGURE 10.1. Buttons presented to children after successful completion of the pain management program at the Pain Clinic of the Children's Hospital of Western Ontario.

we do not know the specific extent to which maturation, gender, parental attitudes, culture, and previous pain experiences shape children's pain perceptions and pain expressions, we do know how to assess and alleviate their pain. A variety of physiological, behavioral, and self-report measures can be used to evaluate distress and pain. There is no one pain measure that is perfectly appropriate for all children and for all types of pain that children experience; instead, there are advantages and disadvantages to each measure. Measures should be selected according to the age of the child and the type of pain that he/she experiences. In evaluating a child's response on any measure, one should consider the child's frame of reference—that is, the nature and extent of his/her previous pain experiences. It is best to be cautious when interpreting children's pain by observing their behaviors and physiological responses, since these do not necessarily covary with the strength of their pain. Moreover, pain intensity cannot be assessed at only a single point in time. Accurate pain assessment involves assessing pain in relation to the child experiencing it and the context in which it is experienced. Serious attention must be focused on children who are retarded or developmentally delayed; their pain needs have long been ignored, and we need to develop sensitive tools for assessing these needs.

Pain assessment is inextricably linked to pain management. Unless we understand the internal and environmental factors that modify a child's pain, our attempts to control it will necessarily be inadequate. The same noxious stimulus does not produce equivalent pains in the same child from time to time or in all children. Consequently, we cannot control pain by gearing our interventions solely to the source of tissue damage. Instead, for maximal efficacy, our interventions must be targeted at the source of tissue damage in relation to the factors that are affecting the nociceptive processing initiated by that tissue damage.

A thorough understanding of children's pain requires an understanding of the nociceptive systems that underlie their perception. These systems provide a logical framework for selecting interventions. Some quite sensible and easy interventions can be adapted from knowledge of the effects of large-fiber stimulation on second-order neurons responding to small-fiber activation (e.g., children rubbing their fingers vigorously and deeply after a finger prick for blood-sampling). Advances in the unraveling of the complexity of specificity, convergence, inhibition, summation, and descending control have important implications for the treatment of children's pain. Principles of pain management must be adapted from the study of nociceptive mechanisms.

The crucial factors for selecting an effective analgesic intervention are to identify the source of noxious stimulation and evaluate the situational, emotional, and behavioral factors that modify the pain. In light of the number of factors that contribute to a child's pain, multistrategy interventions may be most useful. A creative clinical approach, combined with a working knowledge of nociceptive processing, will lead to practical, versatile, and optimal pain control for all children.

Pain Assessment Measures for Children and Parents

Details regarding scoring and administration are available, upon request, from Patricia A. McGrath, PhD, Director, Child Health Research Institute, Children's Hospital of Western Ontario, 800 Commissioners Road East, Box 5375, London, Ontario N6C 2V5, Canada.

General—Acute Pain Assessment: Intake Information

Child's name _____ Date of birth _____ Date _____

Address _____ Telephone (home) _____

_____ (work) _____

Parents' names _____ _____

Completed by Mother __ Father __

General Information

1. Parents: Married/separated/divorced/remarried/widowed (Please circle one.)
   Are you: single?   Yes __ No __
           living common-law? Yes __ No __

2. Parents' principal occupation during last 5 years:
   Mother _____
   Father _____

3. Parents' school level: Mother _____ Father _____

4. What grade is your child in? _____

5. What school does your child attend? _____

6. In general, what is your child's attitude toward school? (Please circle one.)
   Very negative   Negative   Neutral   Positive   Very positive

7. Overall, please indicate the level of your child's grades/academic performance. (Circle one.)
   Nearly failing   Below average   Average   Above average   Superior

8. List your child's favorite pastimes, hobbies, and/or sports.
   _____ _____
   _____ _____
   _____ _____

9. Please list the names, ages, and sex of brothers and sisters in birth order.

	Name	Age	Sex
1.	_____	—	—
2.	_____	—	—
3.	_____	—	—
4.	_____	—	—
5.	_____	—	—

Hospital Experience

10. Hospital experiences (operations and illnesses):

Age (at time)	Reason	Length of stay
1. _____	_____	_____
2. _____	_____	_____

3. _____ _____ _____
4. _____ _____ _____
5. _____ _____ _____

11. General attitude (circle one) toward:

Doctor visits:	Positive	Neutral	Negative
Hospital stays:	Positive	Neutral	Negative
Medical tests:	Positive	Neutral	Negative

12. What does your child usually do when he/she is in pain from a stomachache caused by being nervous or excited? _____
_____
_____

13. Whom does your child usually go to for assistance when he/she is in pain? _____
_____

14. What does your child know about his/her illness (e.g., the nature of the disease and cause)? _____
_____
_____

15. Who generally provides information to the child about his/her illness?_____
_____
_____

Inpatients only—Questions 16, 17, and 18

16. How long has your child been in the hospital? _____
_____

17. When does your family usually come to visit? (time of day, length of visit?) _____
_____
_____

18. When will your child be discharged? _____
_____

19. How does your child know what procedure will take place and when? _____
_____
_____

20. Does your child know about, in general,
    treatment procedures?   Yes _ No _
    necessary medical equipment?   Yes _ No _

21. Does your child talk to you about treatment procedures?
    Yes, frequently ____   Yes, sometimes ____   Not at all ____
    Does your child talk to others about treatment procedures?
    Yes, frequently ____   Yes, sometimes ____   Not at all ____

22. What is the general nature of these conversations?

Complaining ___   Questioning ___

Fearful ___   Other _____

Providing descriptions to others ___   _____

Pain Experiences

23. Has your child had any of the following procedures?   If so, what family members are usually present?

IVs	___	_____
Finger pricks	___	_____
X-rays	___	_____
Injections—i.m.	___	_____
Injections—i.v.	___	_____
Dressing changes	___	_____
Blood samples	___	_____
Other— _____	___	_____
Other— _____	___	_____
Other— _____	___	_____

24. How anxious or worried is your child usually, prior to each of the following procedures? (Circle the most appropriate description of your child's general anxiety.)

	Not at all	Slightly	Moderately	Very	Extremely	Not applicable
IVs	N	S	M	V	E	NA
Finger pricks	N	S	M	V	E	NA
X-rays	N	S	M	V	E	NA
Dressing changes	N	S	M	V	E	NA
Blood samples (vein)	N	S	M	V	E	NA
Injections—i.m.	N	S	M	V	E	NA
Injections—i.v.	N	S	M	V	E	NA
Other— _____	N	S	M	V	E	NA
Other— _____	N	S	M	V	E	NA
Other— _____	N	S	M	V	E	NA

25. How much pain do you think your child experiences during each of the following procedures?

	None	Slight	Moderate	Very much	Extreme	Not applicable
Finger pricks	N	S	M	V	E	NA
Blood samples (vein)	N	S	M	V	E	NA
X-rays	N	S	M	V	E	NA
Injections—i.m.	N	S	M	V	E	NA
Injections—i.v.	N	S	M	V	E	NA
IVs	N	S	M	V	E	NA
Dressing changes	N	S	M	V	E	NA
Other— _____	N	S	M	V	E	NA

Other—_____   N   S   M   V   E   NA
Other—_____   N   S   M   V   E   NA

26. Does your child exhibit any of the following behaviors during procedure? (Specify for which treatments.)

    Nausea   _____

    Crying   _____

    Screaming   _____

    Stalling   _____

    Resisting   _____

    Refusing   _____

    Other   _____

27. Does your child need to be restrained during procedures?   Yes __   No __
If so, how is this usually done? _____
_____

28. How were you initially informed about the Pediatric Pain Program? _____
_____

29. Does your child have any difficulties or problems with treatment that you have not already described? _____
_____
_____

30. Do you have any concerns or questions about the pain management program for your child? _____
_____
_____

General—Acute Pain Assessment: Parent Interview

Part A

Date _____

Child's name _____ Age/sex_____

Information obtained from Mother _____ Father _____ Obtained by _____

1. Rank order of the pain intensity associated with procedures experienced by child (from least to most).

	Mother	Father
1.	_____	_____
2.	_____	_____
3.	_____	_____
4.	_____	_____
5.	_____	_____
6.	_____	_____
7.	_____	_____
8.	_____	_____
9.	_____	_____

2. How does your child respond to each of the following procedures? (Interviewer: Collect information on *behavior* [active, passive; self, others] and *attitudes* [positive, neutral, negative].)

IVs: _____

Finger pricks: _____

X-rays: _____

Dressing changes: _____

Blood sample (vein): _____

Injections—i.m.: _____

Injections—i.v.: _____

Other— _____ : _____

Other— _____ : _____

Other— _____ : _____

Outpatients only—Questions 3, 4, and 5

3. When do you usually come for treatment (day and time)? _____

_____

_____

4. What do you usually do while waiting? _____

_____

_____

5. What does your child usually do while waiting? _____

_____

_____

Part B

6. How anxious are parents in discussing this information?

|⊢——⊣|

 Not at all   Extremely

7. How receptive or supportive are parents to a pain management program?

|⊢——⊣|

 Not at all   Extremely

8. Assess their understanding/knowledge of medical treatments and procedures.

_____

_____

9. What additional support is the child or family receiving (e.g., social work, psychology, etc.)?

_____

_____

_____

General—Acute Pain Assessment: Pre and Post Measures
for Pain Management Program

Name _____ Sex/age _____ Date _____

1. What is it that you have? That is, why do you need treatment? _____

_____

_____

2. What kinds of treatment do you get?

	Voluntary	With prompt
IVs	_____	_____
Finger pricks	_____	_____
X-rays	_____	_____
Injections—i.m.	_____	_____
Injections—i.v.	_____	_____
Dressing changes	_____	_____
Oral medication	_____	_____
Blood samples (vein)	_____	_____
Other— _____	_____	_____
Other— _____	_____	_____
Other— _____	_____	_____

3. What is the purpose for these procedures and what medical equipment is used for each? (Interviewer: Alternate procedure order.)

IVs: _____

_____

Equipment: _____

_____

Dressing changes: _____

_____

Equipment: _____

_____

Injections—i.m.: _____

_____

Equipment: _____

_____

Injections—i.v.: _____

_____

Equipment: _____

_____

Finger pricks: _____

_____

Equipment: _____

_____

Oral medication: _____

_____

Equipment: _____

_____

X-rays: _____

_____

Equipment: _____

_____

Blood samples (vein): _____

_____

Equipment: _____

_____

Other— _____ : _____

_____

Equipment: _____

_____

Other— _____ : _____

_____

Equipment: _____

_____

Other— _____ : _____

_____

Equipment: _____

_____

4a. What kinds of medications do you receive? _____

_____

_____

4b. Where? _____

_____

4c. How often? _____

_____

4d. Who administers it? _____

_____

5. Which face on the face sheet looks the way you feel deep down inside during:
   (Face sheet color: _____)
   Blood samples (vein)   _____
   Finger pricks   _____
   X-rays   _____
   Oral medication   _____
   Dressing changes   _____
   Injections—i.m.   _____
   Injections—i.v.   _____
   IVs   _____
   Other— _____   _____
   Other— _____   _____
   Other— _____   _____

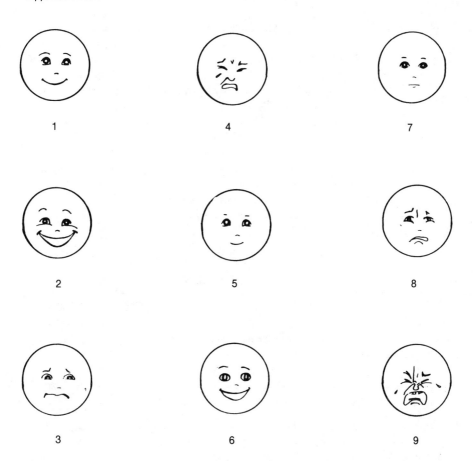

1

4

7

2

5

8

3

6

9

(Three sets of face sheets are used, with faces varying in position. Numbers denote position on sheet, not face value.)

6. What do you do to make the pain go away or to make procedures easier?

_____

_____

_____

7. Can you give me an idea of what happens when you get _____ ? (Interviewer: Specify treatment—to assess child's understanding of his/her own pain behavior.)

_____

_____

_____

8. How sad (depressed) do you feel because of these treatments? (Interviewer: Present treatment procedures in random order.)

|———|

Not at all   Saddest possible

9. How angry do you feel because of these treatments? (Interviewer: Present treatment procedures in random order.)

|———|

Not at all   Angriest possible

10. How afraid do you feel because of these treatments? (Interviewer: Present treatment procedures in random order.)

|———|

Not at all   Most afraid possible

11. How sure/certain are you that you will be able to control the pain someday?

|———|

Not sure   Very sure

12. How much of the pain can you control during _____ ?

|———|

Not at all   Completely

13. How anxious/worried are you during _____ ?

|———|

Not at all   Most anxious possible

14. How much pain do you have during _____ ?

|———|

Not at all   Most pain possible

15. How sad (depressed) do you feel because of your _____ ?

Not at all   Saddest possible

16. How angry do you feel because of your _____ ?

Not at all   Angriest possible

17. How afraid do you feel because of your _____ ?

Not at all   Most afraid possible

18. How anxious/worried are you about your _____ ?

Not at all   Most anxious possible

19. How sure are you that some day you will no longer have this _____ ?

Not at all   Very sure

Oncology—Acute Pain Assessment: Intake Information

Child's name _____   Date of birth _____   Date _____
Address _____   Telephone   (home) _____
_____   (work) _____
Parents' names _____   _____
Completed by   Mother __   Father __

General Information

1. Parents: Married/separated/divorced/remarried/widowed (Please circle one.)
   Are you: single?   Yes __   No __
              living common-law?   Yes __   No __

2. Parents' principal occupation during last 5 years:
   Mother _____
   Father _____

3. Parents' school level: Mother _____   Father _____

4. What grade is your child in? _____

5. What school does your child attend? _____

6. In general, what is your child's attitude toward school? (Please circle one.)
   Very negative   Negative   Neutral   Positive   Very positive

7. Overall, please indicate the level of your child's grades/academic performance.
   (Circle one.)
   Nearly failing   Below average   Average   Above average   Superior

8. List your child's favorite pastimes, hobbies, and/or sports.

   _____   _____
   _____   _____
   _____   _____

9. Please list the names, ages, and sex of brothers and sisters in birth order.

	Name	Age	Sex
1.	_____	__	__
2.	_____	__	__
3.	_____	__	__
4.	_____	__	__
5.	_____	__	__

Hospital Experience

10. Hospital experiences (operations and illnesses):

Age (at time)	Reason	Length of stay
1. _____	_____	_____
2. _____	_____	_____

3. _____ _____ _____

4. _____ _____ _____

5. _____ _____ _____

11. General attitude (circle one) toward:

Doctor visits:	Positive	Neutral	Negative
Hospital stays:	Positive	Neutral	Negative
Medical tests:	Positive	Neutral	Negative

12. What does your child usually do when he/she is in pain from a stomachache caused by being nervous or excited? _____

_____

13. Whom does your child usually go to for assistance when he/she is in pain? _____

_____

14. What does your child know about his/her illness (e.g., the nature of the disease and cause)? _____

_____

15. Who generally provides information to the child about his/her illness?_____

_____

16. Does your child know about the protocol?   Yes _ No _

17. Do you follow the protocol?

Not at all ___ Rarely ___ Occasionally ___ Often ___ All the time ___

18. Does your child follow the protocol?

Not at all ___ Rarely ___ Occasionally ___ Often ___ All the time ___

19. How does your child know what procedure will take place and when? _____

_____

20. Does your child know about, in general,

treatment procedures?   Yes _ No _

necessary medical equipment?   Yes _ No _

21. Does your child talk to you about treatments during the week?

Yes, frequently ___ Yes, sometimes ___ Not at all ___

Does your child talk to others about treatments during the week?

Yes, frequently ___ Yes, sometimes ___ Not at all ___

22. What is the general nature of these conversations?

Complaining ___	Questioning ___
Fearful ___	Other _____
Providing descriptions to others ___	_____

Pain Experiences

23. Has your child had any of the following   If so, what family members are usually
    procedures?   present?
    Lumbar punctures   ___   _____
    Portacatheter use   ___   _____
    IVs   ___   _____
    Finger pricks   ___   _____
    X-rays   ___   _____
    Echocardiograms   ___   _____
    Bone marrow aspirations   ___   _____
    Injections—i.m.   ___   _____
    Injections—i.v.   ___   _____
    Dressing changes   ___   _____
    Blood samples (vein)   ___   _____

    Are there any other procedures not listed above? _____

24. How anxious or worried is your child usually, prior to each of the following proce-
    dures? (Circle the most appropriate description of your child's general anxiety.)

	Not at all	Slightly	Moderately	Very much	Extremely	Not applicable
IVs	N	S	M	V	E	NA
Echocardiograms	N	S	M	V	E	NA
Bone marrow aspirations	N	S	M	V	E	NA
Finger pricks	N	S	M	V	E	NA
X-rays	N	S	M	V	E	NA
Portacatheter use	N	S	M	V	E	NA
Dressing changes	N	S	M	V	E	NA
Blood samples (vein)	N	S	M	V	E	NA
Lumbar punctures	N	S	M	V	E	NA
Injections—i.m.	N	S	M	V	E	NA
Injections—i.v.	N	S	M	V	E	NA
Other— _____	N	S	M	V	E	NA
Other— _____	N	S	M	V	E	NA
Other— _____	N	S	M	V	E	NA

25. How much pain do you think your child experiences during each of the following
    procedures?

	None	Slight	Moderate	Very much	Extreme	Not applicable
Echocardiograms	N	S	M	V	E	NA
Finger pricks	N	S	M	V	E	NA
Lumbar punctures	N	S	M	V	E	NA
Portacatheter use	N	S	M	V	E	NA
Blood samples (vein)	N	S	M	V	E	NA
X-rays	N	S	M	V	E	NA
Injections—i.m.	N	S	M	V	E	NA

Injections—i.v.	N	S	M	V	E	NA
IVs	N	S	M	V	E	NA
Dressing changes	N	S	M	V	E	NA
Bone marrow aspirations	N	S	M	V	E	NA
Other—_____	N	S	M	V	E	NA
Other—_____	N	S	M	V	E	NA
Other—_____	N	S	M	V	E	NA

26. Does your child exhibit any of the following behaviors during procedures? (Specify for which treatments.)

Nausea _____

Crying _____

Screaming _____

Stalling _____

Resisting _____

Refusing _____

Other _____

27. Does your child need to be restrained during procedures?   Yes _ No _
If so, how is this usually done? _____
_____
_____

28. How were you initially informed about the Pediatric Pain Program? _____
_____

29. Does your child have any difficulties or problems with treatment that you have not already described (e.g., preprocedure sleeping difficulties or increased hostility toward brothers and sisters)?_____
_____
_____

30. Do you have any concerns or questions about the pain management program for your child? _____
_____
_____

Oncology—Acute Pain Assessment: Parent Interview

Part A

Date _____

Child's name _____   Age/sex_____

Information obtained from Mother _____ Father _____ Obtained by _____

1. Rank order of the pain intensity associated with oncology procedures experienced by child (from least to most).

	Mother	Father
1.	_____	_____
2.	_____	_____
3.	_____	_____
4.	_____	_____
5.	_____	_____
6.	_____	_____
7.	_____	_____
8.	_____	_____
9.	_____	_____

2. How does your child respond to each of the following procedures? (Interviewer: Collect information on *behavior* [active, passive; self, others] and *attitudes* [positive, neutral, negative].)

   Bone marrow aspirations: _____

   _____

   Finger pricks: _____

   _____

   X-rays: _____

   _____

   Dressing changes: _____

   _____

   Use of portacatheter: _____

   _____

   Injections—i.m.: _____

   _____

   Injections—i.v.: _____

   _____

   IVs: _____

   _____

   Echocardiograms: _____

   _____

   Lumbar punctures: _____

   _____

   Blood samples (vein): _____

   _____

   Other— _____ : _____

   _____

Other— _____ : _____

Other— _____ : _____

3. What do you do when your child has:
Blood samples (vein): _____

Lumbar punctures: _____

Injections—i.m.: _____

Injections—i.v.: _____

IVs: _____

Use of portacatheter: _____

Dressing changes: _____

X-rays: _____

Finger pricks: _____

Echocardiograms: _____

Bone marrow aspirations: _____

Other— _____ : _____

Other— _____ : _____

Other— _____ : _____

4. When do you usually come for treatment (day and time)? _____

5. What do you usually do while waiting? _____

6. What does your child usually do while waiting? _____

Part B

7. How anxious do parents appear in discussing this information?

|——|

   Not at all   Extremely

8. How receptive or supportive are parents to a pain management program?

|——|

   Not at all   Extremely

9. Assess their understanding/knowledge of medical treatments and procedures.

_____
_____
_____

10. What additional support is the child or family getting (e.g., social work, psychology, etc.)?

_____
_____
_____
_____

Oncology—Acute Pain Assessment: Pre and Post Measures
for Pain Management Program

Name _____ Sex/age _____ Date _____

1. What is it that you have? That is, why do you need treatment? _____
   _____
   _____

2. What kinds of treatment do you get?

	Voluntary	With prompt
Portacatheter use	_____	_____
Bone marrow aspirations	_____	_____
Echocardiograms	_____	_____
Blood samples (vein)	_____	_____
IVs	_____	_____
Oral medication	_____	_____
Dressing changes	_____	_____
Finger pricks	_____	_____
X-rays	_____	_____
Lumbar punctures	_____	_____
Injections—i.m.	_____	_____
Injections—i.v.	_____	_____
Other— _____	_____	_____
Other— _____	_____	_____
Other— _____	_____	_____

3. What is the purpose for these procedures and what medical equipment is used for each? (Interviewer: Alternate procedure order.)

   Echocardiograms: _____
   _____

   Equipment: _____
   _____

   IVs: _____
   _____

   Equipment: _____
   _____

   Bone marrow aspirations: _____
   _____

   Equipment: _____
   _____

   Dressing changes: _____
   _____

   Equipment: _____
   _____

   Injections—i.m.: _____
   _____

Equipment: _____

Injections—i.v.: _____

Equipment: _____

Finger pricks: _____

Equipment: _____

X-rays: _____

Equipment: _____

Oral medication: _____

Equipment: _____

Portacatheter use: _____

Equipment: _____

Lumbar punctures: _____

Equipment: _____

Blood samples (vein): _____

Equipment: _____

Other— _____ : _____

Equipment: _____

Other— _____ : _____

Equipment: _____

Other— _____ : _____

Equipment: _____

4a. What kinds of medications do you receive? _____

4b. Where? _____

4c. How often? _____

4d. Who administers it? _____

5. Which face on the face sheet looks the way you feel deep down inside during:
   (Face sheet color: _____)
Blood samples (vein)	_____
Finger pricks	_____
Portacatheter use	_____
Bone marrow aspirations	_____
X-rays	_____
Oral medication	_____
Echocardiograms	_____
Dressing changes	_____
Injections—i.m.	_____
Injections—i.v.	_____
IVs	_____
Lumbar punctures	_____
Other— _____	_____
Other— _____	_____
Other— _____	_____

6. What do you do to make the pain go away or to make procedures easier?
   _____
   _____
   _____

7. Can you give me an idea of what happens when you get _____ ? (Interviewer:
   Specify treatment—to assess child's understanding of his/her own pain behavior.)
   _____
   _____
   _____

8. How sad (depressed) do you feel because of these treatments? (Interviewer: Present
   treatment procedures in random order.)

   |——|

   Not at all   Saddest possible

9. How angry do you feel because of these treatments? (Interviewer: Present treatment
   procedures in random order.)

   |——|

   Not at all   Angriest possible

10. How afraid do you feel because of these treatments? (Interviewer: Present treatment
    procedures in random order.)

    |——|

    Not at all   Most afraid possible

11. How sure/certain are you that you will be able to control the pain someday?

```
├─────────────────────────────────────────────────────────────┤
 Not at all                                              Very sure
```

12. How much of the pain can you control during _____ ?

```
├─────────────────────────────────────────────────────────────┤
 Not at all                                            Completely
```

13. How anxious/worried are you during _____ ?

```
├─────────────────────────────────────────────────────────────┤
 Not at all                                    Most anxious possible
```

14. How much pain do you have during _____ ?

```
├─────────────────────────────────────────────────────────────┤
 Not at all                                      Most pain possible
```

15. How sad (depressed) do you feel because of your disease?

```
├─────────────────────────────────────────────────────────────┤
 Not at all                                        Saddest possible
```

16. How angry do you feel because of your disease?

```
├─────────────────────────────────────────────────────────────┤
 Not at all                                        Angriest possible
```

17. How afraid do you feel because of your disease?

```
├─────────────────────────────────────────────────────────────┤
 Not at all                                      Most afraid possible
```

18. How anxious/worried are you about your disease?

```
├─────────────────────────────────────────────────────────────┤
 Not at all                                    Most anxious possible
```

19. How sure are you that some day you will no longer have this disease?

```
├─────────────────────────────────────────────────────────────┤
 Not at all                                              Very sure
```

Headache History and Pain Information
(To be completed by parent)

Child's name _____ Sex __ Age __
Date of birth _____
Brothers/sisters (names and ages) _____
Form completed by Mother __ Father __ Other _____
Child's school _____ Child's grade __

In general, what is your child's attitude about school? (Please circle one.)
    Very negative   Negative   Neutral   Positive   Very positive
Overall, please indicate the level of your child's grades/academic performance. (Please circle one.)

| Nearly failing | Below average | Average | Above average | Superior |

Has your child's school teacher expressed any concerns regarding academic performance, behavior, or social relationships during the past year? (Please specify.)

_____
_____
_____

List your child's favorite three pastimes, hobbies, extracurricular activities.

_____
_____
_____

Number of school days missed in this school year due to headaches __
Number of school days missed in last month __
Number of doctor's visits in last month because of headaches __
Average frequency of headaches _____
Average duration of headache _____
Parents: Married/separated/divorced/remarried/widowed (Please circle one.)
Parents' principal occupation during last 5 years:
Mother _____
Father _____
Parents' school level: Mother _____ Father _____
Principal residence during last 5 years _____
What causes your child's headaches? _____

Can he/she lessen the pain completely during a headache? _____

What can you do to help your child when he/she has headaches? _____

Is there any family history of regular headaches? (If so, please explain which family member and what type of headaches.) _____

_____
_____

This measure is specific to headaches, but it may be adapted to assess other forms of recurrent and chronic pain.

Do any of your children or other family members have a chronic disease or illness (e.g., diabetes, cancer, etc.)? _____

_____

Do any of your children experience frequent problems with any type of pain (e.g., stomachaches, back pain)? _____

_____

What do you do for yourself when you have a headache? _____

_____

Can you lessen the pain completely when you have a headache? _____

_____

Do any of these trigger your child's headaches? (Respond with A, always; S, sometimes; N, never; D, don't know.)

Foods:
   __ Chocolate
   __ Wheat
   __ Cheese
   __ Sugar
   __ Yeast
   __ Eggs
   __ Meat with nitrates
   __ Other _____

Weather:
   __ Humidity, barometric pressure
   __ Sudden or large temperature shifts
   __ Hot weather
   __ Cold weather
   __ Sun

Emotions:
   __ Anger
   __ Fear
   __ Anxiety, worry
   __ Other _____

Social activities:
   __ Party
   __ Dance
   __ Concert
   __ Movie
   __ Other _____

School:
   __ Class
   __ Tests
   __ Bus
   __ Breaks
   __ Other _____

Other:
   __ Physical activity
   __ Fatigue
   __ Mental concentration
   __ Noise
   __ Siblings

Children's Comprehensive Pain Questionnaire (CCPQ)
(To be administered by trained interviewer)

Part A: Pain History (obtained in interview with parents)

Name _____ Sex _____ Age _____ Date _____
Medical diagnosis _____ Referred by _____ Assessed by _____
Age of child at pain onset _____ Date (mo/yr) _____ Syndrome duration ____
First physician visit re: pain—Date (mo/yr) _____
First diagnosis _____ Intervention_____
Efficacy _____
Number of subsequent health care visits for the pain (chronological order):

	Number	Diagnosis	Intervention/efficacy
Pediatrician/family physician:	_____	_____	_____
Other physicians (specify):	_____	_____	_____
Specialists:	_____	_____	_____
	_____	_____	_____
Emergency room:	_____	_____	_____
	_____	_____	_____
Hospital:	_____	_____	_____
	_____	_____	_____
Other:	_____	_____	_____
	_____	_____	_____

Average frequency of headaches _____ Range _____
Average length of headaches _____ Range _____
Notable changes in frequency or intensity _____

Current frequency _____ Current length _____
Why did you see Dr. _____ at this time? _____
_____

Describe one of your child's usual headaches, and also describe one of his/her worst headaches. (Note: Use the back of the questionnaire if you need more space.)

_____
_____

What medication has your child taken for his/her headaches? (Note: Mark those presently taken with an asterisk and state how effective the medication is.)

This version of the CCPQ specifically assesses headache pain; the instrument has been adapted for many other types of chronic and recurrent pain as well, with the relevant pain problem substituted for the word "headache."

Medication	Efficacy
1. _____	_____
2. _____	_____
3. _____	_____
4. _____	_____
5. _____	_____

Who decides when medication is used, and how is that decision made (i.e., under what conditions)? _____

_____

_____

Part B. Children's Subjective Pain Experience

Average frequency of headaches _____ Range _____

Average length of headaches _____ Range _____

Notable changes in frequency or intensity _____

_____

Current frequency _____ Current length _____

Why did you see Dr. _____ at this time? _____

_____

Describe one of your usual headaches. (Note child's description of the following: where headache occurred; severity; accompanying symptoms; who intervened; duration; probable cause.)

_____

_____

_____

Describe one of your worst headaches. (Note child's description of the following: where headache occurred; severity; accompanying symptoms; who intervened; duration; probable cause.)

_____

_____

_____

Do you usually have any warning that you are going to get a headache?
Yes __ No __ Sometimes __
Verbatim response: _____

_____

When you have a headache, what else is happening to your body? (Note: After child answers, specifically ask about nausea, dizziness, weakness, aura.)

_____

_____

Where is your pain located? Tell me and then show me on these drawings. (Note: Verify by asking child to show on his/her head.) _____

_____

(CHECK AREAS)

HEAD: frontal
            parietal
            temporal
            occipital
            eyes
            other

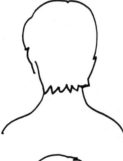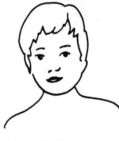

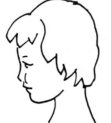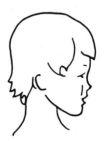

ABDOMINAL :   upper
                  lower
                  L
                  R

LIMB :   arm
             leg
             L
             R

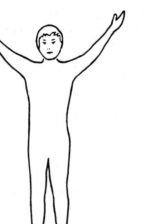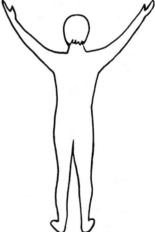

Is it on one side or both sides? (Circle one.)

Unilateral:	usually,	always,	sometimes,	never
Bilateral:	usually,	always	sometimes,	never

Does your pain spread?   Yes __ No __ Where? _____

_____

What words describe your pain? _____

_____

(Prompt, after response:)

   Sharp ___   Aching ___   Stinging ___   Hammering ___   Dull ___

   Throbbing ___   Burning ___   Pounding ___   Cutting ___

When you have a headache, is your pain

steady (the same)?	usually,	always,	sometimes,	never
up and down?	usually,	always,	sometimes,	never
increasing (getting bigger)?	usually,	always,	sometimes,	never

When you have a headache, is there a time in the day or night when it hurts worse? (Inquire, after response, about waking up, morning, afternoon, bedtime, and meals.)

_____

_____

_____

Generally discuss natural temporal variations in frequency or intensity with child (weekdays vs. weekends, sports, school, TV). _____

_____

_____

How much does your head ache? How strong is your pain usually? What words can you use to describe how much your head hurts? _____

_____

Now mark the line to show how strong that is. (Child should have already completed calibration task and used a visual analog scale.)

|———————————————————————————————————|

How sad or depressed do you feel because of your pain?

|———————————————————————————————————|

Why does it make you sad? _____

_____

Why do you think you have headaches? _____

_____

What do your parents think causes them? _____

_____

What do your friends think causes them? _____

_____

How strong is your pain when it hurts the least? _____

_____

Now mark the line to show how strong that is.

|———————————————————————————————————|

Which face on the face sheet looks the way you feel down inside when your pain hurts the most? _

(Face sheet color: _____)

How unpleasant is your pain when it hurts the most?

|————|————————————————————————————————————|

What do you do to reduce the pain when you have a headache?

Method	Efficacy
At school _____	_____
_____	_____
_____	_____
At home _____	_____
_____	_____
_____	_____

Which works best? _____

(Prompt after response, to verify reliance on medication, sleep/rest, withdrawal from mental or physical activity.)

How well does it work? _____

Will any of these cause a headache for you? What causes your pain? (Respond with A, always; S, sometimes; N, never; D, don't know.)

Foods:
_ Chocolate
_ Wheat
_ Cheese
_ Sugar
_ Yeast
_ Eggs
_ Meat with nitrates
_ Other _____

Weather:
_ Humidity, barometric pressure
_ Sudden or large temperature shifts
_ Hot weather
_ Cold weather
_ Sun

Emotions:
_ Anger
_ Fear
_ Anxiety, worry
_ Other _____

Social activities:
_ Party
_ Dance

(Note: After the assessment, indicate whether any of these seem to be "learned pain triggers." Specify why.)

_____
_____
_____

_ Concert
_ Movie
_ Other _____
School:
  _ Class
  _ Tests
  _ Bus
  _ Breaks
  _ Other _____
Other:
  _ Physical activity
  _ Fatigue
  _ Mental concentration
  _ Noise
  _ Siblings

What does your mother/father do for you when you have this pain?

Mother _____

Efficacy _____

Father _____

Efficacy _____

Other—specify significant adult _____

Efficacy _____

How strong is your pain when it hurts the most? _____

Now show me how strong that is.

|——|

Which face on the face sheet looks the way you feel deep down inside when your pain is at its usual strength? _

Now show me how unpleasant or how bothered you are when you have your usual pain.

|——|

How do your brothers and sisters treat you when you have this pain? _____

(Prompt: teasing vs. sympathy.)
How do your friends treat you when you have this pain? _____

(Prompt: teasing vs. sympathy.)
How afraid are you because of this pain?

|——|

Why are you afraid? _____
_____
_____

Who is usually with you when you have a headache? _____
_____

Which face on the face sheet looks the way you feel deep down inside when your pain is least strong? _

How unpleasant is your pain when it hurts the least?

|―――――――――――――――――――――――――|

How angry does your pain make you?

|―――――――――――――――――――――――――|

Why does it make you angry? _____
_____
_____

What kinds of things can't you do because of your pain, when you have _ low-moderate pain or _ strong pain (check pain level that is usual for child)?
(Prompt, after response.)

_____
_____

Are you able to do these things when you have a headache that is _ low-moderate, _ strong? (Y, yes, or N, no, for each.)

	Low-moderate pain	Strong pain
Gym	___	___
Reading	___	___
Schoolwork	___	___
Playing with friends	___	___
Watching TV	___	___
Housework	___	___
Mental games	___	___
Sports	___	___

What good things happen when you have a headache? _____
_____
_____

Do any of those things happen when you have a headache? (Y, yes, or N, no, for each.)

	Low–moderate pain	Strong pain
Leave school	——	——
No homework	——	——
No household responsibilities	——	——
Watch TV	——	——
Listen to music	——	——
No gym	——	——
No sports	——	——
Mom stays home	——	——
Brothers and sisters are quiet	——	——

What is the main reason your pain bothers you? _____
_____

Do you have any other aches and pains? (After child's response, inquire as to abdominal pain, limb pain, lower backaches.) _____
_____

If yes, list age at onset, frequency, duration, intervention, cause, and efficacy.
_____
_____

Can you control—that is, lessen—your pain without medication?

|—————————————————————————————————————|

If so, what do you do? _____
_____

How sure are you that your pain will be reduced some day?

|—————————————————————————————————————|

How much will your pain be reduced?

|—————————————————————————————————————|

How sure/certain are you that your pain will be reduced by this treatment?

|—————————————————————————————————————|

By the way, what's the name for your kind of pain, the medical name?
_____

Also, do you know when your body is really relaxed? Yes __ No __

Give me an example of when you are relaxed. _____
_____
_____

How do you know? _____
_____
_____

Are you relaxed now?   Yes __   No __
How do you know? _____
_____
_____

Are you as relaxed now as you are when (restate event child defined as relaxed)?
Yes __   No __

_____

Maximum/Minimum Pain Questionnaire

Child's code _____ Study _____ Face sheet color _____

We would like to know about your strongest and weakest pain experiences.

1. Please write down what pain or hurt was the strongest for you and mark the line to show us how strong that pain felt to you. Also, choose a face on the face sheet that shows best how you felt deep down inside when you had that pain.

   My strongest pain experience was _____

   _____ when I was __ years old.

   Face: __

   |——|
   Not strong   Strongest possible

2. Now please write down what pain or hurt was your weakest pain experience.

   My smallest or weakest pain experience was _____

   _____ when I was __ years old.

   Face: __

   |——|
   Not strong   Strongest possible

3. In your own words, what is pain?
   Pain is _____

   _____

   _____

Children's Pain Inventory—Intensity (III)

Child's code _____   Study _____

How much does it hurt when . . .

1. you have a stomachache?

|⊢——⊣|

2. you open a birthday present?

|⊢——⊣|

3. you wake up in the morning?

|⊢——⊣|

4. you eat lunch?

|⊢——⊣|

5. you have an injection?

|⊢——⊣|

6. you have your lumbar puncture?

|⊢——⊣|

7. you play in the snow without gloves?

|⊢——⊣|

8. you drop a book on your foot?

|⊢——⊣|

Three pain inventories are used, in which the orders of the questions are randomized. Two versions (III and II) are presented in the Appendix. All are available upon request.

How much does it hurt when . . .

9. your finger is pinched in a drawer?

|———————————————————————————————————————|

10. you are happy?

|———————————————————————————————————————|

11. a bee stings you?

|———————————————————————————————————————|

12. someone teases you?

|———————————————————————————————————————|

13. you get your finger pricked?

|———————————————————————————————————————|

14. while having a great time, your legs get very tired as you bicycle with your friends?

|———————————————————————————————————————|

15. you fall and scrape your knee?

|———————————————————————————————————————|

16. you have a toothache?

|———————————————————————————————————————|

17. you break your arm?

|———————————————————————————————————————|

18. you burn your hand on the stove?

|———————————————————————————————————————|

How much does it hurt when . . .

19. you have a bruise?

|―――――――――――――――――――――――――――――|

20. you have an operation in the hospital?

|―――――――――――――――――――――――――――――|

21. you sleep in a hospital bed?

|―――――――――――――――――――――――――――――|

22. you see your doctor?

|―――――――――――――――――――――――――――――|

23. right now?

|―――――――――――――――――――――――――――――|

24. someone pinches your arm?

|―――――――――――――――――――――――――――――|

25. you have a bone marrow aspiration?

|―――――――――――――――――――――――――――――|

26. you are sad?

|―――――――――――――――――――――――――――――|

27. you get spanked?

|―――――――――――――――――――――――――――――|

28. you have a headache?

|―――――――――――――――――――――――――――――|

How much does it hurt when . . .

29. you have a cold?

|—————————————————————————————————|

30. you have eaten too much candy?

|—————————————————————————————————|

Children's Pain Inventory—Affect (II)

Child's code _____ Study _____ Face sheet color _____

(Note: Interviewer must circle any situations that child has *not* experienced!)

Which face looks the way you would feel . . .

1. when you have a toothache? _
2. when you have a bruise? _
3. when you sleep in a hospital bed? _
4. right now? _
5. when you have a bone marrow aspiration? _
6. when you get spanked? _
7. when you have a cold? _
8. when you break your arm? _
9. when you burn your hand on the stove? _
10. when you have an operation in the hospital? _
11. when you see your doctor? _
12. when someone pinches your arm? _
13. when you are sad? _
14. when you have a headache? _
15. when you've eaten too much candy? _
16. when you have a stomachache? _
17. when you wake up in the morning? _
18. when you have an injection? _
19. when you play in the snow without gloves? _
20. when your finger is pinched in a drawer? _
21. when a bee stings you? _
22. when you get your finger pricked? _
23. when you fall and scrape your knee? _
24. when you open a birthday present? _
25. when you eat lunch? _
26. when you have your lumbar puncture? _
27. when you drop a book on your foot? _
28. when you are happy? _
29. when someone teases you? _
30. when, while having a great time, your legs get very tired as you bicycle with your friends? _

Pain Diary

Child's code _____ Date to be returned _____ Face sheet color _____

For the next month, for *any* pain your child has, please ask him/her to do the following:
1. Indicate the type of pain (e.g., scraped knee, fell and bruised elbow).
2. Choose the face on the face sheet that shows how he/she felt (deep down inside, not necessarily the face the child showed to the world) when he/she had the pain.
3. Mark the line to show how much the pain hurt.
4. Include the date on which the pain occurred.

Type of pain: _____ Face #: _____ Date: _____

Not strong   Strongest possible

Type of pain: _____ Face #: _____ Date: _____

Type of pain: _____ Face #: _____ Date: _____

Type of pain: _____ Face #: _____ Date: _____

Type of pain: _____ Face #: _____ Date: _____

Type of pain: _____ Face #: _____ Date: _____

Type of pain: _____ Face #: _____ Date: _____

Calibration Task and Answer Sheet

Instructions: Present each booklet (two sets of the seven circles are in random order; one circle is centered on each page) to the child twice, and have him/her rate the size of each circle on the accompanying set of visual analog scales. After the child has completed this task, use the values derived from the visual analog scales to determine the mathematical function describing the relationship between perceived circle size and actual circle size.

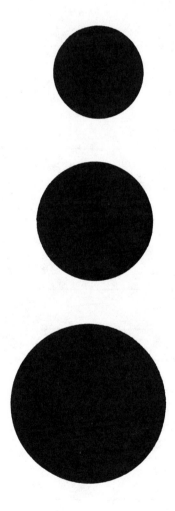

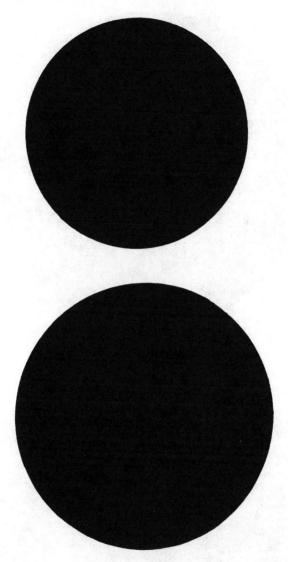

Child's code _____   Date _____   Study _____
Assessor _____

Sets used _____

Calibration task results

	I	II	$\bar{x}$
A = 25	___	___	___
B = 32	___	___	___
C = 42	___	___	___
D = 61	___	___	___
E = 70	___	___	___
F = 85	___	___	___
G = 100	___	___	___

a = ___
b = ___
R^2 = ___
x = 10, y = ___
x = 100, y = ___

References

Abajian, J. C., Mellish, R. W. P., Browne, A. F., Perkins, F. M., Lambert, D. H., & Mazuzan, J. E. (1984). Spinal anesthesia for surgery in the high-risk infant. *Anesthesia and Analgesia, 63,* 359–362.

Abildgaard, C. F. (1984). Progress and problems in hemophilia and von Willebrand's disease. In L. Barness (Ed.), *Advances in pediatrics* (Vol. 31, pp. 137–177). Chicago: Year Book Medical.

Abu-Saad, H. (1984a). Assessing children's responses to pain. *Pain, 19,* 163–171.

Abu-Saad, H. (1984b). Cultural group indicators of pain in children. *Maternal–Child Nursing Journal, 13,* 187–196.

Abu-Saad, H., & Holzmer, W. L. (1981). Measuring children's self-assessment of pain. *Issues in Comprehensive Pediatric Nursing, 5,* 337–349.

Adams, J. E. (1976). Naloxone reversal of analgesia produced by brain stimulation in the human. *Pain, 2,* 161–166.

Akil, H., & Watson, S. J. (1980). The role of endogenous opiates in pain control. In H. W. Kosterlitz & L. Y. Terenius (Eds.), *Pain and society* (pp. 201–222). Weinheim, West Germany: Verlag Chemie.

Akil, H., Watson, S. J., Berger, P. A., & Barchas, J. D. (1978). Endorphins, B-LPH, and ACTH: Biochemical, pharmacological, and anatomical studies. In E. Costa & E. M. Trabucchi (Eds.), *Advances in biochemical psychopharmacology: Vol. 18. The endorphins* (pp. 125–139). New York: Raven Press.

Alcock, D. S., Feldman, W., Goodman, J. T., McGrath, P. J., & Park, J. M. (1985). Evaluation of child life intervention in emergency department suturing. *Pediatric Emergency Care, 1,* 111–115.

Altman, A. J., & Schwartz, A. D. (1983). *Malignant diseases of infancy, childhood, and adolescence.* Philadelphia: W. B. Saunders.

American Academy of Pediatrics, Committee on Drugs. (1977). Guidelines for the ethical conduct of studies to evaluate drugs in pediatric populations. *Pediatrics, 60,* 91–101.

American Academy of Pediatrics, Committee on Fetus and Newborn, Committee on Drugs, Section on Anesthesiology, Section on Surgery. (1987). Neonatal anesthesia. *Pediatrics, 80,* 446.

American Academy of Pediatrics, Committee on Infectious Diseases. (1982). Special report: Aspirin and Reye's syndrome. *Pediatrics, 69,* 810–812.

American Pain Society. (1987). *Principles of analgesic use in the treatment of acute pain and chronic cancer pain: A concise guide to medical practice.* Washington, DC: Author.

American Psychiatric Association. (1980). *Diagnostic and statistical manual of mental disorders* (3rd ed.). Washington, DC: Author.

Anand, K. J. S., & Aynsley-Green, A. (1985). Metabolic and endocrine effects of surgical ligation of patent ductus arteriosus in the human preterm neonate: Are there implications for further improvement of postoperative outcome? *Modern Problems in Paediatrics, 23,* 143–157.

Anand, K. J. S., & Aynsley-Green, A. (1988). Does the newborn infant require potent anaesthesia during surgery? Answers from a randomized trial of halothane anaesthesia. In R. Dubner, G. F. Gebhart, & M. R. Bond (Eds.), *Pain research and clinical management* (Vol. 3., pp. 329–335). Amsterdam: Elsevier.

Anand, K. J. S., Brown, M. J., Bloom, S. R., & Aynsley-Green, A. (1985). Studies on the hormonal regulation of fuel metabolism in the human newborn infant undergoing anaesthesia and surgery. *Hormone Research, 22,* 115–128.

Anand, K. J. S., Brown, M. J., Causon, R. C., Christofides, N. D., Bloom, S. R., & Aynsley-Green, A. (1985). Can the human neonate mount an endocrine and metabolic response to surgery? *Journal of Pediatric Surgery, 20,* 41–48.

Anand, K. J. S., & Hickey, P. R. (1987). Pain and its effects in the human neonate and fetus. *New England Journal of Medicine, 317,* 1321–1329.

Anand, K. J. S., Sippell, W. G., & Aynsley-Green, A. (1987a). Does the newborn infant require anaesthesia during surgery? Answers from a randomised trial of halothane anaesthesia. *Pain* (Suppl. 4), S237.

Anand, K. J. S., Sippell, W. G., & Aynsley-Green, A. (1987b). Randomised trial of fentanyl anaesthesia in preterm babies undergoing surgery: Effects on the stress response. *Lancet, i,* 1987.

Anders, T. F., Sachar, E. J., Kream, J., Roffwarg, H., & Hellman, L. (1971). Behavioral state and plasma cortisol response in the human newborn. *Pediatrics, 46,* 532–537.

Anderson, K. O., Bradley, L. A., Young, L. D., McDaniel, L. K., & Wise, C. M. (1985). Rheumatoid arthritis: Review of psychological factors related to etiology, effects, and treatment. *Psychological Bulletin, 98,* 358–387.

Anderson, K. O., & Masur, F. T. (1983). Psychological preparation for invasive medical and dental procedures. *Journal of Behavioral Medicine, 6,* 1–40.

Andolsek, K., & Novik, B. (1980). Use of hypnosis with children. *Journal of Family Practice, 10,* 503–507.

Andrasik, F., Blanchard, E. B., Edlund, S., & Rosenblum, E. (1982). Autogenic feedback in the treatment of two children with migraine headache. *Child and Family Behavior Therapy, 4,* 13–23.

Andrasik, F., Burke, E. J., Attanasio, V., & Rosenblum, E. L. (1985). Child, parent, and physician reports of a child's headache pain: Relationships prior to and following treatment. *Headache, 25,* 421–425.

Andrasik, F., Kabela, E., Quinn, S., Attanasio, V., Blanchard, E. B., & Rosenblum, E. L. (1988). Psychological functioning of children who have recurrent migraine. *Pain, 34,* 43–52.

Angaut-Petit, D. (1975). The dorsal column system: II. Functional properties and bulbar relay of the post-synaptic fibres of the cat's fasciculus gracilis. *Experimental Brain Research, 22,* 471–493.

Antitch, J. L. (1967). The use of hypnosis in pediatric anesthesia. *Journal of the American Society of Psychosomatic Dentistry and Medicine, 14,* 70–75.

Apley, J. (1958). A common denominator in the recurrent pains of childhood. *Proceedings of the Royal Society of Medicine, 51,* 1023–1024.

Apley, J. (1975). *The child with abdominal pains.* Oxford: Blackwell Scientific.

Apley, J. (1976). Pain in childhood. *Journal of Psychosomatic Research, 20,* 383–389.

Apley, J., & Hale, B. (1973). Children with recurrent abdominal pain: How do they grow up? *British Medical Journal, iii,* 7–9.

Apley, J., Haslam, D. R., & Tulloh, C. G. (1971). Pupillary reaction in children with recurrent abdominal pain. *Archives of Disease in Childhood, 46,* 337–340.

Apley, J., MacKeith, R., & Meadow, R. (1978). *The child and his symptoms: A comprehensive approach.* Oxford: Blackwell Scientific.

Apley, J., & Naish, N. (1958). Recurrent abdominal pains: A field survey of 1,000 school children. *Archives of Disease in Childhood, 33,* 165–170.

Aradine, C. R., Beyer, J. E., & Tompkins, J. M. (1988). Children's pain perceptions before and after analgesia: A study of instrument construct validity and related issues . . . the oucher. *Journal of Pediatric Nursing, 3,* 11-23.

Aristotle. (1902). *Aristotle's psychology: A treatise on the principle of life* (Trans. with introduction and notes by W. A. Hammond). New York: Macmillan. (Original work written ca. 330 B.C.)

Armitage, E. N. (1979). Caudal block in children. *Anaesthesia, 34,* 396.

Armstrong, G. D., & Martinson, I. M. (1980). Death, dying, and terminal care: Dying at home. In J. Kellerman (Ed.), *Psychological aspects of childhood cancer* (pp. 295-311). Springfield, IL: Charles C Thomas.

Aronson, J. (1980). I may be bald but I still have rights. In J. Kellerman (Ed.), *Psychological aspects of childhood cancer* (pp. 184-191). Springfield, IL: Charles C Thomas.

Attanasio, V., Andrasik, P., Burke, E. J., Blake, D. D., Kabela, E., & McCarran, M. S. (1985). Clinical issues in utilizing biofeedback with children. *Clinical Biofeedback and Health, 8,* 134-141.

Attia, J., Ecoffey, C., Sandouk, P., Gross, J. B., & Samii, K. (1986). Epidural morphine in children: Pharmacokinetics and CO_2 sensitivity. *Anesthesiology, 65,* 590-594.

Atweh, S. F., & Kuhar, M. J. (1977). Autoradiographic localization of opiate receptors in rat brain: II. The brain stem. *Brain Research, 129,* 1-12.

Auerbach, S. M. (1979). Preoperative preparation for surgery: A review of recent research and future prospects. In D. J. Oborne, M. M. Gruneberg, & J. R. Eiser (Eds.), *Research in psychology and medicine* (Vol. 2, pp. 344-350). New York: Academic Press.

Bailey, L. M. (1986). Music therapy in pain management. *Journal of Pain and Symptom Management, 1,* 25-28.

Bain, H. W. (1975). Abdominal pain in children. *Primary Care, 2,* 121-133.

Bakke, M. (1976). Effect of acupuncture on the pain perception thresholds of human teeth. *Scandinavian Journal of Dental Research, 84,* 404-408.

Bandura, A. (1976). Effecting change through participant modeling. In J. D. Krumboltz & C. E. Thoresen (Eds.), *Counseling methods* (pp. 248-265). New York: Holt, Rinehart & Winston.

Barber, J. (1979). Utilizing hypnosis in the treatment of pain. In D. J. Oborne, M. M. Gruneberg, & J. R. Eiser (Eds.), *Research in psychology and medicine* (Vol. 1, pp. 35-40). New York: Academic Press.

Barber, J., & Mayer, D. J. (1977). Evaluation of the efficacy and neural mechanism of a hypnotic analgesia procedure in experimental and clinical dental pain. *Pain, 4,* 41-48.

Barber, T. X. (1963). The effects of "hypnosis" on pain: A critical review of experimental and clinical findings. *Psychosomatic Medicine, 25,* 303-333.

Barkas, G., & Duafala, M. E. (1988). Advances in cancer pain management: A review of patient-controlled analgesia. *Journal of Pain and Symptom Management, 3,* 150-160.

Barlow, C. F. (1978). Migraine in childhood. *Research and Clinical Studies in Headache, 5,* 34-46.

Barlow, C. F. (1984). *Clinics in developmental medicine: Vol. 91. Headaches and migraine in childhood.* Philadelphia: J. B. Lippincott.

Barr, R. G. (1981). Recurrent abdominal pain. In S. Gabel (Ed.), *Behavioral problems in childhood: A primary care approach* (pp. 229-241). New York: Grune & Stratton.

Barr, R. G. (1983a). Pain tolerance and developmental change in pain perception. In M. D. Levine, W. B. Carey, A. C. Crocker, & R. T. Gross (Eds.), *Developmental-behavioral pediatrics* (pp. 505-512). Philadelphia: W. B. Saunders.

Barr, R. G. (1983b). Recurrent abdominal pain. In M. D. Levine, W. B. Carey, A. C. Crocker, & R. T. Gross (Eds.), *Developmental-behavioral pediatrics* (pp. 521-528). Philadelphia: W. B. Saunders.

Barr, R. G. (1989). Pain in children. In P. D. Wall & R. Melzack (Eds.), *Textbook of pain* (2nd ed.). Edinburgh: Churchill Livingstone.

Barr, R. G., Levine, M. D., & Watkins J. B. (1979). Recurrent abdominal pain of childhood due to lactose intolerance: A prospective study. *New England Journal of Medicine, 300,* 1449-1452.

Barr, R. G., Levine, M. D., Wilkinson, R. H., & Mulvihill, D. (1979). Chronic and occult stool retention. *Clinical Pediatrics, 18,* 674-686.

Barr, R. G., Watkins, J. B., & Perman, J. A. (1981). Mucosal function and breath hydrogen excretion: Comparative studies in the clinical evaluation of children with nonspecific abdominal complaints. *Pediatrics, 68,* 526-533.

Barrell, J. J., & Price, D. D. (1975). The perception of first and second pain as a function of psychological set. *Perception and Psychophysics, 17,* 163-166.

Barrell, J. J., & Price, D. D. (1977). Two experiential orientations toward a stressful situation and their related somatic and visceral responses. *Psychophysiology, 14,* 517-521.

Basbaum, A. I. (1980). The anatomy of pain and pain modulation. In H. W. Kosterlitz & L. Y. Terenius (Eds.), *Pain and society* (pp. 93-122). Weinheim, West Germany: Verlag Chemie.

Basbaum, A. I., & Fields, H. L. (1978). Endogenous pain control mechanisms: Review and hypothesis. *Annals of Neurology, 4,* 451-462.

Basbaum, A. I., & Fields, H. L. (1984). Endogenous pain control systems: Brainstem spinal pathways and endorphin circuitry. *Annual Review of Neuroscience, 7,* 309-338.

Baum, J. (1977). Epidemiology of juvenile rheumatoid arthritis (JRA). *Arthritis and Rheumatism, 20,* 158-160.

Baxter, D. W., & Olszewski, J. (1960). Congenital universal insensitivity to pain. *Brain, 83,* 381-393.

Beales, J. G. (1979a). Pain in children with cancer. In J. J. Bonica & V. Ventafridda (Eds.), *Advances in pain research and therapy* (Vol. 2, pp. 89-98). New York: Raven Press.

Beales, J. G. (1979b). The effects of attention and distraction on pain among children attending a hospital casualty department. In D. J. Oborne, M. M. Gruneberg, & J. R. Eiser (Eds.), *Research in psychology and medicine* (Vol. 1, pp. 86-90). New York: Academic Press.

Beales, J. G. (1982). The assessment and management of pain in children. In P. Karoly, J. J. Steffen, & D. J. O'Grady (Eds.), *Child health psychology: Concepts and issues* (pp. 154-179). Elmsford, NY: Pergamon Press.

Beales, J. G., Holt, P. J. L., Keen, J. H., & Mellor, V. P. (1983). Children with juvenile chronic arthritis: Their beliefs about their illness and therapy. *Annals of the Rheumatic Diseases, 42,* 481-486.

Beales, J. G., Keen, J. H., & Holt, P. J. L. (1983). The child's perception of the disease and the experience of pain in juvenile chronic arthritis. *Journal of Rheumatology, 10,* 61-65.

Beecher, H. K. (1956). Relationship of significance of wound to pain experienced. *Journal of the American Medical Association, 161,* 1609-1613.

Beecher, H. K. (1959). *The measurement of subjective responses: Quantitative effects of drugs.* New York: Oxford University Press.

Beers, R. F., & Bassett, E. G. (Eds.). (1979). *Mechanisms of pain and analgesic compounds.* New York: Raven Press.

Behbehani, M. M., & Fields, H. L. (1979). Evidence that an excitatory connection between the periaqueductal grey and nucleus raphe magnus mediates stimulation produced analgesia. *Brain Research, 170,* 85-93.

Beitel, R. E., & Dubner, R. (1976). Response of unmyelinated (C) polymodal nociceptors to thermal stimuli applied to monkey's face. *Journal of Neurophysiology, 39,* 1160-1175.

Bell, J., & Bell, C. (1827). *The anatomy and physiology of the human body* (5th American ed.). New York: Collins.

Benitz, W. E., & Tatro, D. S. (1981). *The pediatric drug handbook.* Chicago: Year Book Medical.

Bennett, E. J., Ignacio, A., Patel, K., Grundy, E. M., & Salem, M. R. (1976). Tubocurarine and the neonate. *British Journal of Anaesthesia, 48,* 687-689.

Bennett, G. J., Abdelmoumene, M., Hayashi, H., & Dubner, R. (1980). Physiology and morphology of substantia gelatinosa neurons intracellularly stained with horseradish peroxidase. *Journal of Comparative Neurology, 194,* 808-827.

Bennett, G. J., Abdelmoumene, M., Hayashi, H., Hoffert, M. J., Ruda, M. A., & Dubner, R. (1981). Physiology, morphology, and immunocytology of dorsal horn layer III neurons. *Pain* (Suppl. 1), 291.

Benson, H., Pomeranz, B., & Kutz, I. (1984). The relaxation response and pain. In P. D. Wall & R. Melzack (Eds.), *Textbook of pain* (1st ed., pp. 817-822). Edinburgh: Churchill Livingstone.

Berde, C. B., Holzman, R. S., Sethna, N. F., Dickerson, R. B., & Brustowicz, R. M. (1988). A comparison of methadone and morphine for post-operative analgesia in children and adolescents. *Anesthesiology, 69,* A768.

Berde, C. B., Sethna, N. F., Holzman, R. S., Reidy, P., & Gondek, E. J. (1987). Pharmacokinetics of methadone in children and adolescents in the perioperative period. *Anesthesiology, 67,* A519.

Berg, K. M., Berg, W. K., & Graham, F. K. (1971). Infant heart rate response as a function of stimulus and state. *Psychophysiology, 8,* 30–44.

Berger, H. G. (1974). Somatic pain and school avoidance. *Clinical Pediatrics, 13,* 819–826.

Berger, H. G., Honig, P. J., & Liebman, R. (1977). Recurrent abdominal pain: Gaining control of the symptom. *American Journal of Diseases of Children, 131,* 1340–1344.

Bernstein, B. H., Singsen, B. H., Kent, J. T., Kornreich, H., King, K., Hicks, R., & Hanson, V. (1978). Reflex neurovascular dystrophy in childhood. *Journal of Pediatrics, 93,* 211–215.

Berry, F. R. (1977). Analgesia in patients with fractured shaft of femur. *Anaesthesia, 32,* 576–577.

Besson, J. M. R. (1980). Supraspinal modulation of the segmental transmission of pain. In H. W. Kosterlitz & L. Y. Terenius (Eds.), *Pain and society* (pp. 161–182). Weinheim, West Germany: Verlag Chemie.

Beyer, J. E. (1984). *The Oucher: A user's manual and technical report.* Evanston, IL: Judson.

Beyer, J. E., & Aradine, C. R. (1986). Content validity of an instrument to measure young children's perceptions of the intensity of their pain. *Journal of Pediatric Nursing, 1,* 386–395.

Beyer, J. E., & Aradine, C. R. (1988). Convergent and discriminant validity of a self-report measure of pain intensity for children. *Children's Health Care, 16,* 274–282.

Beyer, J. E., & Byers, M. L. (1985). Knowledge of pediatric pain: the state of the art. *Children's Health Care, 13,* 150–159.

Beyer, J. E., DeGood, D. E., Ashley, L. C., & Russell, G. A. (1983). Patterns of postoperative analgesic use with adults and children following cardiac surgery. *Pain, 17,* 71–81.

Beyer, J. E., & Knapp, T. R. (1986). Methodological issues in the measurement of children's pain. *Children's Health Care, 14,* 233–241.

Bibace, R., & Walsh, M. E. (1979). Developmental stages of children's conceptualizations of illness. In G. C. Stone, F. Cohen, & N. E. Adler (Eds.), *Health psychology: A handbook* (pp. 285–301). San Francisco: Jossey-Bass.

Bibace, R., & Walsh, M. E. (1980). Development of children's concept of illness. *Pediatrics, 66,* 912–917.

Bille, B. (1962). Migraine in school children. *Acta Paediatrica Scandinavica, 51* (Suppl. 136), 1–151.

Bille, B. (1981). Migraine in childhood and its prognosis. *Cephalalgia, 1,* 71–75.

Bille, B. (1982). Migraine in childhood. *Panminerva Medica–Europa Medica, 24,* 57–62.

Binger, C. M., Ablin, A. R., Feuerstein, R. C., Kushner, J. H., Zoger, S., & Mikkelsen, C. (1969). Childhood leukemia: Emotional impact on the patient and family. *New England Journal of Medicine, 280,* 414–418.

Black, P. R., Welch, K. J., & Eraklis, A. J. (1986). Juxtapancreatic intestinal duplications with pancreatic ductal communication: A cause of pancreatitis and recurrent abdominal pain in childhood. *Journal of Pediatric Surgery, 21,* 257–261.

Blevens, K., Buchino, J. J., & Fellows, R. (1984). A child with chronic abdominal pain and leg weakness. *Journal of Pediatrics, 105,* 329–332.

Blix, M. (1884). Experimentelle beitrage zur losung der frage über die specifische energieder hautnerven. *Zeitschrift für Biologie, 20,* 141–160.

Bloch, G. J. (1980). *Mesmerism: A translation of the original medical and scientific writings of F. A. Mesmer, M.D.* Los Altos, CA: William Kaufmann.

Blom, G. E., & Nicholls, G. (1954). Emotional factors in children with rheumatoid arthritis. *American Journal of Orthopsychiatry, 24,* 588–601.

Boehncke, H. (1970). Pain analysis in childhood. In R. Janzen (Ed.), *Pain analysis* (pp. 73–81). Bristol, England: John Wright.

Bond, B., & Stevens, S. S. (1969). Cross-modality matching of brightness to loudness by 5-year-olds. *Perception and Psychophysics, 6,* 337–339.

Bond, M. R. (1980). The suffering of severe intractable pain. In H. W. Kosterlitz & L. Y. Terenius (Eds.), *Pain and society* (pp. 53–62). Weinheim, West Germany: Verlag Chemie.

Bond, M. R. (1984). *Pain: Its nature, analysis and treatment.* Edinburgh: Churchill Livingstone.

Bond, M. R. (1985). Cancer pain: Psychological substrates and therapy. In H. L. Fields, R. Dubner, & F. Cervero (Eds.), *Advances in pain research and therapy* (Vol. 9, pp. 559–567). New York: Raven Press.

Bonica, J. J. (1953). *The management of pain.* Philadelphia: Lea & Febiger.

Bonica, J. J. (1977). Neurophysiologic and pathologic aspects of acute and chronic pain. *Archives of Surgery, 112,* 750–761.

Bonica, J. J. (1979a). Introduction to management of pain of advanced cancer. In J. J. Bonica & V. Ventafridda (Eds.), *Advances in pain research and therapy* (Vol. 2, pp. 115–130). New York: Raven Press.

Bonica, J. J. (1979b). Introduction to nerve blocks. In J. J. Bonica & V. Ventafridda (Eds.), *Advances in pain research and therapy* (Vol. 2, pp. 303–310). New York: Raven Press.

Bonica, J. J. (1980). Pain research and therapy: Past and current status and future needs. In L. K. Y. Ng & J. J. Bonica (Eds.), *Pain, discomfort and humanitarian care* (pp. 1–46). Amsterdam: Elsevier/North-Holland.

Bonica, J. J. (1984). Management of cancer pain. *Recent Results in Cancer Research, 89,* 13–27.

Bonica, J. J. (1985). Treatment of cancer pain: Current status and future needs. In H. L. Fields, R. Dubner, & F. Cervero (Eds.), *Advances in pain research and therapy* (Vol. 9, pp. 589–616). New York: Raven Press.

Bonica, J. J., Liebeskind, J. C., & Albe-Fessard, D. G. (Eds.). (1979). *Advances in pain research and therapy* (Vol. 3). New York: Raven Press.

Boone, J. E. (1983). Viral arthritis. In M. E. Gershwin & D. L. Robbins (Eds.), *Musculoskeletal diseases of children* (pp. 339–366). New York: Grune & Stratton.

Boone, J. E., Baldwin, J., & Levine, C. (1974). Juvenile rheumatoid arthritis. *Pediatric Clinics of North America, 21,* 885–915.

Boring, E. G. (1942). *Sensation and perception in the history of experimental psychology.* New York: Appleton-Century-Crofts.

Botney, M., & Fields, H. L. (1983). Amitriptyline potentiates morphine analgesia by a direct action on the central nervous system. *Annals of Neurology, 13,* 160–164.

Bouckoms, A. J. (1984). Psychosurgery. In P. D. Wall & R. Melzack (Eds.), *Textbook of pain* (pp. 666–676). Edinburgh: Churchill Livingstone.

Bowler, G. M. R., Wildsmith, J. A., & Scott, D. B. (1986). Epidural administration of local anesthetics. In M. J. Cousins & G. D. Phillips (Eds.), *Acute pain management* (pp. 187–236). New York: Churchill Livingstone.

Bowsher, D. (1957). Termination of the central pain pathway in man: The conscious appreciation of pain. *Brain, 80,* 606–622.

Bowyer, S. L., & Hollister, J. R. (1984). Limb pain in childhood. *Pediatric Clinics of North America, 31,* 1053–1081.

Bradley, L. A., Prokop, C. K., Gentry, W. D., Van der Heide, L. H., & Prieto, E. J. (1981). Assessment of chronic pain. In C. K. Prokop & L. A. Bradley (Eds.), *Medical psychology: Contributions to behavioral medicine* (pp. 91–117). New York: Academic Press.

Bramwell, R. G. B., Bullen, C., & Radford, P. (1982). Caudal block for post-operative analgesia in children. *Anaesthesia, 37,* 1024–1028.

Bray, R. J. (1983). Postoperative analgesia provided by morphine infusion in children. *Anaesthesia, 38,* 1075–1078.

Bray, R. J., Beeton, C., Hinton, W., & Seviour, J. A. (1986). Plasma morphine levels produced by continuous infusion in children. *Anaesthesia, 41,* 753–755.

Brenning, R. (1960). "Growing pains." *Acta Societatis Medicorum Upsaliensis, 65,* 185–201.

Brescia, F. J. (1987a). An overview of pain and symptom management in advanced cancer. *Journal of Pain and Symptom Management, 2,* S7–S11.

Brescia, F. J. (1987b). Introduction: A short course on the management of cancer pain. *Journal of Pain and Symptom Management, 2,* S5.

Brewer, E. J., Jr., Giannini, E. H., & Barkley, E. (1980). Gold therapy in the management of juvenile rheumatoid arthritis. *Arthritis and Rheumatism, 23,* 404–411.

Bromage, P. R. (1984). Epidural anaesthetics and narcotics. In P. D. Wall & R. Melzack (Eds.), *Textbook of pain* (pp. 558–565). Edinburgh: Churchill Livingstone.

Browder, J., & Gallagher, J. P. (1948). Dorsal cordotomy for painful phantom limb. *Annals of Surgery, 128,* 456–469.

Brown, A. G., & Fyffe, R. E. W. (1981). Form and function of dorsal horn neurones with axons ascending the dorsal column in cat. *Journal of Physiology, 321,* 31–47.

Brown, J. K. (1977). Migraine and migraine equivalents in children. *Developmental Medicine and Child Neurology, 19,* 683–692.

Brown, R. E., Jr., & Broadman, L. M. (1987). Patient-controlled analgesia (PCA) for postoperative pain control in adolescents. *Anesthesia and Analgesia, 66,* S22.

Brown, T. C. K. (1985). Local and regional anaesthesia in children. *Anaesthesia, 40,* 407–409.

Browne, W. J., Mally, M. A., & Kane, R. P. (1960). Psychosocial aspects of hemophilia: A study of twenty-eight hemophilic children and their families. *American Journal of Orthopsychiatry, 30,* 730–740.

Brunnquell, D., & Hall, M. D. (1982). Issues in the psychological care of pediatric oncology patients. *American Journal of Orthopsychiatry, 52,* 32–44.

Bryan-Brown, C. W. (1986). Development of pain management in critical care. In M. J. Cousins & G. D. Phillips (Eds.), *Acute pain management* (pp. 1–19). Edinburgh: Churchill Livingstone.

Buck, E.D., & Bodensteiner, J. (1981). Thoracic cord tumor appearing as recurrent abdominal pain. *American Journal of Diseases of Children, 135,* 574–575.

Buda, F. B., & Joyce, R. P. (1979). Successful treatment of atypical migraine of childhood with anticonvulsants. *Military Medicine, 144,* 521–523.

Burke, E. C., & Peters, G. A. (1956). Migraine in childhood: A preliminary report. *AMA Journal of Diseases of Children, 92,* 330–336.

Burrows, G. D., Elton, D., & Stanley, G. V. (Eds.). (1987). *Handbook of chronic pain management.* Amsterdam: Elsevier.

Burton, L. (1974). Tolerating the intolerable: The problems facing parents and children following diagnosis. In L. Burton (Ed.), *Care of the child facing death* (pp. 16–38). London: Routledge & Kegan Paul.

Bush, G. H., & Stead, A. L. (1962). The use of D-tubocurarine in neonatal anaesthesia. *British Journal of Anaesthesia, 34,* 721–728.

Byrne, W. J., Arnold, W. C., Stannard, M. W., & Redman, J. F. (1985). Ureteropelvic junction obstruction presenting with recurrent abdominal pain: Diagnosis by ultrasound. *Pediatrics, 76,* 934–937.

Cadman, D., Boyle, M., & Offord, D. R. (1988). The Ontario Child Health Study: Social adjustment and mental health of siblings of children with chronic health problems. *Journal of Developmental and Behavioral Pediatrics, 9,* 117–121.

Cairns, N. U., Clark, G. M., Smith, S. D., & Lansky, S. B. (1979). Adaptation of siblings to childhood malignancy. *Journal of Pediatrics, 95,* 484–487.

Calabro, J. J. (1981). Juvenile rheumatoid arthritis: Mode of onset as key to early diagnosis and management. *Postgraduate Medicine, 70,* 120–133.

Calabro, J. J. (1988). Juvenile rheumatoid arthritis. *Clinics in Pediatric Medicine and Surgery, 5,* 57–75.

Calabro, J. J., Wachtel, A. E., Holgerson, W.B., & Repice, M. M. (1976). Growing pains: Fact or fiction? *Postgraduate Medicine, 59,* 66–72.

Campbell, J. D. (1975). Illness is a point of view: The development of children's concepts of illness. *Child Development, 46,* 92–100.

Campos, J. J. (1976). Heart rate: A sensitive tool for the study of emotional development in the infant. In L. P. Lipsitt (Ed.), *Developmental psychobiology* (pp. 1–31). Hillsdale, NJ: Erlbaum.

Campos, J. J., Emde, R. N., Gaensbauer, T., & Henderson, C. (1975). Cardiac and behavioral interrelationships in the reactions of infants to strangers. *Developmental Psychology, 11*, 589–601.

Cannon, J. T., Liebeskind, J. C., & Frenk, H. (1978). Neural and neurochemical mechanisms of pain inhibition. In R. A. Sternbach (Ed.), *The psychology of pain* (pp. 27–47). New York: Raven Press.

Caradang, M. L. A., Folkins, C. H., Hines, P. A., & Steward, M. S. (1979). The role of cognitive level and sibling illness in children's conceptualizations of illness. *American Journal of Orthopsychiatry, 49*, 474–481.

Casey, K. L. (1980). Supraspinal mechanisms in pain: The reticular formation. In H. W. Kosterlitz & L. Y. Terenius (Eds.), *Pain and society* (pp. 183–200). Weinheim, West Germany: Verlag Chemie.

Cassidy, J. T. (1982a). Basic concepts of drug therapy. In J. T. Cassidy (Ed.), *Textbook of pediatric rheumatology* (pp. 99–129). New York: Wiley.

Cassidy, J. T. (1982b). Definition and classification of rheumatic diseases in children. In J. T. Cassidy (Ed.), *Textbook of pediatric rheumatology* (pp. 1–13). New York: Wiley.

Cassidy, J. T. (1982c). Juvenile rheumatoid arthritis. In J. T. Cassidy (Ed.), *Textbook of pediatric rheumatology* (pp. 169–281). New York: Wiley.

Cataldo, M. F., Russo, D. C., Bird, B. L., & Varni, J. (1980). Assessment and management of chronic disorders. In J. M. Ferguson & C. B. Taylor (Eds.), *The comprehensive handbook of behavioral medicine: Vol. 3. Extended applications and issues* (pp. 67–95). New York: Spectrum.

Cervero, F., Iggo, A., & Ogawa, H. (1976). Nociceptor-driven dorsal horn neurones in the lumbar spinal cord of the cat. *Pain, 2*, 5–24.

Chapman, C. R. (1980). The measurement of pain in man. In H. W. Kosterlitz & L. Y. Terenius (Eds.), *Pain and society* (pp. 339–354). Weinheim, West Germany: Verlag Chemie.

Chapman, C. R., & Benedetti, C. (1977). Analgesia following transcutaneous electrical stimulation and its partial reversal by a narcotic antagonist. *Life Sciences, 21*, 1645–1648.

Chapman, C. R., & Turner, J. A. (1986). Psychological control of acute pain in medical settings. *Journal of Pain and Symptom Management, 1*, 9–20.

Chapman, W. P., & Jones, C. M. (1944). Variations in cutaneous and visceral pain sensitivity in normal subjects. *Journal of Clinical Investigations, 23*, 81–91.

Charache, S. (1981). Treatment of sickle cell anemia. *Annual Review of Medicine, 32*, 195–206.

Charlesworth, W. R. (1982). An ethological approach to research on facial expressions. In C. E. Izard (Ed.), *Measuring emotions in infants and children* (pp. 317–334). New York: Cambridge University Press.

Chaves, J. F., & Barber, T. X. (1976). Acupuncture analgesia: A six-factor theory. In M. Weisenberg & B. Tursky (Eds.), *Pain: New perspectives in therapy and research* (pp. 43–66). New York: Plenum Press.

Christensen, M. F., & Mortensen, O. (1975). Long-term prognosis in children with recurrent abdominal pain. *Archives of Disease in Childhood, 50*, 110–114.

Chutorian, A. M. (1978). Migrainous syndromes in children. In R. A. Thompson & J. R. Green (Eds.), *Pediatric neurology and neurosurgery* (pp. 183–204). New York: Spectrum.

Cioppa, F. J., & Thal, A.D. (1975). Hypnotherapy in a case of juvenile rheumatoid arthritis. *American Journal of Clinical Hypnosis, 18*, 105–110.

Clarke, S., & Radford, M. (1986). Topical anaesthesia for venepuncture. *Archives of Disease in Childhood, 61*, 1132–1134.

Classification of chronic pain. (1986). *Pain* (Suppl. 3), S1–S225.

Cleeland, C. S. (1987). Nonpharmacological management of cancer pain. *Journal of Pain and Symptom Management, 2*, S23–S28.

Cleeland, C. S., Shacham, S., Dahl, J. L., & Orrison, W. (1984). CSF β-endorphin and the severity of pain. *Neurology, 34*, 378–380.

Clement-Jones, V., McLoughlin, L., Tomlin, S., Besser, G. M., Rees, L. H., & Wen, H. L. (1980). Increased beta-edorphin but not met-enkephalin levels in human cerebrospinal fluid after acupuncture for recurrent pain. *Lancet, ii*, 946–949.

Cleveland, S. E., Reitman, E. E., & Brewer, E. J., Jr. (1965). Psychological factors in juvenile rheumatoid arthritis. *Arthritis and Rheumatism, 8*, 1152-1158.

Clifton, R. K., Graham, F. K., & Hatton, H. M. (1968). Newborn heart-rate response and response habituation as a function of stimulus duration. *Journal of Experimental Child Psychology, 6*, 265-278.

Clifton, R. K., & Meyers, W. J. (1969). The heart-rate response of four-month-old infants to auditory stimuli. *Journal of Experimental Child Psychology, 7*, 122-135.

Cohen, S. N. (1980). Ethics of drug research in children. In S. J. Yaffe (Ed.), *Pediatric pharmacology: Therapeutic principles in practice* (pp. 93-100). New York: Grune & Stratton.

Cole, T. B., Sprinkle, R. H., Smith, S. J., & Buchanan, G. R. (1986). Intravenous narcotic therapy for children with severe sickle cell pain crisis. *American Journal of Diseases of Children, 140*, 1255-1259.

Coleman, W. L. (1984). Recurrent chest pain in childhood. *Pediatric Clinics of North America, 31*, 1007-1026.

Collins, C., Koren, G., Crean, P., Klein, J., Roy, W. L., & Macleod, S. M. (1985). Fentanyl pharmacokinetics and hemodynamic effects in preterm infants during ligation of patent ductus arteriosus. *Anesthesia and Analgesia, 64*, 1078-1080.

Collins, G. L. (1965). Pain sensitivity and ratings of childhood experience. *Perceptual and Motor Skills, 21*, 349-350.

Collins, W. F., Nulsen, F. E., & Randt, C. T. (1960). Relation of peripheral nerve fiber size and sensation in man. *Archives of Neurology, 3*, 381-385.

Combrinck-Graham, L., Gursky, E. J., & Saccar, C. L. (1980). Psychoactive agents. In S. J. Yaffe (Ed.), *Pediatric pharmacology: Therapeutic principles in practice* (pp. 455-478). New York: Grune & Stratton.

Congdon, P. J., & Forsythe, W. I. (1979). Migraine in childhood: A study of 300 children. *Developmental Medicine and Child Neurology, 21*, 209-216.

Conrad, P. (1980). Painful legs: The GP's dilemma. *Australian Family Physician, 9*, 691-694.

Cooperman, A. M., Hall, B., Mikalacki, K., Hardy, R., & Sadar, E. (1977). Use of transcutaneous electrical stimulation in the control of postoperative pain. *American Journal of Surgery, 133*, 185-187.

Cornaglia, C., Massimo, L., Haupt, R., Melodia, A., Sizemore, W., & Benedetti, C. (1984). Incidence of pain in children with neoplastic diseases. *Pain* (Suppl. 2), 28.

Cousins, M. M., & Mather, L. E. (1984). Intrathecal and epidural administration of opioids. *Anesthesiology, 61*, 276-310.

Cox, B. M., Goldstein, A., & Li, C. H. (1976). Opioid activity of a peptide, β-lipotropin-(61-91), derived from β-lipotropin. *Proceedings of the National Academy of Sciences, USA, 73*, 1821-1823.

Coyle, N., Mauskop, A., Maggard, J., & Foley, K. M. (1986). Continuous subcutaneous infusions of opiates in cancer patients with pain. *Oncology Nursing Forum, 13*, 53-57.

Craig, K. D. (1975). Social modelling determinants of pain processes. *Pain, 1*, 375-378.

Craig, K. D. (1978). Social modeling influences on pain. In R. A. Sternbach (Ed.), *The psychology of pain* (pp. 73-109). New York: Raven Press.

Craig, K. D. (1980). Ontogenetic and cultural influences on the expression of pain in man. In H. W. Kosterlitz & L. Y. Terenius (Eds.), *Pain and society* (pp. 37-52). Weinheim, West Germany: Verlag Chemie.

Craig, K. D. (1983). Modeling and social learning factors in chronic pain. In J. J. Bonica, U. Lindblom, & A. Iggo (Eds.), *Advances in pain research and therapy* (Vol. 5, pp. 813-827). New York: Raven Press.

Craig, K. D. (1984). Emotional aspects of pain. In P. D. Wall & R. Melzack (Eds.), *Textbook of pain* (pp. 153-161). Edinburgh: Churchill Livingstone.

Craig, K. D., & Best, J. A. (1977). Perceived control over pain: Individual differences and situational determinants. *Pain, 3*, 127-135.

Craig, K. D., Grunau, R. V. E., & Branson, S. M. (1988). Age-related aspects of pain: pain in children. In R. Dubner, G. F. Gebhart, & M. R. Bond (Eds.), *Pain research and clinical management* (Vol. 3, pp. 317-328). Amsterdam: Elsevier.

Craig, K. D., McMahon, R. J., Morison, J. D., & Zaskow, C. (1984). Developmental changes in infant pain expression during immunization injections. *Social Science and Medicine, 19,* 1331-1337.

Craig, Y. (1974). 'The care of our dying child'—a parent offers some personal observations based on recollection. In L. Burton (Ed.), *Care of the child facing death* (pp. 87-100). London: Routledge & Kegan Paul.

Crasilneck, H. B., & Hall, J. A. (1973). Clinical hypnosis in problems in pain. *American Journal of Clinical Hypnosis, 15,* 153-161.

Crasilneck, H. B., & Hall, J. A. (1975). *Clinical hypnosis: Principles and applications.* New York: Grune & Stratton.

Cullen, K. J., & Macdonald, W. B. (1963). The periodic syndrome: Its nature and prevalence. *Medical Journal of Australia, 2,* 167-173.

Cullen, S. C. (1958). Hypno-induction techniques in pediatric anesthesia. *Anesthesiology, 19,* 279-281.

Cyriax, J. (1984). Vertebral manipulation. In P. D. Wall & R. Melzack (Eds.), *Textbook of pain* (pp. 725-734). Edinburgh: Churchill Livingstone.

Dahlquist, L. M., Gil, K. M., Armstrong, F. D., Ginsberg, A., & Jones, B. (1985). Behavioral management of children's distress during chemotherapy. *Journal of Behavior Therapy and Experimental Psychiatry, 16,* 325-329.

Dahlstrom, B., Bolme, P., Feychting, H., Noack, G., & Paalzow, L. (1979). Morphine kinetics in children. *Clinical Pharmacology and Therapeutics, 26,* 354-365.

Dallenbach, K. M. (1939). Pain: History and present status. *Journal of Psychiatry, 52,* 331-347.

Daniels, E. (1962). The hypnotic approach in anesthesia for children. *American Journal of Clinical Hypnosis, 4,* 244-248.

D'Apolito, K. (1984). The neonate's response to pain. *American Journal of Maternal/Child Nursing, 9,* 256-257.

Darwin, E. (1794). *Zoonomia.* London: J. Johnson.

Dash, J. (1980). Hypnosis for symptom amelioration. In J. Kellerman (Ed.), *Psychological aspects of childhood cancer* (pp. 215-230). Springfield, IL: Charles C Thomas.

Davis, J. R., Vichinsky, E. P., & Lubin, B. H. (1980). Current treatment of sickle cell disease. *Current Problems in Pediatrics, 10,* 1-64.

Dennis, S. G., & Melzack, R. (1977). Pain-signalling systems in the dorsal and ventral spinal cord. *Pain, 4,* 97-132.

Descartes, R. (1972). *L'homme (Treatise on man)* (T. S. Hall, Trans.). Cambridge, MA: Harvard University Press. (Original work published 1664)

DeSousa, A. L., Kalsbeck, J. E., Mealey, J., Jr., Campbell, R. L., & Hockey, A. (1979). Intraspinal tumors in children: A review of 81 cases. *Journal of Neurosurgery, 51,* 437-445.

Deubner, D. C. (1977). An epidemiologic study of migraine and headache in 10-20 year olds. *Headache, 17,* 173-179.

deVeber, L. L. (1986, October). *Cancer pain in children.* Paper presented at the 6th World Congress on the Terminally Ill, Montreal.

Devor, M. (1984). The pathophysiology and anatomy of damaged nerve. In P. D. Wall & R. Melzack (Eds.), *Textbook of pain* (pp. 49-64). Edinburgh: Churchill Livingstone.

Diamond, C. A., & Matthay, K. K. (1988). Childhood acute lymphoblastic leukemia. *Pediatric Annals, 17,* 156-170.

Diamond, S. (1979). Biofeedback and headache. *Headache, 19,* 180-184.

Diamond, S., & Montrose, D. (1984). The value of biofeedback in the treatment of chronic headache: A four-year retrospective study. *Headache, 24,* 5-18.

Dieckmann, G., & Witzmann, A. (1982). Initial and long-term results of deep brain stimulation for chronic intractable pain. *Applied Neurophysiology, 45,* 167-172.

Dietrich, S. L. (1976). Musculoskeletal problems. In M. W. Hilgartner (Ed.), *Hemophilia in children* (pp. 59-70). Littleton, MA: Publishing Sciences Group.

DiLeo, J. H. (1977). *Child development: Analysis and synthesis.* New York: Brunner/Mazel.

Dimson, S. B. (1971). Transit time related to clinical findings in children with recurrent abdominal pain. *Pediatrics, 47,* 666-674.

Dionne, R. A. (1986). Methodological needs and pharmacological research with adult dental patients. *Anesthesia Progress, 33,* 50-54.

Dionne, R. A., Campbell, R. A., Cooper, S. A., Hall, D. L., & Buckingham, B. (1983). Suppression of postoperative pain by preoperative administration of ibuprofen in comparison to placebo acetaminophen and acetaminophen plus codeine. *Journal of Clinical Pharmacology, 23,* 37-43.

Dodd, E., Wang, J. M., & Rauck, R. L. (1988). Patient controlled analgesia for post-surgical pediatric patients ages 6-16 years. *Anesthesiology, 69,* A372.

Dolgin, M. J., & Katz, E. R. (1988). Conditioned aversions in pediatric cancer patients receiving chemotherapy. *Journal of Developmental and Behavioral Pediatrics, 9,* 82-85.

Dolgin, M. J., Katz, E. R., Doctors, S. R., & Siegel, S. E. (1986). Caregivers' perceptions of medical compliance in adolescents with cancer. *Journal of Adolescent Health Care, 7,* 22-27.

Dolgin, M. J., Katz, E. R., McGinty, K., & Siegel, S. E. (1985). Anticipatory nausea and vomiting in pediatric cancer patients. *Pediatrics, 75,* 547-552.

Downes, J. J., & Betts, E. K. (1977). Anesthesia for the critically ill infant. *Refresher Courses in Anesthesiology, 5,* 47-69.

Downes, J. J., & Raphaely, R. C. (1973). Pediatric anesthesia and intensive care. *Pennsylvania Medicine, 76,* 57-61.

Drotar, D. (1977). Family oriented intervention with the dying adolescent. *Journal of Pediatric Psychology, 2,* 68-71.

Drotar, D. (1981). Psychological perspectives in chronic childhood illness. *Journal of Pediatric Psychology, 6,* 211-228.

Dubner, R. (1980). Peripheral and central mechanisms of pain. In L. K. Y. Ng & J. J. Bonica (Eds.), *Pain, discomfort and humanitarian care* (pp. 61-82). Amsterdam: Elsevier/North-Holland.

Dubner, R., & Bennett, G. J. (1983). Spinal and trigeminal mechanisms of nociception. *Annual Review of Neuroscience, 6,* 381-418.

Dubner, R., Gebhart, G. F., & Bond, M. R. (Eds.). (1988). *Pain research and clinical management* (Vol. 3). Amsterdam: Elsevier.

Dubner, R., Hoffman, D. S., & Hayes, R. L. (1981). Neuronal activity in medullary dorsal horn of awake monkeys trained in a thermal discrimination task: III. Task-related responses and their functional role. *Journal of Neurophysiology, 46,* 444-464.

Dubner, R., Ruda, M. A., Miletic, V., Hoffert, M. J., Bennett, G. J., Nishikawa, N., & Coffield, J. (1984). Neural circuitry mediating nociception in the medullary and spinal dorsal horns. In L. Kruger & J. C. Liebeskind (Eds.), *Advances in pain research and therapy* (Vol. 6, pp. 151-166). New York: Raven Press.

Dubuisson, D. (1984). Root surgery. In P. D. Wall & R. Melzack (Eds.), *Textbook of pain* (pp. 590-600). Edinburgh: Churchill Livingstone.

Duchamp, M. (1832). Maladies de la croissance. In F. G. Levrault (Ed.), *Mémoires de médecine practique.* Paris: Jean-Frederic Lobstein. (Original work published 1823)

Duncan, A. (1985). The postoperative period. *Clinics in Anaesthesiology, 3,* 619-632.

Dundee, J. W., & Loan, W. B. (1983). Assessment of analgesic drugs. In N. E. Williams & H. Wilson (Eds.), *International encyclopedia of pharmacology and therapeutics: Section 112. Pain and its management* (pp. 79-88). Elmsford, NY: Pergamon Press.

Dunn, D. K., & Jannetta, P. J. (1973, February). Evaluation of chronic pain in children. *Current Problems in Surgery,* pp. 64-72.

Dunn-Geier, B. J., McGrath, P. J., Rourke, B. P., Latter, J., & D'Astous, J. (1986). Adolescent chronic pain: The ability to cope. *Pain, 26,* 23-32.

Dunton, D. H. (1970). The child's concept of death. In B. Schoenberg, A. C. Carr, D. Peretz, & A. H. Kutscher (Eds.), *Loss and grief: Psychological management in medical practice* (pp. 355-361). New York: Columbia University Press.

Dworkin, S. F., & Chen, A. C. N. (1981). Cognitive modification of pain by varying context, expectation, information, and suggestion. *Pain* (Suppl. 1), S69.

Dworkin, S. F., Chen, A. C. N., Schubert, M. M., & Clark, D. W. (1984). Cognitive modification of pain: Information in combination with N$_2$O. *Pain, 19*, 338-351.

Dworkin, S. F., Schubert, M. M., Chen, A. C. N., & Clark, D. W. (1986). Psychological preparation influences nitrous oxide analgesia: Replication of laboratory findings in a clinical setting. *Oral Surgery, Oral Medicine, Oral Pathology, 61*, 108-112.

Dyck, P. J., Lambert, E. H., & Nichols, P. C. (1971). Quantitative measurement of sensation related to compound action potential and number and sizes of myelinated and unmyelinated fibres of sural nerve in health, Friedrich's ataxia, hereditary sensory neuropathy and tabes dorsalis. In A. Remond & W. A. Cobb (Eds.), *Handbook of electroencephalography and clinical neurophysiology* (Vol. 9, pp. 83-118). Amsterdam: Elsevier.

Dyck, P. J., Lambert, E. H., & O'Brien, P. C. (1976). Pain in peripheral neuropathy related to rate and kind of fibre degeneration. *Neurology, 26*, 466-471.

Egermark-Eriksson, I. (1982). Prevalence of headache in Swedish schoolchildren. *Acta Paediatrica Scandinavica, 71*, 135-140.

Ekeke, G. I. (1987). Sickle cell disease: Some haematological changes in steady state and crisis. *Biomedica Biochimica Acta, 46*, 197-201.

Ekman, P., & Friesen, W. V. (1969). The repertoire of non-verbal behavior: Categories, origins, usage, and coding. *Semiotica, 1*, 49-98.

Ekman, P., & Oster, H. (1979). Facial expressions of emotion. *Annual Review of Psychology, 30*, 527-554.

Eland, J. M. (1974). *Children's communication of pain*. Unpublished master's thesis, University of Iowa.

Eland, J. M. (1982). Minimizing injection pain associated with prekindergarten immunizations. *Issues in Comprehensive Pediatric Nursing, 5*, 361-372.

Eland, J. M. (1983). Children's pain: Developmentally appropriate efforts to improve identification of source, intensity and relevant intervening variables. In G. Felton & M. Albert (Eds.), *Nursing research: A monograph for non-nurse researchers* (pp. 64-79). Iowa City: University of Iowa Press.

Eland, J. M. (1985). The role of the nurse in children's pain. In K. King (Ed.), *Recent advances in nursing* (pp. 29-45). Edinburgh: Churchill Livingstone.

Eland, J. M., & Anderson, J. E. (1977). The experience of pain in children. In A. K. Jacox (Ed.), *Pain: A source book for nurses and other health professionals* (pp. 453-471). Boston: Little, Brown.

Elkins, G. R., & Carter, B. D. (1981). Use of a science fiction-based imagery technique in child hypnosis. *American Journal of Clinical Hypnosis, 23*, 274-277.

Ellenberg, L., Kellerman, J., Dash, J., Higgins, G., & Zeltzer, L. (1980). Use of hypnosis for multiple symptoms in an adolescent girl with leukemia. *Journal of Adolescent Health Care, 1*, 132-136.

Elliott, C. H., & Olson, R. A. (1983). The management of children's distress in response to painful medical treatment for burn injuries. *Behaviour Research and Therapy, 21*, 675-683.

Epstein, M. H., & Harris, J., Jr. (1978). Children with chronic pain: Can they be helped? *Pediatric Nursing, 4*, 42-44.

Ernst, A. R., Routh, D. K., & Harper, D. C. (1984). Abdominal pain in children and symptoms of somatization disorder. *Journal of Pediatric Psychology, 9*, 77-86.

Eyres, R. L., Bishop, W., Oppenheim, R. C., & Brown, T. C. K. (1983a). Plasma bupivacaine concentrations in children during caudal epidural analgesia. *Anaesthesia and Intensive Care, 11*, 20-22.

Eyres, R. L., Bishop, W., Oppenheim, R. C., & Brown, T. C. K. (1983b). Plasma lignocaine concentrations following topical laryngeal application. *Anaesthesia and Intensive Care, 11*, 23-26.

Eyres, R. L., Hastings, C., Brown, T. C. K., & Oppenheim, R. C. (1986). Plasma bupivacaine concentrations following lumbar epidural anaesthesia in children. *Anaesthesia and Intensive Care, 14*, 131-134.

Eyres, R. L., Kidd, J., Oppenheim, R., & Brown, T. C. K. (1978). Local anaesthetic plasma levels in children. *Anaesthesia and Intensive Care, 1*, 243-247.

Farrell, M. K. (1984). Abdominal pain. *Pediatrics, 74*, 955-957.

Feifel, N. (Ed.). (1959). *The meaning of death*. New York: McGraw-Hill.

Feldman, W., McGrath, P., Hodgson, C., Ritter, H., & Shipman, R. T. (1985). The use of dietary fiber in the management of simple, childhood, idiopathic, recurrent, abdominal pain. *American Journal of Diseases of Children, 139,* 1216–1218.

Fenichel, G. M. (1981). Migraine in children. In A. J. Moss (Ed.), *Pediatrics update: Reviews for physicians* (pp. 25–41). New York: Elsevier.

Fentress, D. W., Masek, B.J., Mehegan, J. E., & Benson, H. (1986). Biofeedback and relaxation-response training in the treatment of pediatric migraine. *Developmental Medicine and Child Neurology, 28,* 139–146.

Feuerstein, M., Barr, R. G., Francoeur, T. E., Houle, M., & Rafman, S. (1982). Potential biobehavioral mechanisms of recurrent abdominal pain in children. *Pain, 13,* 287–298.

Field, P. (1981). A phenomenological look at giving an injection. *Journal of Advanced Nursing, 6,* 291–296.

Field, T. (1982). Behavioral and cardiovascular activity during interactions between "high-risk" infants and adults. In P. Karoly, J. J. Steffen, & D. J. O'Grady (Eds.), *Child health psychology: Concepts and issues* (pp. 180–210). Elmsford, NY: Pergamon Press.

Fields, H. L. (1985). Neural mechanisms of opiate analgesia. In H. L. Fields, R. Dubner, & F. Cervero (Eds.), *Advances in pain research and therapy* (Vol. 9, pp. 479–486). New York: Raven Press.

Fields, H. L., & Basbaum, A. I. (1978). Brain stem control of spinal pain-transmission neurons. *Annual Review of Physiology, 40,* 217–248.

Fields, H. L., & Basbaum, A. I. (1984). Endogenous pain control mechanisms. In P. D. Wall & R. Melzack (Eds.), *Textbook of pain* (pp. 142–152). Edinburgh: Churchill Livingstone.

Fields, H. L., Basbaum, A. I., Clanton, C. H., & Anderson, S. D. (1977). Nucleus raphe magnus inhibition of spinal cord dorsal horn neurons. *Brain Research, 126,* 441–453.

Fields, H. L., Dubner, R., & Cervero, F. (Eds.). (1985). *Advances in pain research and therapy* (Vol. 9). New York: Raven Press.

Finholt, D. A., Stirt, J. A., & DiFazio, C. A. (1985). Epidural morphine for postoperative analgesia in pediatric patients. *Anesthesia and Analgesia, 64,* 211.

Fisichelli, V. R., Karelitz, S., & Haber, A. (1969). The course of induced crying activity in the neonate. *Journal of Psychology, 73,* 183–191.

Fisichelli, V. R., Karelitz, S., Fisichelli, R. M., & Cooper, J. (1974). The course of induced crying activity in the first year of life. *Journal of Pediatric Research, 8,* 921–928.

Fitzgerald, B. (1976). Intravenous regional anaesthesia in children. *British Journal of Anaesthesia, 48,* 485–486.

Fitzgerald, M. (1981). A study of the cutaneous afferent input to substantia gelatinosa. *Neuroscience, 6,* 2229–2237.

Fitzgerald, M. (1982). The contralateral input to the dorsal horn of the spinal cord in the decerebrate spinal rat. *Brain Research, 236,* 275–287.

Flannery, R. B., Jr., Sos, J., & McGovern, P. (1981). Ethnicity as a factor in the expression of pain. *Psychosomatics, 22,* 39–50.

Flavell, J. H. (1963). *The developmental psychology of Jean Piaget.* Princeton, NJ: Van Nostrand.

Fletcher, A. B. (1987). Pain in the neonate. *New England Journal of Medicine, 317,* 1347–1348.

Foerster, O., & Gagel, O. (1931). Die Vorderseitenstrangdurchschneidung beim Menschen: Eine klinisch-patho-physiologisch-anatomische Studie. *Zeitschrift für die Gesamte Neurologie und Psychiatrie, 138,* 1–92.

Foley, K. M. (1979). Pain syndromes in patients with cancer. In J. J. Bonica & V. Ventafridda (Eds.), *Advances in pain research and therapy* (Vol. 2, pp. 59–75). New York: Raven Press.

Foley, K. M. (1985). Pharmacologic approaches to cancer pain management. In H. L. Fields, R. Dubner, & F. Cervero (Eds.), *Advances in pain research and therapy* (Vol. 9, pp. 629–653). New York: Raven Press.

Foley, K. M. (1987). Cancer pain syndromes. *Journal of Pain and Symptom Management, 2,* S13–S17.

Forbes, C. D. (1984). Clinical aspects of hemophilias and their treatment. In O. D. Ratnoff & C. D. Forbes (Eds.), *Disorders of hemostasis* (pp. 177–239). New York: Grune & Stratton.

Fordyce, W. E. (1976a). Direct and positive reinforcement of pain behavior. In *Behavioral methods for chronic pain and illness* (pp. 46–73). St. Louis: C. V. Mosby.

Fordyce, W. E. (1976b). Exercise and the increase in activity level. In *Behavioral methods for chronic pain and illness* (pp. 168–183). St. Louis: C. V. Mosby.

Fordyce, W. E. (1976c). Pain as a clinical problem. In *Behavioral methods for chronic pain and illness* (pp. 11–25). St. Louis: C. V. Mosby.

Fordyce, W. E. (1978). Learning processes in pain. In R. A. Sternbach (Ed.), *The psychology of pain* (pp. 49–72). New York: Raven Press.

Foreman, R. D., Beall, J. E., Applebaum, A. E., Coulter, J. D., & Willis, W. D. (1976). Effects of dorsal column stimulation on primate spinothalamic tract neurons. *Journal of Neurophysiology, 39,* 534–546.

Forsythe, W. I., Gillies, D., & Sills, M. A. (1984). Propanolol ('Inderal') in the treatment of childhood migraine. *Developmental Medicine and Child Neurology, 26,* 737–741.

Fowler-Kerry, S., & Lander, J. (1987). Management of injection pain in children. *Pain, 30,* 169–175.

Fox, E. J., & Melzack, R. (1976). Transcutaneous electrical stimulation and acupuncture: Comparison of treatment for low-back pain. *Pain, 2,* 141–148.

Frid, M., & Singer, G. (1979). Hypnotic analgesia in conditions of stress is partially reversed by naloxone. *Psychopharmacology, 63,* 211–215.

Friedrich, W. N. (1977). Ameliorating the psychological impact of chronic physical disease on the child and family. *Journal of Pediatric Psychology, 2,* 26–31.

Friesen, R. H., & Henry, D. B. (1986). Cardiovascular changes in preterm neonates receiving isoflurane, halothane, fentanyl, and ketamine. *Anesthesiology, 64,* 238–242.

Frodi, A. M., & Lamb, M. E. (1978). Sex differences in responsiveness to infants: A developmental study of psychophysiological and behavioral responses. *Child Development, 49,* 1182–1188.

Fromm, E., & Shor, R. E. (Eds.). (1979). *Hypnosis: Developments in research and new perspectives.* Chicago: Aldine.

Frydman, M. (1980). Perception of illness severity and psychiatric symptoms in parents of chronically ill children. *Journal of Psychosomatic Research, 24,* 361–369.

Furman, R. A. (1970). The child's reaction to death in the family. In B. Schoenberg, A. C. Carr, D. Peretz, & A. H. Kutscher (Eds.), *Loss and grief: Psychological management in medical practice* (pp. 70–86). New York: Columbia University Press.

Gaal, J. M., Goldsmith, L., & Needs, R. E. (1980, November). *The use of hypnosis, as an adjunct to anesthesia, to reduce pre- and post-operative anxiety in children.* Paper presented at the annual meeting of the American Society of Clinical Hypnosis, Minneapolis.

Gaffney, A. (1984). *Pain: Perspective in childhood.* Unpublished doctoral dissertation, University College, Cork, Ireland.

Gaffney, A. (1988). How children describe pain: A study of words and analogies used by 5–14 year-olds. In R. Dubner, G. F. Gebhart, & M. R. Bond (Eds.), *Pain research and clinical management* (Vol. 3, pp. 341–347). Amsterdam: Elsevier.

Gaffney, A., & Dunne, E. A. (1986). Developmental aspects of children's definitions of pain. *Pain, 26,* 105–117.

Gaffney, A., & Dunne, E. A. (1987). Children's understanding of the causality of pain. *Pain, 29,* 91–104.

Gaffney, A., & Gaffney, P. R. (1987). Recurrent abdominal pain in children and the endogenous opiates: A brief hypothesis. *Pain, 30,* 217–219.

Galdston, R. (1972). The burning and the healing of children. *Psychiatry, 35,* 57–66.

Galler, J. R., Neustein, S., & Walker, W. A. (1980). Clinical aspects of recurrent abdominal pain in children. In L. A. Barnes (Ed.), *Advances in pediatrics* (Vol. 27, pp. 31–53). Chicago: Year Book Medical.

Gardner, G. G. (1976). Childhood, death, and human dignity: Hypnotherapy for David. *International Journal of Clinical and Experimental Hypnosis, 24,* 122–139.

Gardner, G. G., & Olness, K. (1981). *Hypnosis and hypnotherapy in children.* New York: Grune & Stratton.

Gascon, G. G. (1984). Chronic and recurrent headaches in children and adolescents. *Pediatric Clinics of North America, 31,* 1027-1051.

Gasser, H. S. (1943). Pain-producing impulses in peripheral nerves. *Proceedings of the Association for Research in Nervous and Mental Disease, 23,* 44-62.

Gaw, A. C., Chang, L. W., & Shaw, L.-C. (1975). Efficacy of acupuncture on osteoarthritic pain: A controlled double-blind study. *New England Journal of Medicine, 293,* 375-378.

Gelfand, S. (1963). The relationship of birth order to pain tolerance. *Journal of Clinical Psychology, 19,* 406.

Gescheider, G. A. (1976). *Psychophysics: Method and theory.* Hillsdale, NJ: Erlbaum.

Gewanter, H. L., Roghmann, K. J., & Baum, J. (1983). The prevalence of juvenile arthritis. *Arthritis and Rheumatism, 26,* 599-603.

Ghia, J. N., Mao, W., Toomey, T. C., & Gregg, J. M. (1976). Acupuncture and chronic pain mechanisms. *Pain, 2,* 285-299.

Gildea, J. H., & Quirk, T. R. (1977). Assessing the pain experience in children. *Nursing Clinics of North America, 12,* 631-637.

Gladtke, E. (1983). Use of antipyretic analgesics in the pediatric patient. *American Journal of Medicine, 75,* 121-126.

Glaser, J. P., & Engel, G. L. (1977). Psychodynamics, psychophysiology and gastrointestinal symptomatology. *Clinics in Gastroenterology, 6,* 507-531.

Glazer, E. J., & Basbaum, A. I. (1981). Immunohistochemical localization of leucine-enkephalin in the spinal cord of the cat: Enkephalin-containing marginal neurons and pain modulation. *Journal of Comparative Neurology, 196,* 377-389.

Glennon, B., & Weisz, J. R. (1978). An observational approach to the assessment of anxiety in young children. *Journal of Consulting and Clinical Psychology, 46,* 1246-1257.

Glenski, J. A., Warner, M. A., Dawson, B., & Kaufman, B. (1984). Postoperative use of epidurally administered morphine in children and adolescents. *Mayo Clinic Proceedings, 59,* 530-533.

Gobel, S. (1979). Neural circuitry in the substantia gelatinosa of Rolando: Anatomical insights. In J. J. Bonica, J. C. Liebeskind, & D. G. Albe-Fessard (Eds.), *Advances in pain research and therapy* (Vol. 3, pp. 175-195). New York: Raven Press.

Gobel, S., Falls, W. M., Bennett, G. J., Abdelmoumene, M., Hayashi, H., & Humphrey, E. (1980). An EM analysis of the synaptic connections of horseradish peroxidase-filled stalked cells and islet cells in the substantia gelatinosa of adult cat spinal cord. *Journal of Comparative Neurology, 194,* 781-807.

Gogan, J. L., Koocher, G. P., Foster, D. J., & O'Malley, J. E. (1977). Impact of childhood cancer on siblings. *Health and Social Work, 2,* 42-57.

Gogan, J. L., O'Malley, J. E., & Foster, P. J. (1977). Treating the pediatric cancer patient: A review. *Journal of Pediatric Psychology, 2,* 42-48.

Goldscheider, A. (1884). Die spezifische energieder gefuhlsnerven der haut. *Monatschefte für praktische Dermatologie, III,* 198-208.

Goldstein, A., Tachibana, S., Lowney, L. I., Hunkapiller, M., & Hood, L. (1979). Dynorphin (1-13), an extraordinarily potent opioid peptide. *Proceedings of the National Academy of Sciences USA, 76,* 6666-6670.

Gottfried, A. W., & Gaiter, J. L. (Eds.). (1985). *Infant stress under intensive care environmental neonatology.* Baltimore: University Park Press.

Gracely, R. H. (1980). Pain measurement in man. In L. K. Y. Ng & J. J. Bonica (Eds.), *Pain, discomfort and humanitarian care* (pp. 111-137). Amsterdam: Elsevier/North-Holland.

Gracely, R. H., McGrath, P. A., & Dubner, R. (1978). Ratio scales of sensory and affective verbal pain descriptors. *Pain, 5,* 5-18.

Graham, F. K. (1956). Behavioral differences between normal and traumatized newborns: I. The test procedures. *Psychological Monographs: General and Applied, 70,* 1-16.

Graham, F. K., Matarazzo, R. G., & Caldwell, B. M. (1956). Behavioral differences between normal and traumatized newborns: II. Standardization, reliability and validity. *Psychological Monographs: General and Applied, 70,* 17-33.

Gray, M. L., & Crowell, D. H. (1968). Heart rate changes to sudden peripheral stimuli in the human during early infancy. *Journal of Pediatrics, 72,* 807-814.

Green, M. (1967). Diagnosis and treatment: Psychogenic, recurrent, abdominal pain. *Pediatrics, 40,* 84-89.

Greenberg, J., Ohene-Frempong K., Halus, J., Way, C., & Schwartz, E. (1983). Trial of low doses of aspirin as prophylaxis in sickle cell disease. *Journal of Pediatrics, 102,* 781-784.

Gross, S. C., & Gardner, G. G. (1980). Child pain: Treatment approaches. In W. L. Smith, H. Merskey, & S. C. Gross (Eds.), *Pain: Meaning and management* (pp. 127-142). New York: SP Medical and Scientific Books.

Grunau, R. V. E., & Craig, K. D. (1987). Pain expression in neonates: Facial action and cry. *Pain, 28,* 395-410.

Gruner, O. C. (1930). *A treatise on the* Canon of medicine *of Avicenna.* London: Luzac.

Guenthner, E. E., Hilgartner, M. W., Miller, C. H., & Vienne, G. (1980). Hemophilic arthropathy: Effect of home care on treatment patterns and joint disease. *Journal of Pediatrics, 97,* 378-382.

Guilbaud, G., Besson, J.-M., Oliveras, J. L., & Liebeskind, J. C. (1973). Suppression by LSD of the inhibitory effect exerted by dorsal raphe stimulation on certain spinal cord interneurons in the cat. *Brain Research, 61,* 417-422.

Guilbaud, G., Peschanski, M., & Besson, J.-M. (1984). Experimental data related to nociception and pain at the supraspinal level. In P. D. Wall & R. Melzack (Eds.), *Textbook of pain* (pp. 110-118). Edinburgh: Churchill Livingstone.

Gunnar, M. R. (1986, April). *The organization of "stress" responses in the newborn.* Paper presented at the International Conference for Infant Studies, Symposium on Stress and Coping, Los Angeles.

Gunnar, M., Fisch, R. O., Korsvik, S., & Donhowe, J. (1981). The effects of circumcision on serum cortisol and behavior. *Psychoneuroendocrinology, 6,* 269-276.

Gunnar, M. R., Fisch, R. O., & Malone, S. (1984). The effects of a pacifying stimulus behavioral and adrenocortical responses to circumcision. *Journal of the American Academy of Child Psychiatry, 23,* 34-38.

Gunnar, M. R., Isensee, J., & Fust, L. S. (1987). Adrenocortical activity and the Brazelton Neonatal Assessment Scale: Moderating effects of the newborn's biobehavioral status. *Child Development, 58,* 1448-1458.

Gunnar, M. R., Malone, S., Vance, G., & Fisch, R. O. (1985). Coping with aversive stimulation in the neonatal period: Quiet sleep and plasma cortisol levels during recovery from circumcision. *Child Development, 56,* 824-834.

Gunnar, M. R., Wall, L., & DeBoer, J. (1985). *A psychoendocrine study of stress versus distress.* Poster presentation at the meeting of the Society for Research in Child Development, Toronto.

Gunsberger, M. (1973). Acupuncture in the treatment of sore throat symptomatology. *American Journal of Chinese Medicine, 1,* 337-340.

Gybels, J. M. (1979). Electrical stimulation of the central gray for pain relief in humans: A critical review. In J. J. Bonica, J. C. Liebeskind, & D. G. Albe-Fessard (Eds.), *Advances in pain research and therapy* (Vol. 3, pp. 499-509). New York: Raven Press.

Haft, H., Ransohoff, J., & Carter, S. (1959). Spinal cord tumors in children. *Pediatrics, 23,* 1152-1159.

Hahn, Y. S., & McLone, D. G. (1984). Pain in children with spinal cord tumors. *Child's Brain, 11,* 36-46.

Hain, W. R., & Mason, J. S. (1986). Analgesia for children. *British Journal of Hospital Medicine, 36,* 375-378.

Hall, K., & Stride, E. (1954). The varying response to pain in psychiatric disorders: A study in abnormal psychology. *British Journal of Medical Psychology, 27,* 48-60.

Hallin, R. G., & Torebjork, H. E. (1976). Studies on cutaneous A and C fibre afferents, skin nerve blocks and perception. In Y. Zotterman (Ed.), *Sensory functions of the skin in primates* (pp. 137-148). Oxford: Pergamon Press.

Hammond, D. L. (1985). Pharmacology of central pain-modulating networks (biogenic amines and nonopioid analgesics). In H. L. Fields, R. Dubner, & F. Cervero (Eds.), *Advances in pain research and therapy* (Vol. 9, pp. 499-511). New York: Raven Press.

Hammond, D. L., & Yaksh, T. L. (1981). Peripheral and central pathways in pain. *Pharmacology and Therapeutics, 14,* 459-475.

Han, J. S., & Terenius, L. (1982). Neurochemical basis of acupuncture analgesia. *Annual Review of Pharmacology and Toxicology, 22,* 193-220.

Hanson, V. (1983). Juvenile rheumatoid arthritis. In J. Umbreit (Ed.), *Physical disabilities and health impairments: An introduction* (pp. 240-249). Columbus, OH: Charles E. Merrill.

Hardy, J. D., Wolff, H. G., & Goodell, H. (1952). *Pain and reactions.* Baltimore: Williams & Wilkins.

Harpin, V. A., & Rutter, N. (1982). Development of emotional sweating in the newborn infant. *Archives of Disease in Childhood, 57,* 691-695.

Harpin, V. A., & Rutter, N. (1983). Making heel pricks less painful. *Archives of Disease in Childhood, 58,* 226-228.

Hart, F. A. (1974). Pain in osteoarthrosis. *Practitioner, 212,* 244-250.

Hartman, G. A. (1981). Hypnosis as an adjuvant in the treatment of childhood cancer. In J. J. Spinetta & P. Deasy-Spinetta (Eds.), *Living with childhood cancer* (pp. 143-152). St. Louis: C. V. Mosby.

Haslam, D. R. (1969). Age and the perception of pain. *Psychonomic Science, 15,* 86-87.

Hassan, S. Z. (1977). Caudal anesthesia in infants. *Anesthesia and Analgesia, 56,* 686-689.

Hawksley, J. C. (1931). Race, rheumatism and growing pains. *Archives of Disease in Childhood, 6,* 303-306.

Hawksley, J. C. (1938). The incidence and significance of "growing pains" in children and adolescents. *Journal of the Royal Institute of Public Health and Hygiene, 1,* 798-805.

Hawksley, J. C. (1939). The nature of growing pains and their relation to rheumatism in children and adolescents. *British Medical Journal, i,* 155-157.

Hayes, R. L., Dubner, R., & Hoffman, D. S. (1981). Neuronal activity in medullary dorsal horn of awake monkeys trained in a thermal discrimination task: II. Behavioral modulation of responses to thermal and mechanical stimuli. *Journal of Neurophysiology, 46,* 428-443.

Hayes, R. L., Price, D. D., & Dubner, R. (1979). Behavioral and physiological studies of sensory coding and modulation of trigeminal nociceptive input. In J. J. Bonica, J. C. Liebeskind, & D. G. Albe-Fessard (Eds.), *Advances in pain research and therapy* (Vol. 3, pp. 219-243). New York: Raven Press.

Health and Welfare Canada. (1984). *Cancer pain: A monograph on the management of cancer pain* (A report of the Expert Advisory Committee on the Management of Severe Chronic Pain in Cancer Patients to the Honourable Monique Begin, Minister of National Health and Welfare). Ottawa: Author.

Heisel, J. S. (1972). Life changes as etiologic factors in juvenile rheumatoid arthritis. *Journal of Psychosomatic Research, 16,* 411-420.

Henoch, M. J., Batson, J. W., & Baum, J. (1978). Psychosocial factors in juvenile rheumatoid arthritis. *Arthritis and Rheumatism, 21,* 229-233.

Herrera, H., Simmons, M. K., & French, A. P. (1983). Psychological and social considerations in the care of the chronically ill child. In M. E. Gershwin & D. L. Robbins (Eds.), *Musculoskeletal diseases of children* (pp. 25-41). New York: Grune & Stratton.

Hester, N. K. (1979). The preoperational child's reaction to immunization. *Nursing Research, 28,* 250-255.

Hilgard, E. R. (1969). Pain as a puzzle for psychology and physiology. *American Psychologist, 24,* 103-113.

Hilgard, E. R. (1973). A neodissociation interpretation of pain reduction in hypnosis. *Psychological Review, 80,* 396-411.

Hilgard, E. R., & Hilgard, J. R. (1983). *Hypnosis in the relief of pain.* Los Altos, CA: William Kaufmann.

Hilgard, J. R., & LeBaron, S. (1982). Relief of anxiety and pain in children and adolescents with cancer: Quantitative measures and clinical observations. *International Journal of Clinical and Experimental Hypnosis, 30,* 417-442.

Hilgard, J. R., & LeBaron, S. (1984). *Hypnotherapy of pain in children with cancer.* Los Altos, CA: William Kaufmann.

Hilgartner, M. W. (Ed.). (1976a). *Hemophilia in children*. Littleton, MA: Publishing Sciences Group.

Hilgartner, M. W. (1976b). Current therapy. In M. W. Hilgartner (Ed.), *Hemophilia in children* (pp. 151–170). Littleton, MA: Publishing Sciences Group.

Hill, O. W., & Blendis, L. (1967). Physical and psychological evaluation of 'non-organic' abdominal pain. *Gut, 8*, 221–229.

Hillier, L. M., & McGrath, P. A. (1987). Cognitive-behavioral approach to the management of acute pain in children. *Pain* (Suppl. 4), S236.

Hockenberry, M. J., & Bologna-Vaughan, S. (1985). Preparation for intrusive procedures using noninvasive techniques in children with cancer: State of the art vs. new trends. *Cancer Nursing, 8*, 97–102.

Hodges, K., Kline, J. J., Barbero, G., & Flanery, R. (1985). Depressive symptoms in children with recurrent abdominal pain and in their families. *Journal of Pediatrics, 107*, 622–626.

Hodges, K., Kline, J. J., Barbero, G., & Woodruff, C. (1985). Anxiety in children with recurrent abdominal pain and their parents. *Psychosomatics, 26*, 859–866.

Hoelscher, T. J., & Lichstein, K. L. (1984). Behavioral assessment and treatment of child migraine: Implications for clinical research and practice. *Headache, 24*, 94–103.

Hoffman, D. S., Dubner, R., Hayes, R. L., & Medlin, T. P. (1981). Neuronal activity in medullary dorsal horn of awake monkeys trained in a thermal discrimination task: I. Responses to innocuous and noxious thermal stimuli. *Journal of Neurophysiology, 46*, 409–427.

Holguin, J., & Fenichel, G. (1967). Migraine. *Journal of Pediatrics, 70*, 290–297.

Hosobuchi, Y. (1980). The majority of unmyelinated afferent axons in human ventral roots probably conduct pain. *Pain, 8*, 167–180.

Houde, R. W. (1979). Systemic analgesics and related drugs: Narcotic analgesics. In J. J. Bonica & V. Ventafridda (Eds.), *Advances in pain research and therapy* (Vol. 2, pp. 263–273). New York: Raven Press.

Houle, M., McGrath, P. A., Moran, G., & Garrett, O. J. (1988). Efficacy of hypnosis- and relaxation-induced analgesia on two dimensions of pain for cold pressor and electrical tooth pulp stimulation. *Pain, 33*, 241–251.

Householder, G. T. (1985). Intolerance to aspirin and the nonsteroidal anti-inflammatory drugs. *Journal of Oral and Maxillofacial Surgery, 43*, 333–337.

Houts, A. C. (1982). Relaxation and thermal feedback treatment of child migraine headache: A case study. *American Journal of Clinical Biofeedback, 5*, 154–157.

Hughes, J., Smith, T. W., Kosterlitz, H. W., Fothergill, L. A., Morgan, B. A., & Morris, H. R. (1975). Identification of two related pentapeptides from the brain with potent opiate agonist activity. *Nature, 258*, 577–579.

Hughes, M. C., & Zimin, R. (1978). Children with psychogenic abdominal pain and their families: Management during hospitalization. *Clinical Pediatrics, 17*, 569–573.

Huskisson, E. C. (1974). Measurement of pain. *Lancet, ii*, 1127–1131.

Huskisson, E. C. (1984). Non-narcotic analgesics. In P. D. Wall & R. Melzack (Eds.), *Textbook of pain* (pp. 505–513). Edinburgh: Churchill Livingstone.

Hyams, J. S. (1982). Chronic abdominal pain caused by sorbitol malabsorption. *Journal of Pediatrics, 100*, 772–773.

Iggo, A. (1980). Segmental neurophysiology of pain control. In H. W. Kosterlitz & L. Y. Terenius (Eds.), *Pain and society* (pp. 123–140). Weinheim, West Germany: Verlag Chemie.

Illingworth, R. S. (1982). Limp, limb and joint pains. In *Common symptoms of disease in children* (pp. 239–251). Oxford: Blackwell Scientific.

International Association for the Study of Pain, Subcommittee on Taxonomy. (1979). Pain terms: A list with definitions and notes on usage. *Pain, 6*, 249–252.

Ivey, J., Brewer, E. J., & Giannini, E. H. (1981). Psychosocial functioning in children with juvenile rheumatoid arthritis. *Arthritis and Rheumatism, 24*, S100.

Izard, C. E. (1982). Measuring emotions in human development. In C. E. Izard (Ed.), *Measuring emotions in infants and children* (pp. 3–20). New York: Cambridge University Press.

Izard, C. E., & Doughtery, L. M. (1982). Two complementary systems for measuring facial expressions in infants and children. In C. E. Izard (Ed.), *Measuring emotions in infants and children* (pp. 97-126). New York: Cambridge University Press.

Izard, C. E., Hembree, E. A., Dougherty, L. M., & Spizzirri, C. C. (1983). Changes in facial expressions of 2- to 19-month-old infants following acute pain. *Developmental Psychology, 19,* 418-426.

Izard, C. E., Huebner, R. R., Risser, D., McGinnes, G. C., & Dougherty, L. M. (1980). The young infant's ability to produce discrete emotion expressions. *Developmental Psychology, 16,* 132-140.

Jackson, D. N. (1976). *The Basic Personality Inventory.* London, Ontario: Research Psychologists Press.

Jackson, D. N., MacLennan, R. N., Erdle, S. W. P., Holden, R. R., Lalonde, R. N., & Thompson, G. R. (1986). Clinical judgments of depression. *Journal of Clinical Psychology, 42,* 136-145.

Jacobs, J. C. (1982). Juvenile rheumatoid arthritis. In J. A. Downey & N. L. Low (Eds.), *The child with disabling illness: Principles of rehabilitation* (pp. 3-27). New York: Raven Press.

Jacobson, E. (1938). *Progressive relaxation.* Chicago: University of Chicago Press.

Jacobson, L. (1984). Intrathecal and extradural narcotics. In C. Benedetti, C. R. Chapman, & G. Moricca (Eds.), *Advances in pain research and therapy* (Vol. 7, pp. 199-236). New York: Raven Press.

Jacox, A. K. (1980). The assessment of pain. In W. L. Smith, H. Merskey, & S. C. Gross (Eds.), *Pain: Meaning and management* (pp. 75-88). New York: SP Medical and Scientific Books.

Jaffe, J. H., & Martin, W. R. (1980). Narcotic analgesics and antagonists. In A. G. Gilman, L. S. Goodman, & A. Gilman (Eds.), *The pharmacological basis of therapeutics* (pp. 245-283). New York: Macmillan.

Janig, W. (1984). Neurophysiological mechanisms of cancer pain. *Recent Results in Cancer Research, 89,* 45-58.

Janik, J. S., & Ein, S. H. (1979). Normal intestinal rotation with non-fixation: A cause of chronic abdominal pain. *Journal of Pediatric Surgery, 14,* 670-674.

Jay, G. W., & Tomasi, L. G. (1981). Pediatric headaches: A one year retrospective analysis. *Headache, 21,* 5-9.

Jay, S. M., Elliott, C. H., Katz, E., & Siegel, S. E. (1987). Cognitive-behavioral and pharmacologic interventions for children's distress during painful medical procedures. *Journal of Consulting and Clinical Psychology, 55,* 860-865.

Jay, S. M., Elliott, C. H., Ozolins, M., Olson, R. A., & Pruitt, S. D. (1985). Behavioural management of children's distress during painful medical procedures. *Behaviour Research and Therapy, 23,* 513-552.

Jay, S. M., Elliott, C., & Varni, J. W. (1986). Acute and chronic pain in adults and children with cancer. *Journal of Consulting and Clinical Psychology, 54,* 601-607.

Jay, S. M., Ozolins, M., Elliott, C. H., & Caldwell, S. (1983). Assessment of children's distress during painful medical procedures. *Health Psychology, 2,* 133-147.

Jeans, M. E. (1983a). Pain in children: A neglected area. In P. Firestone, P. J. McGrath, & W. Feldman (Eds.), *Advances in behavioral medicine for children and adolescents* (pp. 23-37). Hillsdale, NJ: Erlbaum.

Jeans, M. E. (1983b). The measurement of pain in children. In R. Melzack (Ed.), *Pain measurement and assessment* (pp. 183-189. New York: Raven Press.

Jeans, M. E., & Gordon, D. J. (1981). An investigation of the developmental characteristics of the concept of pain. *Pain* (Suppl. 1), S11.

Jensen, B. H. (1981). Caudal block for post-operative pain relief in children with genital operations: A comparison between bupivacaine and morphine. *Acta Anaesthesiologica Scandinavica, 25,* 373-375.

Jensen, T. S., Krebs, B., Neilsen, J., & Rasmussen, P. (1984). Non-painful phantom limb phenomena in amputees: Incidence, clinical characteristics and temporal course. *Acta Neurologica Scandinavica, 70,* 407-414.

Jerrett, M. D. (1985). Children and their pain experience. *Children's Health Care, 14,* 83-89.

Jerrett, M. D., & Evans, K. (1986). Children's pain vocabulary. *Journal of Advanced Nursing, 11,* 403-408.

Jessup, B. A. (1984). Biofeedback. In P. D. Wall & R. Melzack (Eds.), *Textbook of pain* (pp. 776–786). Edinburgh: Churchill Livingstone.

Johnson, J. E. (1973). Effects of accurate expectations about sensations on the sensory and distress components of pain. *Journal of Personality and Social Psychology, 27,* 261–275.

Johnson, J. E., Dabbs, J. M., Jr., & Leventhal, H. (1970). Psychosocial factors in the welfare of surgical patients. *Nursing Research, 19,* 18–29.

Johnson, J. E., Kirchoff, K. T., & Endress, M. P. (1975). Altering children's distress behavior during orthopedic cast removal. *Nursing Research, 24,* 404–410.

Johnson, J. E., Leventhal, H., & Dabbs, J. M., Jr. (1971). Contributions of emotional and instrumental response processes in adaptation to surgery. *Journal of Personality and Social Psychology, 20,* 55–64.

Johnston, C. C. (1987). Acoustical attributes of infant pain cries: Discriminating features. *Pain* (Suppl. 4), S233.

Johnston, C. C., & O'Shaughnessy, D. (1988). Acoustical attributes of infant pain cries: Discriminating features. In R. Dubner, G. F. Gebhart, & M. R. Bond (Eds.), *Pain research and clinical management* (Vol. 3, pp. 336–340). Amsterdam: Elsevier.

Johnston, C. C., & Strada, M. E. (1986). Acute pain response in infants: A multidimensional description. *Pain, 24,* 373–382.

Jordon, M. K., & O'Grady, D. J. (1982). Children's health beliefs and concepts: Implications for child health care. In P. Karoly, J. J. Steffen, & D. J. O'Grady (Eds.), *Child health psychology: Concepts and issues* (pp. 58–76). Elmsford, NY: Pergamon Press.

Kaiko, R. F. (1980). Age and morphine analgesia in cancer patients with postoperative pain. *Clinical Pharmacology and Therapeutics, 28,* 823–826.

Kaiser, A. D. (1927). Incidence of rheumatism, chorea and heart disease in tonsillectomized children. *Journal of the American Medical Association, 89,* 2239–2245.

Kalnins, I. V. (1977). The dying child: A new perspective. *Journal of Pediatric Psychology, 2,* 39–41.

Kalnins, I. V., & Love, R. (1982). Children's concepts of health and illness—and implications for health education: An overview. *Health Education Quarterly, 9,* 104–115.

Kalwinsky, D. K., Mirro, J., & Dahl, G. V. (1988). Biology and therapy of childhood acute nonlymphocytic leukemia. *Pediatric Annals, 17,* 172–190.

Kane, K., & Taub, A. (1975). A history of local electrical analgesia. *Pain, 1,* 125–138.

Kanner, R. M. (1987). Pharmacological management of pain and symptom control in cancer. *Journal of Pain and Symptom Management, 2,* S19–S22.

Kaptchuk, T. J. (1983). *The web that has no weaver: Understanding Chinese medicine.* New York: Congdon & Weed.

Karoly, P., Steffen, J. J., & O'Grady, D. J. (Eds.). (1982). *Child health psychology: Concepts and issues.* Elmsford, NY: Pergamon Press.

Katz, E. R. (1980). Illness impact and social reintegration. In J. Kellerman (Ed.), *Psychological aspects of childhood cancer* (pp. 14–46). Springfield, IL: Charles C Thomas.

Katz, E. R., & Jay, S. M. (1984). Psychological aspects of cancer in children, adolescents, and their families. *Clinical Psychology Review, 4,* 525–542.

Katz, E. R., Kellerman, J., & Ellenberg, L. (1987). Hypnosis in the reduction of acute pain and distress in children with cancer. *Journal of Pediatric Psychology, 12,* 379–394.

Katz, E. R., Kellerman, J., Rigler, D., Williams, K. O., & Siegel, S. E. (1977). School intervention with pediatric cancer patients. *Journal of Pediatric Psychology, 2,* 72–76.

Katz, E. R., Kellerman, J., & Siegel, S. E. (1980). Behavioral distress in children with cancer undergoing medical procedures: Developmental considerations. *Journal of Consulting and Clinical Psychology, 48,* 356–365.

Katz, E. R., Kellerman, J., & Siegel, S. E. (1981). Anxiety as an affective focus in the clinical study of acute behavioral distress: A reply to Shacham and Daut. *Journal of Consulting and Clinical Psychology, 49,* 470–471.

Katz, E. R., Sharp, B., Kellerman, J., Marston, A. R., Hershman, J. M., & Siegel, S. E. (1982). Beta-endorphin immunoreactivity and acute behavioral distress in children with leukemia. *Journal of Nervous and Mental Disease, 170,* 72-77.

Katz, E. R., Varni, J. W., & Jay, S. M. (1984). Behavioral assessment and management of pediatric pain. *Progress in Behavior Modification, 18,* 163-193.

Kavanagh, C. (1983a). A new approach to dressing change in the severely burned child and its effect on burn-related psychopathology. *Heart and Lung, 12,* 612-619.

Kavanagh, C. (1983b). Alternative approach to burned children. *American Journal of Psychiatry, 140,* 268.

Kavanagh, C. (1983c). Psychological intervention with the severely burned child: Report of an experimental comparison of two approaches and their effects on psychological sequelae. *Journal of the American Academy of Child Psychiatry, 22,* 145-156.

Kay, B. (1974). Forum: Caudal block for post-operative pain relief in children. *Anaesthesia, 29,* 610-614.

Keefe, F. J., & Bradley, L. A. (1984). Behavioral and psychological approaches to the assessment and treatment of chronic pain. *General Hospital Psychiatry, 6,* 49-54.

Keele, K. D. (1957). *Anatomies of pain.* Springfield, IL: Charles C Thomas.

Kellerman, J. S. (1979). Psychological intervention in pediatric cancer: A look toward the future. In D. J. Oborne, M. M. Gruneberg, & J. R. Eiser (Eds.), *Research in psychology and medicine* (Vol. 2, pp. 394-400). New York: Academic Press.

Kellerman, J. (Ed.). (1980a). *Psychological aspects of childhood cancer.* Springfield, IL: Charles C Thomas.

Kellerman, J. (1980b). Comprehensive psychosocial care of the child with cancer: Description of a program. In J. Kellerman (Ed.), *Psychological aspects of childhood cancer* (pp. 195-214). Springfield, IL: Charles C Thomas.

Kellerman, J. (1980c). Night terrors in a leukemic child. In J. Kellerman (Ed.), *Psychological aspects of childhood cancer* (pp. 283-288). Springfield, IL: Charles C Thomas.

Kellerman, J. (1980d). Prognostic expectation and magical thinking. In J. Kellerman (Ed.), *Psychological aspects of childhood cancer* (pp. 292-294). Springfield, IL: Charles C Thomas.

Kellerman, J., & Varni, J. W. (1982). Pediatric hematology/oncology. In D. C. Russo & J. Varni (Eds.), *Behavioral pediatrics: Research and practice* (pp. 67-100). New York: Plenum Press.

Kellerman, J., Zeltzer, L., Ellenberg, L., & Dash, J. (1983). Adolescents with cancer: Hypnosis for the reduction of the acute pain and anxiety associated with medical procedures. *Journal of Adolescent Health Care, 4,* 85-90.

Kempthorne, P. M., & Brown, T. C. K. (1984). Nerve blocks around the knee in children. *Anaesthesia and Intensive Care, 12,* 14-17.

Kenshalo, D. R., Jr., Giesler, G. J., Jr., Leonard, R. B., & Willis, W. D. (1980). Responses of neurons in primate ventral posterior lateral nucleus to noxious stimuli. *Journal of Neurophysiology, 43,* 1594-1614.

Kenshalo, D. R., Jr., & Isensee, O. (1980). Responses of primate SI cortical neurons to noxious stimuli. *Society for Neuroscience Abstracts, 6,* 245.

Kerr, F. W. L. (1980). The structural basis of pain: Circuitry and pathways. In L. K. Y. Ng & J. J. Bonica (Eds.), *Pain, discomfort and humanitarian care* (pp. 49-60). Amsterdam: Elsevier/North-Holland.

Khan, M. (1983). The burned patient. In E. A. M. Frost & I. C. Andrews (Eds.), *International anesthesiology clinics: Vol. 21. Recovery room care* (pp. 127-137). Boston: Little, Brown.

Kirschner, B. S. (1988). Inflammatory bowel disease in children. *Pediatric Clinics of North America, 35,* 189-208.

Kirya, C., & Werthmann, M. W. (1978). Neonatal circumcision and penile dorsal nerve block: A painless procedure. *Journal of Pediatrics, 92,* 998-1000.

Koch, C., & Melchior, J. C. (1969). Headache in childhood: A five year material from a pediatric university clinic. *Danish Medical Bulletin, 16,* 109-144.

Koch, C. R., Hermann, J., & Donaldson, M. H. (1974). Supportive care of the child with cancer and his family. *Seminars in Oncology, 1,* 81-86.

Kofinas, G. D., Kofinas, A. D., & Tavakoli, F. M. (1985). Maternal and fetal β-endorphin release in response to the stress of labor and delivery. *American Journal of Obstetrics and Gynecology, 152,* 56-59.

Koocher, G. P. (1980). Initial consultations with the pediatric cancer patient. In J. Kellerman (Ed.), *Psychological aspects of childhood cancer* (pp. 231-237). Springfield, IL: Charles C Thomas.

Koocher, G. P., & Berman, S. J. (1983). Life threatening and terminal illness in childhood. In M. D. Levine, W. B. Carey, A. C. Crocker, & R. T. Gross (Eds.), *Developmental-behavioral pediatrics* (pp. 488-501). Philadelphia: W. B. Saunders.

Koocher, G. P., & O'Malley, J. E. (Eds.). (1981). *The Damocles syndrome: Psychosocial consequences of surviving childhood cancer.* New York: McGraw-Hill.

Kopel, F. B., Kim, I. C., & Barbero, G. J. (1967). Comparison of rectosigmoid motility in normal children, children with recurrent abdominal pain, and children with ulcerative colitis. *Pediatrics, 39,* 539-545.

Kosterlitz, H. W., & McKnight, A. T. (1980). Endorphins and enkephalins. *Advances in Internal Medicine, 26,* 1-36.

Krainick, J.-U., & Thoden, U. (1984). Dorsal column stimulation. In P. D. Wall & R. Melzack (Eds.), *Textbook of pain* (pp. 701-705). Edinburgh: Churchill Livingstone.

Kruger, L., & Liebeskind, J. C. (Eds.). (1984). *Advances in pain research and therapy* (Vol. 6). New York: Raven Press.

Krupp, G. R., & Friedman, A. P. (1953). Migraine in children. *American Journal of Diseases of Children, 87,* 146-150.

Kumazawa, T., & Perl, E. R. (1978). Excitation of marginal and substantia gelatinosa neurons in the primate spinal cord: Indications of their place in dorsal horn functional organization. *Journal of Comparative Neurology, 177,* 417-434.

Kupst, M. J., Schulman, J. L., Honig, G., Maurer, H., Morgan, E., & Fochtman, D. (1982). Family coping with childhood leukemia: One year after diagnosis. *Journal of Pediatric Psychology, 7,* 157-174.

Kupst, M. J., Schulman, J. L., Maurer, H., Honig, G., Morgan, E., & Fochtman, D. (1984). Coping with pediatric leukemia: A two-year study. *Journal of Pediatric Psychology, 9,* 149-163.

Kurylyszyn, N., McGrath, P. J., Cappelli, M., & Humphreys, P. (1986). Children's drawings: What can they tell us about intensity of pain? *Clinical Journal of Pain, 2,* 155-158.

Kuttner, L., & LePage, T. (1989). Face scales for the assessment of pediatric pain: A critical review. *Canadian Journal of Behavioural Science, 21,* 198-209.

Kuttner, L., Bowman, M., & Teasdale, M. (1988). Psychological treatment of distress, pain and anxiety for young children with cancer. *Journal of Developmental and Behavioral Pediatrics, 9,* 374-381.

Laaksonen, A.-L., & Laine, V. (1961). A comparative study of joint pain in adult and juvenile rheumatoid arthritis. *Annals of the Rheumatic Diseases, 20,* 386-387.

LaBaw, W. L. (1973). Adjunctive trance therapy with severely burned children. *International Journal of Child Psychotherapy, 2,* 80-92.

LaBaw, W. L. (1975). Auto-hypnosis in haemophilia. *Haematologia, 9,* 103-110.

LaBaw, W. L., Holton, C., Tewell, K., & Eccles, D. (1975). The use of self-hypnosis by children with cancer. *American Journal of Clinical Hypnosis, 17,* 233-238.

Labbe, E. L., & Williamson, D. A. (1983). Temperature biofeedback in the treatment of children with migraine headaches. *Journal of Pediatric Psychology, 8,* 317-326.

Labbe, E. L., & Williamson, D. A. (1984). Treatment of childhood migraine using autogenic feedback training. *Journal of Consulting and Clinical Psychology, 52,* 968-976.

Lacouture, P. G., Gaudreault, P., & Lovejoy, F. H. (1984). Chronic pain in childhood: A pharmacologic approach. *Pediatric Clinics of North America, 31,* 1133-1151.

Lai, C.-W., Ziegler, D. K., Lansky, L. L., & Torres, F. (1982). Hemiplegic migraine in childhood: Diagnostic and therapeutic aspects. *Journal of Pediatrics, 101,* 696-699.

Lamour, Y., Willer, J.-C., & Guilbaud, G. (1982). Neuronal responses to noxious stimulation in rat somatosensory cortex. *Neuroscience Letters, 29,* 35-40.

Lang, M., & Tisher, M. (1978). *Children's Depression Scale: C.D.S. (9–16 Years). Research Addition.* Melbourne: Australian Council for Educational Research.

Lanzkowsky, P. (1980). *Pediatric hematology–oncology: A treatise for the clinician.* New York: McGraw-Hill.

Larsson, B., & Melin, L. (1986). Chronic headaches in adolescents: Treatment in a school setting with relaxation training as compared with information-contact and self-registration. *Pain, 25,* 325–336.

Lascari, A. D., & Stebbens, J. A. (1973). The reactions of families to childhood leukemia. *Clinical Pediatrics, 12,* 210–214.

Laska, E. M., Sunshine, A., Mueller, F., Elvers, W. B., Siegel, C., & Rubin, A. (1984). Caffeine as an analgesic adjuvant. *Journal of the American Medical Association, 251,* 1711–1718.

Lavigne, J. V., & Ryan, M. (1979). Psychologic adjustment of siblings of children with chronic illness. *Pediatrics, 63,* 616–627.

Lavigne, J. V., Schulein, M. J., & Hahn, Y. S. (1986a). Psychological aspects of painful medical conditions in children: I. Developmental aspects and assessment. *Pain, 27,* 133–146.

Lavigne, J. V., Schulein, M. J., & Hahn, Y. S. (1986b). Psychological aspects of painful medical conditions in children: II. Personality factors, family characteristics and treatment. *Pain, 27,* 147–169.

LeBaron, S., & Zeltzer, L. (1984). Assessment of acute pain and anxiety in children and adolescents by self-reports, observer reports, and a behavior checklist. *Journal of Consulting and Clinical Psychology, 52,* 729–738.

LeBars, D., Dickenson, A. H., & Besson, J.-M. (1979). Diffuse noxious inhibitory controls (DNIC): II. Lack of effect on non-convergent neurones, supraspinal involvement and theoretical implications. *Pain, 6,* 305–327.

Lebenthal, E., Rossi, T. M., Nord, K. S., & Branski, D. (1981). Recurrent abdominal pain and lactose absorption in children. *Pediatrics, 67,* 828–832.

Lehmann, J. F., & deLateur, B. J. (1982a). Cryotherapy. In J. F. Lehmann (Ed.), *Therapeutic heat and cold* (pp. 563–602). Baltimore: Williams & Wilkins.

Lehmann, J. F., & deLateur, B. J. (1982b). Therapeutic heat. In J. F. Lehmann (Ed.), *Therapeutic heat and cold* (pp. 404–562). Baltimore: Williams & Wilkins.

Lehmann, J. F., & deLateur, B. J. (1984). Ultrasound, shortwave, microwave, superficial heat and cold in the treatment of pain. In P. D. Wall & R. Melzack (Eds.), *Textbook of pain* (pp. 717–724). Edinburgh: Churchill Livingstone.

Lehmann, J. F., Warren, C. G., & Scham, S. M. (1974). Therapeutic heat and cold. *Clinical Orthopaedics and Related Research, 99,* 207–245.

Leo, K. C. (1983). Use of electrical stimulation at acupuncture points for the treatment of reflex sympathetic dystrophy in a child: A case report. *Physical Therapy, 63,* 957–959.

Levenson, P. M., Copeland, D. R., Morrow, J. R., Pfefferbaum, B., & Silberberg, Y. (1983). Disparities in disease-related perceptions of adolescent cancer patients and their parents. *Journal of Pediatric Psychology, 8,* 33–45.

Levine, J. D., & Gordon, N. C. (1982). Pain in prelingual children and its evaluation by pain-induced vocalization. *Pain, 14,* 85–93.

Levine, M. D. (Ed.). (1984). Symposium on recurrent pain in children. *Pediatric Clinics of North America, 31,* 947–1135.

Levine, M. D., & Rappaport, L. A. (1984). Recurrent abdominal pain in school children: The loneliness of the long-distance physician. *Pediatric Clinics of North America, 31,* 969–992.

Levine, M. N., Sackett, D. L., & Bush, H. (1986). Heroin versus morphine for cancer pain? *Archives of Internal Medicine, 146,* 353–356.

Levine, P. H., & Zeltzer, L. (1985). *Control of pain.* New York: National Hemophilia Foundation.

Levinson, J. E., & Shear, E. S. (1983). Patient management: A comprehensive concerned continuum of care. In M. E. Gershwin & D. L. Robbins (Eds.), *Musculoskeletal diseases of children* (pp. 43–53). New York: Grune & Stratton.

Lewis, C., Knopf, D., Chastain-Lorber, K., Ablin, A., Zoger, S., Matthay, K., Glasser, M., & Pantell, R. (1988). Patient, parent, and physician perspectives on pediatric oncology rounds. *Journal of Pediatrics, 112,* 378-384.

Lewis, T. (1942). *Pain.* London: Macmillan.

Li, F. P., & Bader, J. L. (1987). Epidemiology of cancer in childhood. In D. G. Nathan & F. A. Oski (Eds.), *Hematology of infancy and childhood* (Vol. 2, pp. 918-941). Philadelphia: W. B. Saunders.

Liebman, W. M. (1978). Recurrent abdominal pain in children: A retrospective survey of 119 patients. *Clinical Pediatrics, 17,* 149-153.

Light, A. R., & Perl, E. R. (1979a). Reexamination of the dorsal root projection to the spinal dorsal horn including observations on the differential termination of coarse and fine fibers. *Journal of Comparative Neurology, 186,* 117-132.

Light, A. R., & Perl, E. R. (1979b). Spinal termination of functionally identified primary afferent neurons with slowly conducting myelinated fibers. *Journal of Comparative Neurology, 186,* 133-150.

Linn, S., Beardslee, W., & Patenaude, A. F. (1986). Puppet therapy with pediatric bone marrow transplant patients. *Journal of Pediatric Psychology, 11,* 37-46.

Linton, S. J. (1982). A critical review of behavioural treatments for chronic benign pain other than headache. *British Journal of Clinical Psychology, 21,* 321-337.

Linton, S. J. (1986). Behavioural remediation of chronic pain: A status report. *Pain, 24,* 125-141.

Lipton, E. L., Steinschneider, A., & Richmond, J. B. (1965). The autonomic nervous system in early life. *New England Journal of Medicine, 273,* 147-153.

Lipton, S. (1984). Percutaneous cordotomy. In P. D. Wall & Melzack (Eds.), *Textbook of pain* (pp. 632-638). Edinburgh: Churchill Livingstone.

Litt, I. F., Cuskey, W. R., & Rosenberg, A. (1982). Role of self-esteem and autonomy in determining medication compliance among adolescents with juvenile rheumatoid arthritis. *Pediatrics, 69,* 15-17.

Littlejohns, D. W., & Vere, D. W. (1981). The clinical assessment of analgesic drugs. *British Journal of Clinical Pharmacology, 11,* 319-332.

Livingston, W. K. (Ed.). (1976). *Pain mechanisms: A physiologic interpretation of causalgia and its related states.* New York: Plenum Press. (Original work published 1943)

Loeser, J. D. (1980). Nonpharmacologic approaches to pain relief. In L. K. Y. Ng & J. J. Bonica (Eds.), *Pain, discomfort and humanitarian care* (pp. 275-292). Amsterdam: Elsevier/North-Holland.

Lollar, D. J., Smits, S.J., & Patterson, D. L. (1982). Assessment of pediatric pain: An empirical perspective. *Journal of Pediatric Psychology, 7,* 267-277.

London, P., & Cooper, L. M. (1969). Norms of hypnotic susceptibility in children. *Developmental Psychology, 1,* 113-124.

Long, D. M., Erickson, D., Campbell, J., & North, R. (1981). Electrical stimulation of the spinal cord and peripheral nerves for pain control. *Applied Neurophysiology, 44,* 207-217.

Long, D. M., & Hagfors, N. (1975). Electrical stimulation in the nervous system: The current status of electrical stimulation of the nervous system for relief of pain. *Pain, 1,* 109-123.

Lourey, C. J., & McDonald, I. H. (1973). Caudal anaesthesia in infants and children. *Anaesthesia and Intensive Care, 1,* 547-548.

Ludvigsson, J. (1974). Propranolol used in prophylaxis of migraine in children. *Acta Neurologica Scandinavica, 50,* 109-115.

Lunn, J. N. (1979). Postoperative analgesia after circumcision: A randomised comparison between caudal analgesia and intramuscular morphine in boys. *Anaesthesia, 34,* 552-554.

Lusher, J. M. (1987). Diseases of coagulation: The fluid phase. In D. G. Nathan & F. A. Oski (Eds.), *Hematology of infancy and childhood* (Vol. 2, pp. 1293-1342). Philadelphia: W. B. Saunders.

Lynn, B., & Perl, E. R. (1977). Failure of acupuncture to produce localised analgesia. *Pain, 3,* 339-351.

Macdonald, A. (1984). *Acupuncture: From ancient art to modern medicine.* London: George Allen & Unwin.

MacKeith, R., & O'Neill, D. (1951). Recurrent abdominal pain in children. *Lancet, ii,* 278-282.

Magendie, F. (1822a). Expériences sur les fonctions des racines des nerfs qui naissent de la moelle épinière. *Journal of Physiology and Experimental Pathology, 2,* 366-371.

Magendie, F. (1822b). Expériences sur les fonctions des racines des nerfs rachidiens. *Journal of Physiology and Experimental Pathology, 2,* 276-279.

Magni, G., Carli, M., deLeo, D., Tshilolo, M., & Zanesco, L. (1986). Longitudinal evaluations of psychological distress in parents of children with malignancies. *Acta Paediatrica Scandinavica, 75,* 283-288.

Marshall, D. G. (1967). Diagnosis and treatment: Recurrent abdominal pain in children—a surgeon's viewpoint. *Pediatrics, 40,* 1024-1026.

Masek, B. J., Russo, D. C., & Varni, J. W. (1984). Behavioral approaches to the management of chronic pain in children. *Pediatric Clinics of North America, 31,* 1113-1131.

Mather, L. E., & Cousins, M. J. (1986). Local anaesthetics: Principles of use. In M. J. Cousins & G. D. Phillips (Eds.), *Acute pain management* (pp. 105-131). New York: Churchill Livingstone.

Mather, L. E., & Mackie, J. (1983). The incidence of postoperative pain in children. *Pain, 15,* 271-282.

Mather, L. E., & Phillips, G. D. (1986). Opioids and adjuvants: Principles of use. In M. J. Cousins & G. D. Phillips (Eds.), *Acute pain management* (pp. 77-103). New York: Churchill Livingstone.

Mattsson, A. (1972). Long-term physical illness in childhood: A challenge to psychosocial adaptation. *Pediatrics, 50,* 801-811.

Mayer, D. J., & Liebeskind, J. C. (1974). Pain reduction by focal electrical stimulation of the brain: An anatomical and behavioural analysis. *Brain Research, 68,* 73-93.

Mayer, D.J., & Price, D. D. (1976). Central nervous system mechanisms of analgesia. *Pain, 2,* 379-404.

Mayer, D. J., Price, D. D., & Becker, D. P. (1975). Neurophysiological characterization of the anterolateral spinal cord neurons contributing to pain perception in man. *Pain, 1,* 51-58.

Mayer, D. J., Price, D. D., & Rafii, A. (1977). Antagonism of acupuncture analgesia in man by the narcotic antagonist naloxone. *Brain Research, 121,* 368-372.

McAnarney, E. R., Pless, I. B., Satterwhite, B., & Friedman, S. B. (1974). Psychological problems of children with chronic juvenile arthritis. *Pediatrics, 53,* 523-528.

McCaffery, M. (1979). *Nursing management of the patient with pain.* Philadelphia: J. B. Lippincott.

McCaffery, M., & Beebe, A. (1989). *Pain: Clinical manual for nursing practice.* St. Louis: C. V. Mosby.

McCue, K. (1980). Preparing children for medical procedures. In J. Kellerman (Ed.), *Psychological aspects of childhood cancer* (pp. 238-256). Springfield, IL: Charles C Thomas.

McGrath, P. A. (1983). Biologic basis of pain and analgesia: The role of situational variables in pain control. *Anesthesia Progress, 30,* 137-146.

McGrath, P. A. (1987a). The management of chronic pain in children. In G. D. Burrows, D. Elton, & G. V. Stanley (Eds.), *Handbook of chronic pain management* (pp. 205-216). Amsterdam: Elsevier.

McGrath, P. A. (1987b). The multidimensional assessment and management of recurrent pain syndromes in children and adolescents. *Behaviour Research and Therapy, 25,* 251-262.

McGrath, P. A. (1987c). An assessment of children's pain: A review of behavioral, physiological, and direct scaling techniques. *Pain, 31,* 147-176.

McGrath, P. A., Brooke, R. I., & Varkey, M. (1981). Analgesic efficacy and subject expectation for clinical and experimental pain. *Pain* (Suppl. 1), S13.

McGrath, P. A., & deVeber, L. L. (1986a). The management of acute pain evoked by medical procedures in children with cancer. *Journal of Pain and Symptom Management, 1,* 145-150.

McGrath, P. A., & deVeber, L. L. (1986b). Helping children cope with painful procedures. *American Journal of Nursing, 86,* 1278-1279.

McGrath, P. A., deVeber, L. L., & Hearn, M. T. (1983). Modulation of acute pain and anxiety for pediatric oncology patients. *Conference Proceedings, American Pain Society,* Abstract 93.

McGrath, P. A., deVeber, L. L., & Hearn, M. T. (1985). Multidimensional pain assessment in children. In H. L. Fields, R. Dubner, & F. Cervero (Eds.), *Advances in pain research and therapy* (Vol. 9, pp. 387-393). New York: Raven Press.

McGrath, P. A., & Hillier, L. M. (1989). The undertreatment of pain in children: an overview. *Pediatrician, 16,* 6-15.

McGrath, P. A., & Hinton, G. G. (1987). The assessment and management of recurrent headaches in children. *Pain* (Suppl. 4), S235.

McGrath, P. A., Sharav, Y., Dubner, R., & Gracely, R. H. (1981). Masseter inhibitory periods and sensations evoked by electrical tooth pulp stimulation. *Pain, 10,* 1-17.

McGrath, P. J. (1983). Migraine headaches in children and adolescents. In P. Firestone, P. J. McGrath, & W. Feldman (Eds.), *Advances in behavioral medicine for children and adolescents* (pp. 39-57). Hillsdale, NJ: Erlbaum.

McGrath, P. J., Dunn-Geier, J., Cunningham, S. J., Brunette, R., D'Astous, J., Humphreys, P., Latter, J., & Keene, D. (1986). Psychological guidelines for helping children cope with chronic benign intractable pain. *Clinical Journal of Pain, 1,* 229-233.

McGrath, P. J., & Feldman, W. (1986). Clinical approach to recurrent abdominal pain in children. *Journal of Developmental and Behavioral Pediatrics, 7,* 56-61.

McGrath, P. J., Johnson, G., Goodman, J. T., Schillinger, J., Dunn, J., & Chapman, J.-A. (1985). CHEOPS: A behavioral scale for rating postoperative pain in children. In H. L. Fields, R. Dubner, & F. Cervero (Eds.), *Advances in pain research and therapy* (Vol. 9, pp. 395-402). New York: Raven Press.

McGrath, P. J., & Unruh, A. (1987). *Pain in children and adolescents.* Amsterdam: Elsevier.

McGraw, M. B. (1941). Neural maturation as exemplified in the changing reactions of the infant to pinprick. *Child Development, 12,* 31-42.

McGraw, M. B. (1945). *The neuromuscular maturation of the human infant.* New York: Hafner.

McKeever, P. (1983). Siblings of chronically ill children: A literature review with implications for research and practice. *American Journal Orthopsychiatry, 53,* 209-217.

McNichol, L. R. (1985). Sciatic nerve block for children. *Anaesthesia, 40,* 410-414.

Means, L. J., Allen, H. M., Lookabill, S. J., & Krishna, G. (1988). Recovery room initiation of patient-controlled analgesia in pediatric patients. *Anesthesiology, 69,* A772.

Mehler, W. R. (1962). The anatomy of the so-called "pain tract" in man: An analysis of the course and distribution of the ascending fibers of the fasciculus anterolateralis. In J. D. French & R. W. Porter (Eds.), *Basic research in paraplegia* (pp. 26-55). Springfield, IL: Charles C Thomas.

Meichenbaum, D., & Turk, D. (1976). The cognitive-behavioral management of anxiety, anger, and pain. In P. O. Davidson (Ed.), *The behavioral management of anxiety, depression, and pain* (pp. 1-34). Montreal: Book Center.

Meignier, M., Souron, R., & LeNeel, J.-C. (1983). Postoperative dorsal epidural analgesia in the child with respiratory disabilities. *Anesthesiology, 59,* 473-475.

Melamed, B. G. (1980). Behavioral psychology in pediatrics. In S. Rachman (Ed.), *Contributions to medical psychology* (Vol. 2, pp. 255-288). Oxford: Pergamon Press.

Melamed, B. G., Robbins, R. L., & Graves, S. (1982). Preparation for surgery and medical procedures. In D. C. Russo & J. W. Varni (Eds.), *Behavioral pediatrics: Research and practice* (pp. 225-267). New York: Plenum Press.

Melamed, B. G., & Siegel, L. J. (1975). Reduction of anxiety in children facing hospitalization and surgery by use of filmed modeling. *Journal of Consulting and Clinical Psychology, 43,* 511-521.

Melamed, B. G., & Siegel, L. J. (Eds.). (1980). *Behavioral medicine: Vol. 6. Practical applications in health care.* New York: Springer.

Melamed, B. G., Yurcheson, R., Fleece, E. L., Hutcherson, S., & Hawes, R. (1978). Effects of film modeling on the reduction of anxiety-related behaviors in individuals varying in level of previous experience in the stress situation. *Journal of Consulting and Clinical Psychology, 46,* 1357-1367.

Melzack, R. (1961). The perception of pain. *Scientific American, 204,* 41-49.

Melzack, R. (1973). *The puzzle of pain.* New York: Basic Books.

Melzack. R. (1976). Pain: Past, present and future. In M. Weisenberg & B. Tursky (Eds.), *Pain: New perspectives in therapy and research* (pp. 135-145). New York: Plenum Press.

Melzack, R. (Ed.). (1983). *Pain measurement and assessment.* New York: Raven Press.

Melzack, R. (1984). Acupuncture and related forms of folk medicine. In P. D. Wall & R. Melzack (Eds.), *Textbook of pain* (pp. 691-700). Edinburgh: Churchill Livingstone.

Melzack, R., & Dennis, S. G. (1978). Neurophysiological foundations of pain. In R. A. Sternbach (Ed.), *The psychology of pain* (pp. 1-26). New York: Raven Press.

Melzack, R., Ofiesh, J. G., & Mount, B. M. (1976). The Brompton mixture: Effects on pain in cancer patients. *Canadian Medical Association Journal, 115,* 125-129.

Melzack, R., & Wall, P. D. (1965). Pain mechanisms: A new theory. *Science, 150,* 971-978.

Melzack, R., & Wall, P. D. (1982). *The challenge of pain.* New York: Penguin Books.

Mennie, A. T. (1974). The child in pain. In L. Burton (Ed.), *Care of the child facing death* (pp. 49-59). London: Routledge & Kegan Paul.

Merskey, H. (1968). Psychological aspects of pain. *Postgraduate Medical Journal, 44,* 297-306.

Merskey, H. (1970). On the development of pain. *Headache, 10,* 116-123.

Merskey, H. (1975). Pain, learning and memory. *Journal of Psychosomatic Research, 19,* 319-324.

Merskey, H. (1987). Pain, personality and psychosomatic complaints. In G. D. Burrows, D. Elton, & G. V. Stanley (Eds.), *Handbook of chronic pain management* (pp. 137-146). Amsterdam: Elsevier.

Michael, B. E., & Copeland, D. R. (1987). Psychosocial issues in childhood cancer: An ecological framework for research. *American Journal of Pediatric Hematology/Oncology, 9,* 73-83.

Michael, M. I., & Williams, J. M. (1952). Migraine in children. *Journal of Pediatrics, 41,* 18-24.

Michelsson, K., Jarvenpaa, A.-L., & Rinne, A. (1983). Sound spectrographic analysis of pain cry in preterm infants. *Early Human Development, 8,* 141-149.

Michener, W. M. (1981). An approach to recurrent abdominal pain in children. *Primary Care, 8,* 277-283.

Miles, F. (1984). Pituitary destruction. In P. D. Wall & R. Melzack (Eds.), *Textbook of pain* (pp. 656-665). Edinburgh: Churchill Livingstone.

Miller, A. J., & Kratochwill, T. R. (1979). Reduction of frequent stomach ache complaints by time out. *Behavior Therapy, 10,* 211-218.

Millichap, J. G. (1978). Recurrent headaches in 100 children. *Child's Brain, 4,* 95-105.

Minuchin, S., Baker, L., Rosman, B. L., Liebman, R., Milman, L., & Todd, T. C. (1975). A conceptual tool of psychosomatic illness in children: Family organization and family therapy. *Archives of General Psychiatry, 32,* 1031-1038.

Miser, A. W., Davis, D. M., Hughes, C. S., Mulne, A. F., & Miser, J. S. (1983). Continuous subcutaneous infusion of morphine in children with cancer. *American Journal of Diseases of Children, 137,* 383-385.

Miser, A. W., Dothage, J. A., Wesley, R. A., & Miser, J. S. (1987). The prevalence of pain in a pediatric and young adult cancer population. *Pain, 29,* 73-83.

Miser, A.W., McCalla, J., Dothage, J. A., Wesley, M., & Miser, J. S. (1987). Pain as a presenting symptom in children and young adults with newly diagnosed malignancy. *Pain, 29,* 85-90.

Miser, A. W., Miser, J. S., & Clark, B. S. (1980). Continuous intravenous infusion of morphine sulfate for control of severe pain in children with terminal malignancy. *Journal of Pediatrics, 96,* 930-932.

Mitchell, A. A., Lovejoy, F. H., Slone, D., & Shapiro, S. (1982). Acetaminophen and aspirin. *American Journal of Diseases of Children, 136,* 976-979.

Mitchell, S. W. (1965). *Injuries of nerves and their consequences.* New York: Dover. (Original work published 1871)

Monks, R., & Merskey, H. (1984). Psychotropic drugs. In P. D. Wall & R. Melzack (Eds.), *Textbook of pain* (pp. 526-537). Edinburgh: Churchill Livingstone.

Morrow, G. R., Carpenter, P. J., & Hoagland, A. C. (1984). The role of social support in parental adjustment to pediatric cancer. *Journal of Pediatric Psychology, 9,* 317-329.

Moss, H. A., & Nannis, E. D. (1980). Psychological effects of central nervous system treatment of children with acute lymphocytic leukemia. In J. Kellerman (Ed.), *Psychological aspects of childhood cancer* (pp. 171-183). Springfield, IL: Charles C Thomas.

Moulin, D. E., & Coyle, N. (1986). Spinal opioid analgesics and local anesthetics in the management of chronic cancer pain. *Journal of Pain and Symptom Management, 1,* 79-86.

Muller, E., Hollien, H., & Murry, T. (1974). Perceptual responses to infant crying: Identification of cry types. *Journal of Child Language, 1,* 89–95.

Muller, J. (1842). *Elements of physiology.* Taylor, Schmerzenburg.

Murray, A. D. (1979). Infant crying as an elicitor of parental behavior: An examination of two models. *Psychological Bulletin, 86,* 191–215.

Murry, T., Amundson, P., & Hollien, H. (1977). Acoustical characteristics of infant cries: Fundamental frequency. *Journal of Child Language, 4,* 321–328.

Nagy, M. H. (1959). The child's view of death. In H. Feifel (Ed.), *The meaning of death* (pp. 79–98). New York: McGraw-Hill.

Naish, J. M., & Apley, J. (1951). 'Growing pains': A clinical study of nonarthritic limb pains in children. *Archives of Disease in Childhood, 26,* 134–140.

Natapoff, J. N. (1978). Children's views of health: A developmental study. *American Journal of Public Health, 68,* 995–1000.

National surveillance for Reye syndrome, 1981: Update, Reye syndrome and salicylate usage. (1982, February 12). *Morbidity and Mortality Weekly Report, 31,* 53–56; 61.

Neuhauser, C., Amsterdam, B., Hines, P., & Steward, M. (1978). Children's concepts of healing: Cognitive development and locus of control factors. *American Journal of Orthopsychiatry, 48,* 335–341.

Neuman, G. G., & Hansen, D. D. (1980). The anaesthetic management of preterm infants undergoing ligation of patent ductus arteriosus., *Canadian Anaesthetists' Society Journal, 27,* 248–253.

Newburger, P. E., & Sallan, S. E. (1981). Chronic pain: Principles of management. *Journal of Pediatrics, 98,* 180–189.

Ng, L. K. Y., & Bonica, J. J. (Eds.). (1980). *Pain, discomfort and humanitarian care.* Amsterdam: Elsevier/North-Holland.

Nocella, J., & Kaplan, R. M. (1982). Training children to cope with dental treatment. *Journal of Pediatric Psychology, 7,* 175–178.

Noordenbos, W. (1959). *Pain: Problems pertaining to the transmission of nerve impulses which give rise to pain; preliminary statement.* Amsterdam: Elsevier.

Notermans, S. L. H., & Tophoff, M. (1967). Sex differences in pain tolerance and pain appreciation. *Psychiatria, Neurologia, Neurochirurgia, 70,* 23–29.

Nover, R. A. (1973). Pain and the burned child. *Journal of the American Academy of Child Psychiatry, 12,* 499–505.

O'Brien, J. P. (1984). Orthopaedic surgery. In P. D. Wall & R. Melzack (Eds.), *Textbook of pain* (pp. 608–614). Edinburgh: Churchill Livingstone.

Obrist, P. A., Light, K. C., & Hastrup, J. L. (1982). Emotion and the cardiovascular system: A critical perspective. In C. E. Izard (Ed.), *Measuring emotions in infants and children* (pp. 299–316). New York: Cambridge University Press.

O'Connor, J., & Bensky, D. (Eds.). (1981). *Acupuncture: A comprehensive text.* Chicago: Shanghai College of Traditional Medicine.

O'Hara, M., McGrath, P. J., D'Astous, J., & Vair, C. A. (1987). Oral morphine versus injected meperidine (Demerol) for pain relief in children after orthopedic surgery. *Journal of Pediatric Orthopedics, 7,* 78–82.

Olness, K. (1981a). Hypnosis in pediatric practice. *Current Problems in Pediatrics, 12,* 1–47.

Olness, K. (1981b). Imagery (self-hypnosis) as adjunct therapy in childhood cancer: Clinical experience with 25 patients. *American Journal of Pediatric Hematology/Oncology, 3,* 313–321.

Olness, K., & Gardner, G. G. (1978). Some guidelines for uses of hypnotherapy in pediatrics. *Pediatrics, 62,* 228–233.

Olness, K., & MacDonald, J. (1981). Self-hypnosis and biofeedback in the management of juvenile migraine. *Journal of Developmental and Behavioral Pediatrics, 2,* 168–170.

Olness, K., Wain, H. J., & Ng, L. (1980). A pilot study of blood endorphins in children using self-hypnosis. *Journal of Developmental and Behavioral Pediatrics, 1,* 187–188.

Orne, M. T. (1980). Nonpharmacological approaches to pain relief: Hypnosis, biofeedback, placebo effects. In L. K. Y. Ng & J. J. Bonica (Eds.), *Pain, discomfort and humanitarian care* (pp. 253–274). Amsterdam: Elsevier/North-Holland.

Orne, M. T. (1983). Hypnotic methods for managing pain. In J. J. Bonica, U. Lindblom, & A. Iggo (Eds.), *Advances in pain research and therapy* (Vol. 5, pp. 847–856). New York: Raven Press.

Orne, M. T., & Dinges, D. F. (1984). Hypnosis. In P. D. Wall & R. Melzack (Eds.), *Textbook of pain* (pp. 806–816). Edinburgh: Churchill Livingstone.

Oster, J. (1972a). Growing pain. *Danish Medical Bulletin, 19*, 72–79.

Oster, J. (1972b). Recurrent abdominal pain, headache and limb pains in children and adolescents. *Pediatrics, 50*, 429–436.

Oster, J., & Nielsen, A. (1972). Growing pains. *Acta Paediatrica Scandinavica, 61*, 329–334.

Ostwald, P. (1972). The sounds of infancy. *Developmental Medicine and Child Neurology, 14*, 350–361.

Owens, M. E. (1984). Pain in infancy: Conceptual and methodological issues. *Pain, 20*, 213–230.

Owens, M. E. (1986). Assessment of infant pain in clinical settings. *Journal of Pain and Symptom Management, 1*, 29–31.

Owens, M. E., & Todt, E. H. (1984). Pain in infancy: Neonatal reaction to a heel lance. *Pain, 20*, 77–86.

Pain, anesthesia, and babies. (1987). *Lancet, ii*, 543–544.

Papatheophilou, R., Jeavons, P. M., & Disney, M. E. (1972). Recurrent abdominal pain: A clinical and electroencephalographic study. *Developmental Medicine and Child Neurology, 14*, 31–44.

Passo, M. H. (1982). Aches and limb pain. *Pediatric Clinics of North America, 29*, 209–219.

Payne, B., & Norfleet, M. A. (1986). Chronic pain and the family: A review. *Pain, 26*, 1–22.

Perl, E. R. (1968). Myelinated afferent fibres innervating the primate skin and their response to noxious stimuli. *Journal of Physiology, 197*, 593–615.

Perl, E. R. (1980). Afferent basis of nociception and pain: Evidence from the characteristics of sensory receptors and their projections to the spinal dorsal horn. In J. J. Bonica (Ed.), *Pain* (pp. 19–45). New York: Raven Press.

Perl, E. R. (1984). Characterization of nociceptors and their activation of neurons in the superficial dorsal horn: First steps for the sensation of pain. In L. Kruger & J. C. Liebeskind (Eds.), *Advances in pain research and therapy* (Vol. 6, pp. 23–51). New York: Raven Press.

Perl, E. R. (1985). Unraveling the story of pain. In H. L. Fields, R. Dubner, & F. Cervero (Eds.), *Advances in pain research and therapy* (Vol. 9, pp. 1–29). New York: Raven Press.

Perrin, E. C., & Gerrity, P. S. (1981). There's a demon in your belly: Children's understanding of illness. *Pediatrics, 67*, 841–849.

Perry, S. W., Cella, D. F., Falkenberg, J., Heidrich, G., & Goodwin, C. (1987). Pain perception in burn patients with stress disorders. *Journal of Pain and Symptom Management, 2*, 29–33.

Perry, S. W., & Heidrich, G. (1982). Management of pain during debridement: A survey of U.S. burn units. *Pain, 13*, 267–280.

Pert, C. B., & Snyder, S. H. (1973). Opiate receptor: Demonstration in nervous tissue. *Science, 179*, 1011–1014.

Peterson, H. A. (1977). Leg aches. *Pediatric Clinics of North America, 24*, 731–736.

Peterson, L., & Shigetomi, C. (1981). The use of coping techniques to minimize anxiety in hospitalized children. *Behavior Therapy, 12*, 1–14.

Petrovich, D. V. (1957). The Pain Apperception Test: A preliminary report. *Journal of Psychology, 44*, 339–346.

Petrovich-Bartell, N., Cowan, N., & Morse, P. A. (1982). Mothers' perceptions of infant distress vocalizations. *Journal of Speech and Hearing Research, 25*, 371–376.

Petty, R. E. (1982). Epidemiology and genetics of the rheumatic diseases of childhood. In J. T. Cassidy (Ed.), *Textbook of pediatric rheumatology* (pp. 15–45). New York: Wiley.

Piaget, J., & Inhelder, B. (1969). *The psychology of the child.* New York: Basic Books.

Piquard-Gauvain, A., Rodary, C., Rezvani, A., & Lemerle, J. (1984). Establishment of a new rating scale for the evaluation of pain in young children (2–6 years) with cancer. *Pain* (Suppl. 2), S25.

Platt, O. S., & Nathan, D. G. (1987). Sickle cell disease. In D. G. Nathan & F. A. Oski (Eds.), *Hematology of infancy and childhood* (Vol. 1, pp. 655–698). Philadelphia: W. B. Saunders.

Pless, I. B. (1983). Effects of chronic illness on adjustment: Clinical implications. In P. Firestone, P. J. McGrath, & W. Feldman (Eds.), *Advances in behavioral medicine for children and adolescents* (pp. 1–21). Hillsdale, NJ: Erlbaum.

Pless, I. B., & Roghmann, K. J. (1971). Chronic illness and its consequences: Observations based on three epidemiologic surveys. *Journal of Pediatrics, 79,* 351–359.

Pless, I. B., Roghmann, K., & Haggerty, R. J. (1972). Chronic illness, family functioning, and psychological adjustment: A model for the allocation of preventive mental health services. *International Journal of Epidemiology, 1,* 271–277.

Pomeranz, B., Cheng, R., & Law, P. (1977). Acupuncture reduces electrophysiological and behavioral responses to noxious stimuli: Pituitary is implicated. *Experimental Neurology, 54,* 172–178.

Porter, F. L., Porges, S. W., & Marshall, R. E. (1988). Newborn pain cries and vagal tone: Parallel changes in response to circumcision. *Child Development, 59,* 495–505.

Porter, J., & Jick, H. (1980). Addiction rate in patients treated with narcotics. *New England Journal of Medicine, 302,* 123.

Postone, N. (1987). Phantom limb pain: A review. *International Journal of Psychiatry in Medicine, 17,* 57–70.

Pothmann, R., & Goepel, R. (1984). Comparison of the visual analog scale (VAS) and a Smiley analog scale (SAS) for the evaluation of pain in children. *Pain* (Suppl. 2), S25.

Potter, P. C., & Roberts, M. C. (1984). Children's perceptions of chronic illness: The roles of disease symptoms, cognitive development, and information. *Journal of Pediatric Psychology, 9,* 13–27.

Poznanski, E. O. (1976). Children's reactions to pain: A psychiatrist's perspective. *Clinical Pediatrics, 15,* 1114–1119.

Pratt, K. C. (1954). The neonate. In L. Carmichael (Ed.), *Manual of child psychology* (2nd ed., pp. 215–291). New York: Wiley.

Prensky, A. L. (1976). Migraine and migrainous variants in pediatric patients. *Pediatric Clinics of North America, 23,* 461–471.

Prensky, A. L., & Sommer, D. (1979). Diagnosis and treatment of migraine in children. *Neurology, 29,* 506–510.

Price, D. D. (1984a). Dorsal horn mechanisms of pain. In R. A. Davidoff (Ed.), *The handbook of the spinal cord* (pp. 751–777). New York: Marcel Dekker.

Price, D. D. (1984b). Role of psychophysics, neuroscience, and experimental analysis in the study of pain. In L. Kruger & J. C. Liebeskind (Eds.), *Advances in pain research and therapy* (Vol. 6, pp. 341–355). New York: Raven Press.

Price, D.D. (1988). *Psychological and neural mechanisms of pain.* New York: Raven Press.

Price, D. D., & Barber, J. (1987). An analysis of factors that contribute to the efficacy of hypnotic analgesia. *Journal of Abnormal Psychology, 96,* 46–51.

Price, D. D., Barrell, J. J., & Gracely, R. H. (1980). A psychophysical analysis of experiential factors that selectively influence the affective dimension of pain. *Pain, 8,* 137–149.

Price, D. D., & Dubner, R. (1977). Neurons that subserve the sensory-discriminative aspects of pain. *Pain, 3,* 307–338.

Price, D. D., Dubner, R., & Hu, J. W. (1976). Trigeminothalamic neurons in nucleus caudalis responsive to tactile, thermal, and nociceptive stimulation of monkey's face. *Journal of Neurophysiology, 39,* 936–953.

Price, D. C., Hayashi, H., Dubner, R., & Ruda, M. A. (1979). Functional relationships between neurons of marginal and substantia gelatinosa layers of primate dorsal horn. *Journal of Neurophysiology, 42,* 1590–1608.

Price, D. D., Hayes, R. L., Ruda, M., & Dubner, R. (1978). Spatial and temporal transformations of input to spinothalamic tract neurons and their relation to somatic sensations. *Journal of Neurophysiology, 41,* 933–947.

Price, D. D., Hu, J. W., Dubner, R., & Gracely, R. H. (1977). Peripheral suppression of first pain and central summation of second pain evoked by noxious heat pulses. *Pain, 3,* 57–68.

Price, D. D., & Mayer, D. J. (1974). Physiological laminar organization of the dorsal horn of *M. mulatta*. *Brain Research, 79,* 321-325.

Price, D. D., McGrath, P. A., Rafii, A., & Buckingham, B. (1983). The validation of visual analogue scales as ratio scale measures for chronic and experimental pain. *Pain, 17,* 45-56.

Price, D. D., Rafii, A., Watkins, L. R., & Buckingham, B. (1984). A psychophysical analysis of acupuncture analgesia. *Pain, 19,* 27-42.

Pringle, M. L. K., Butler, N. R., & Davie, R. (1966). *11,000 seven-year-olds: First report of the National Child Development Study.* London: Longmans, Green.

Procacci, P. (1980). History of the pain concept. In H. W. Kosterlitz & L. Y. Terenius (Eds.), *Pain and society* (pp. 3-12). Weinheim, West Germany: Verlag Chemie.

Prugh, D. G., & Kisley, A. J. (1982). Psychosocial aspects of pediatrics and psychiatric disorders. In C. H. Kemp, H. K. Silver, & D. O'Brien (Eds.), *Current pediatric diagnosis and treatment* (pp. 638-670). Los Altos, CA: Lange Medical.

Purcell-Jones, G., Dorman, F., & Sumner, E. (1988). Paediatric anaesthetists' perceptions of neonatal and infant pain. *Pain, 33,* 181-187.

Ramón y Cajal, S. (1982). *Degeneration and regeneration of the nervous system.* New York: Hafner. (Original work published 1928)

Ramsden, R., Friedman, B., & Williamson, D. A. (1983). Treatment of childhood headaches reports with contingency management procedures. *Journal of Clinical Child Psychology, 12,* 202-206.

Rapoport, J. L., & Mikelsen, E. J. (1978). Antidepressants. In J. Werry (Ed.), *Pediatric psychopharmacology* (pp. 208-233). New York: Brunner/Mazel.

Ratcliff, R. N., & Kempthorne, P. M. (1983). Temporary tibial nerve block: Adjunct to inhibitory plasters in the physiotherapy management of equinus in severely head injured children. *Australian Journal of Physiotherapy, 29,* 119-125.

Ravenscroft, K. (1982). The burn unit. *Psychiatric Clinics of North America, 5,* 419-432.

Reichmanis, M., & Becker, R. O. (1977). Relief of experimentally-induced pain by stimulation at acupuncture loci: A review. *Comparative Medicine East and West, 5,* 281-288.

Reilly, T. P., Hasazi, J. E., & Bond, L. A. (1982). Children's conceptions of death and personal mortality. *Journal of Pediatric Psychology, 8,* 21-31.

Reynolds, D. V. (1969). Surgery in the rat during electrical analgesia induced by focal brain stimulation. *Science, 164,* 444-445.

Richards, M. P., Bernal, J. F., & Brackbill, Y. (1976). Early behavioral differences: Gender or circumcision. *Developmental Psychobiology, 9,* 89-95.

Richards, T. (1985). Can a fetus feel pain? *British Medical Journal, 291,* 1220-1221.

Richardson, D. E., & Akil, H. (1977a). Pain reduction by electrical brain stimulation in man: Part 1. Acute administration in periaqueductal and periventricular sites. *Journal of Neurosurgery, 47,* 178-183.

Richardson, D. E., & Akil, H. (1977b). Pain reduction by electrical brain stimulation in man: Part 2. Chronic self-administration in the periventricular gray matter. *Journal of Neurosurgery, 47,* 184-194.

Richardson, P. H., & Vincent, C. A. (1986). Acupuncture for the treatment of pain: A review of evaluative research. *Pain, 24,* 15-40.

Richter, I. L., McGrath, P. J., Humphreys, P. J., Goodman, J. T., Firestone, P., & Keene, D. (1986). Cognitive and relaxation treatment of paediatric migraine. *Pain, 25,* 195-203.

Richter, N. C. (1984). The efficacy of relaxation training with children. *Journal of Abnormal Child Psychology, 12,* 319-344.

Ringel, R. L., & Kluppel, D. D. (1964). Neonatal crying—a normative study. *Folia Phoniatria, 16,* 1-9.

Rivara, F. P., Parish, R. A., & Mueller, B. A. (1986). Extremity injuries in children: Predictive value of clinical findings. *Pediatrics, 78,* 803-807.

Robinson, S., & Gregory, G. A. (1981). Fentanyl–air–oxygen anesthesia for ligation of a patent ductus arteriosus in preterm infants. *Anesthesia and Analgesia, 60,* 331-334.

Rodgers, B. M., Webb, C. J., Stergios, D., & Newman, B. M. (1988). Patient-controlled analgesia in pediatric surgery. *Journal of Pediatric Surgery, 23,* 259-262.

Rogalsky, R. J., Black, G. B., & Reed, M. H. (1986). Orthopedic manifestations of leukemia in children. *Journal of Bone and Joint Surgery, 68,* 494-501.

Rogers, A. G. (1986a). Changing the route of administration in children. *Journal of Pain and Symptom Management, 1,* 33.

Rogers, A. G. (1986b). The availability of narcotics and attitudes towards their use. *Journal of Pain and Symptom Management,* 1, 157-158.

Ross, D. M. (1984). Thought-stopping: A coping strategy for impending feared events. *Issues in Comprehensive Pediatric Nursing, 7,* 83-89.

Ross, D. M., & Ross, S. A. (1982). *A study of the pain experience in children* (Final Report, Ref. No. 1 R01 HD13672-01). Bethesda, MD: National Institute of Child Health and Human Development.

Ross, D. M., & Ross, S. A. (1984a). Childhood pain: The school-aged child's viewpoint. *Pain, 20,* 179-191.

Ross, D. M., & Ross, S. A. (1984b). Teaching the child with leukemia to cope with teasing. *Issues in Pediatric Nursing, 7,* 59-66.

Ross, D. M., & Ross, S. A. (1984c). The importance of type of question, psychological climate and subject set in interviewing children about pain. *Pain, 19,* 71-79.

Ross, D. M., & Ross, S. A. (1985). Pain instruction with third- and fourth-grade children: A pilot study. *Journal of Pediatric Psychology, 10,* 55-63.

Ross, D. M., & Ross, S. A. (1988). *Childhood pain: Current issues, research, and management.* Baltimore: Urban & Schwarzenberg.

Ross, S. A. (1984). Impending hospitalization: Timing of preparation for the school-aged child. *Children's Health Care, 12,* 187-189.

Roth, G. J., & Majerus, P. W. (1975). The mechanism of the effect of aspirin on human platelets: I. Acetylation of a particulate fraction protein. *Journal of Clinical Investigation, 56,* 624-632.

Rothner, A. D. (1979). Headaches in children: A review. *Headache, 19,* 156-162.

Rothner, A. D. (1983). Diagnosis and management of headache in children and adolescents. *Neurologic Clinics, 1,* 511-526.

Rozzell, M. S., Hijazi, M., & Pack, B. (1983). The painful episode. *Nursing Clinics of North America, 18,* 185-199.

Rubin, L. S., Barbero, G. J., & Sibinga, M. S. (1967). Pupillary reactivity in children with recurrent abdominal pain. *Psychosomatic Medicine, 29,* 111-120.

Ruda, M. A. (1982). Opiates and pain pathways: Demonstration of enkephalin synapses on dorsal horn projection neurons. *Science, 215,* 1523-1525.

Ruggeri, S. B., Athreya, B. H., Doughty, R., Gregg, J. R., & Das, M. M. (1982). Reflex sympathetic dystrophy in children. *Clinical Orthopaedics and Related Research, 163,* 225-230.

Sagi, A. (1981). Mothers' and non-mothers' identification of infant cries. *Infant Behavior and Development, 4,* 37-40.

Sallan, S. E., & Weinstein, H. J. (1987). Childhood acute leukemia. In D. G. Nathan & F. A. Oski (Eds.), *Hematology of infancy and childhood* (Vol. 2, pp. 1028-1063). Philadelphia: W. B. Saunders.

Sanders, S. H. (1979). Behavioral assessment and treatment of clinical pain: Appraisal and current status. In M. Herson, R. M. Eisler, & P. M. Miller (Eds.), *Progress in behavior modification* (Vol. 8, pp. 249-291). New York: Academic Press.

Sank, L. I., & Biglan, A. (1974). Operant treatment of a case of recurrent abdominal pain in a 10-year-old boy. *Behavior Therapy, 5,* 677-681.

Saunders, C. (1981). Current views on pain relief and terminal care. In J. Swerdlowa (Ed.), *The therapy of pain* (pp. 215-241). Lancaster, England: MTP Press.

Savedra, M. (1976). Coping with pain: Strategies of severely burned children. *Maternal-Child Nursing Journal, 5,* 197-203.

Savedra, M., Gibbons, P. T., Tesler, M., Ward, J. A., & Wegner, C. (1982). How do children describe pain? A tentative assessment. *Pain, 14,* 95-104.

Savedra, M., Tesler, M., Ward, J. A., Holzemer, W., & Wilkie, D. (1987). Children's preference for pain intensity scales. *Pain* (Suppl. 4), S234.

Savedra, M., Tesler, M. D., Ward, J. A., Wegner, C., & Gibbons, P. T. (1981). Description of the pain experience: A study of school-age children. *Issues in Comprehensive Pediatric Nursing, 5*, 373–380.

Scarr, S., & Salapatek, P. (1970). Patterns of fear development during infancy. *Merrill–Palmer Quarterly, 16*, 53–90.

Scarr-Salapatek, S. (1976). Comments on "Heart rate: A sensitive tool for the study of emotional development in the infant." In L. P. Lipsitt (Ed.), *Developmental psychobiology* (pp. 32–34). Hillsdale, NJ: Erlbaum.

Schachter, S. (1959). *The psychology of affiliation.* Stanford, CA: Stanford University Press.

Schafer, D. W. (1975). Hypnosis use on a burn unit. *International Journal of Clinical and Experimental Hypnosis, 23*, 1–14.

Schechter, N. L. (1984). Recurrent pains in children: An overview and an approach. *Pediatric Clinics of North America, 31*, 949–968.

Schechter, N. L. (1985). Pain and pain control in children. *Current Problems in Pediatrics, 15*, 1–67.

Schechter, N. L., & Allen, D. A. (1986). Physicians' attitudes toward pain in children. *Journal of Developmental and Behavioral Pediatrics, 7*, 350–354.

Schechter, N. L., Allen D. A., & Hanson, K. (1986). Status of pediatric pain control: A comparison of hospital analgesic usage in children and adults. *Pediatrics, 77*, 11–15.

Schechter, N. L., Berrien, F. B., & Katz, S. M. (1988). The use of patient-controlled analgesia in adolescents with sickle cell pain crisis: A preliminary report. *Journal of Pain and Symptom Management, 3*, 109–113.

Schludermann, E., & Zubek, J. P. (1962). Effect of age on pain sensitivity. *Perceptual and Motor Skills, 14*, 295–301.

Schowalter, J. E. (1970). The child's reaction to his own terminal illness. In B. Schoenberg, A. C. Carr, D. Peretz, & A. H. Kutscher (Eds.), *Loss and grief: Psychological management in medical practice* (pp. 51–69). New York: Columbia University Press.

Schuler, D., Polcz, A., Revesz, T., Koos, R., Bakos, M., & Gal, N. (1981). Psychological late effects of leukemia in children and their prevention. *Medical and Pediatric Oncology, 9*, 191–194.

Schulte-Steinberg, O. (1980). Neural blockade for pediatric surgery. In M. J. Cousins & P. O. Bridenbaugh (Eds.), *Neural blockade in clinical anesthesia and management of pain* (pp. 503–523). Philadelphia: J. B. Lippincott.

Schulte-Steinberg, O., & Rahlfs, V. W. (1978). Caudal anesthesia in children. *Anesthesiology, 49*, 372–373.

Schultz, N. V. (1971). How children perceive pain. *Nursing Outlook, 19*, 670–673.

Scott, P. J., Ansell, B. M., & Huskisson, E. C. (1977). Measurement of pain in juvenile chronic polyarthritis. *Annals of the Rheumatic Diseases, 36*, 186–187.

Scott, R. (1978)."It hurts red": A preliminary study of children's perception of pain. *Perceptual and Motor Skills, 47*, 787–791.

Scott, R. B. (1982). The management of pain in children with sickle cell disease. In R. B. Scott (Ed.), *Advances in the pathophysiology, diagnosis, and treatment of sickle cell disease* (pp. 47–58). New York: Alan R. Liss.

Scott, R. D., Sarokhan, A. J., & Dalziel, R. (1984). Total hip and total knee arthoplasty in juvenile rheumatoid arthritis. *Clinical Orthopaedics and Related Research, 182*, 90–98.

Scott, R. D., & Sledge, C. B. (1981). The surgery of juvenile rheumatoid arthritis. In W. N. Kelly, E. D. Harris, S. Ruddy, & C. B. Sledge (Eds.), *Textook of rheumatology* (pp. 2014–2019). Philadelphia: W. B. Saunders.

Sedlackova, E. (1964). Analyse acoustique de la voix du nouveau-nés. *Folia Phoniatrica, 16*, 44–58.

Seham, M., & Hilbert, E. H. (1933). Muscular rheumatism in childhood. *American Journal of Diseases of Children, 46*, 826–853.

Sehnert, K. W. (1980). On teaching self-care to children. In T. Ferguson (Ed.), *Medical self-care: Access to health tools* (pp. 199–202). New York: Summit Books.

Seltzer, Z., & Devor, M. (1979). Epaptic transmission in chronically damaged peripheral nerves. *Neurology, 29,* 1061-1064.

Sergis-Deavenport, E., & Varni, J. W. (1983). Behavioral assessment and management of adherence to factor replacement therapy in hemophilia. *Journal of Pediatric Psychology, 8,* 367-377.

Shacham, S., & Daut, R. (1981). Anxiety or pain: What does the scale measure? *Journal of Consulting and Clinical Psychology, 49,* 468-469.

Shapiro, L. A., Jedeikin, R. J., Shalev, D., & Hoffman, S. (1984). Epidural morphine analgesia in children. *Anesthesiology, 61,* 210-212.

Shapiro, M. J. (1939). Differential diagnosis of nonrheumatic "growing pains" and subacute rheumatic fever. *Journal of Pediatrics, 14,* 315-322.

Sherman, E. D. (1943). Sensitivity to pain. *Canadian Medical Association Journal, 48,* 437-441.

Sherman, E. D., & Robillard, E. (1960). Sensitivity to pain in the aged. *Canadian Medical Association Journal, 83,* 944-947.

Shinnar, S., & D'Souza, B. J. (1981). The diagnosis and management of headaches in childhood. *Pediatric Clinics of North America, 29,* 79-94.

Shorkey, C. T., & Taylor, J. E. (1973). Management of maladaptive behavior of a severely burned child. *Child Welfare, 52,* 543-547.

Shukla, G. D., Sahu, S. C., Tripathi, R. P., & Gupta, D. K. (1982). Phantom limb: A phenomenological study. *British Journal of Psychiatry, 141,* 54-58.

Siegel, L. J., & Peterson, L. (1980). Stress reduction in young dental patients through coping skills and sensory information. *Journal of Consulting and Clinical Psychology, 48,* 785-787.

Siegel, L. J., & Peterson, L. (1981). Maintenance effects of coping skills and sensory information on young children's response to repeated dental procedures. *Behavior Therapy, 12,* 530-535.

Siegel, S. E. (1980). The current outlook for childhood cancer: The medical background. In J. Kellerman (Ed.), *Psychological aspects of childhood cancer* (pp. 5-13). Springfield, IL: Charles C Thomas.

Sillanpaa, M. (1976). Prevalence of migraine and other headache in Finnish children starting school. *Headache, 16,* 288-290.

Sillanpaa, M. (1977). Clonidine prophylaxis of childhood migraine and other vascular headache: A double blind study of 57 children. *Headache, 17,* 28-31.

Sillanpaa, M. (1983). Changes in the prevalence of migraine and other headaches during the first seven school years. *Headache, 23,* 15-19.

Simeonsson, R. J., Buckley, L., & Monson, L. (1979). Conceptions of illness causality in hospitalized children. *Journal of Pediatric Psychology, 4,* 77-84.

Simmel, M. L. (1961). The absence of phantoms for congenitally missing limbs. *American Journal of Psychology, 74,* 467-470.

Simmel, M. L. (1962). Phantom experiences following amputation in childhood. *Journal of Neurology, Neurosurgery and Psychiatry, 25,* 69-78.

Simon, E. J., Hiller, J. M., & Edelman, I. (1973). Stereospecific binding of the potent narcotic analgesic [³H]etorphine to rat-brain homogenate. *Proceedings of the National Academy of Sciences USA, 70,* 1947-1949.

Sjolund, B. H., & Bjorklund, A. (Eds.). (1982). *Brain stem control of spinal mechanisms.* Amsterdam: Elsevier.

Sjolund, B. H., & Eriksson, M. B. E. (1979). The influence of naloxone on analgesia produced by peripheral conditioning stimulation. *Brain Research, 173,* 295-301.

Sjolund, B. H., & Eriksson, M. B. E. (1980). Stimulation techniques in the management of pain. In H. W. Kosterlitz & L. Y. Terenius (Eds.), *Pain and society* (pp. 415-430). Weinheim, West Germany: Verlag Chemie.

Skinner, H. A., Steinhauer, P. D., & Santa-Barbara, J. (1983). The Family Assessment Measure. *Canadian Journal of Community Mental Health, 2,* 91-105.

Slavin, L. A. (1981). Evolving psychosocial issues in the treatment of childhood cancer: A review. In G. P. Koocher & J. E. O'Malley (Eds.), *The Damocles syndrome: Psychosocial consequences of surviving childhood cancer* (pp. 1-30). New York: McGraw-Hill.

Smith, J. B., & Willis, A. L. (1971). Aspirin selectively inhibits prostaglandin production in human platelets. *Nature: New Biology, 231,* 235-237.

Snyder, S. H. (1977). Opiate receptors and internal opiates. *Scientific American, 236,* 44-56.

Solomon, R. A., Viernstein, M. C., & Long, D. M. (1980). Reduction of postoperative pain and narcotic use by transcutaneous electrical nerve stimulation. *Surgery, 87,* 142-146.

Sourkes, B. M. (1980a). "All the things that I don't like about having leukemia": Children's lists. In J. Kellerman (Ed.), *Psychological aspects of childhood cancer* (pp. 289-291). Springfield, IL: Charles C Thomas.

Sourkes, B. M. (1980b). Siblings of the pediatric cancer patient. In J. Kellerman (Ed.), *Psychological aspects of childhood cancer* (pp. 47-69). Springfield, IL: Charles C Thomas.

Spangfort, E. (1984). Disc surgery. In P. D. Wall & R. Melzack (Eds.), *Textbook of pain* (pp. 601-607). Edinburgh: Churchill Livingstone.

Spielberger, C. D., Edwards, C. D., Lushenc, R. E., Montuori, J., & Platzek, D. (1973). *Preliminary test manual for the State-Trait Anxiety Inventory for Children.* Palo Alto, CA: Consulting Psychologists Press.

Spielberger, C. D., Gorsuch, R. L., & Lushene, R. E. (1970). *Manual for the State-Trait Anxiety Inventory ("Self-Evaluation Questionnaire").* Palo Alto, CA: Consulting Psychologists Press.

Spinetta, J. J. (1980). Disease-related communication: How to tell. In J. Kellerman (Ed.), *Psychological aspects of childhood cancer* (pp. 257-269). Springfield, IL: Charles C Thomas.

Spinetta, J. J. (1981a). Adjustment and adaptation in children with cancer. In J. J. Spinetta & P. Deasy-Spinetta (Eds.), *Living with childhood cancer* (pp. 5-23). St. Louis: C. V. Mosby.

Spinetta, J. J. (1981b). Living with childhood cancer. In J. J. Spinetta & P. Deasy-Spinetta (Eds.), *Living with childhood cancer* (pp. 3-4). St. Louis: C. V. Mosby.

Spinetta, J. J., & Deasy-Spinetta, P. (Eds.). (1981a). *Living with childhood cancer.* St. Louis: C. V. Mosby.

Spinetta, J. J., & Deasy-Spinetta, P. (1981b). Talking with children who have life threatening illness. In J. J. Spinetta & P. Deasy-Spinetta (Eds.), *Living with childhood cancer* (pp. 234-252). St. Louis: C. V. Mosby.

Spinetta, J. J., & Maloney, L. J. (1975). Death anxiety in the outpatient leukemic child. *Pediatrics, 56,* 1034-1037.

Spinetta, J. J., Rigler, D., & Karon, M. (1973). Anxiety in the dying child. *Pediatrics, 52,* 841-845.

Spoerel, W. E. (1975). Acupuncture analgesia in China. *American Journal of Chinese Medicine, 3,* 359-368.

Steinherz, P. G. (1987). Acute lymphoblastic leukemia of childhood. *Hematology/Oncology Clinics of North America, 1,* 549-566.

Steinhorn, S. C., & Myers, M. H. (1981). Progress in the treatment of childhood acute leukemia: A review. *Medical and Pediatric Oncology, 9,* 333-346.

Sternbach, R. A. (1968). *Pain: A psychophysiological analysis.* New York: Academic Press.

Sternbach, R. A. (Ed.). (1978). *The psychology of pain.* New York: Raven Press.

Sternbach, R. A. (1980). Psychological techniques in the management of pain. In H. W. Kosterlitz & L. Y. Terenius (Eds.), *Pain and society* (pp. 431-444). Weinheim, West Germany: Verlag Chemie.

Sternbach, R. A. (1984). Behaviour therapy. In P. D. Wall & R. Melzack (Eds.), *Textbook of pain* (pp. 800-805). Edinburgh: Churchill Livingstone.

Stevens, B., Hunsberger, M., & Browne, G. (1987). Pain in children: Theoretical, research, and practice dilemmas. *Journal of Pediatric Nursing, 2,* 154-166.

Stewart, M. L. (1977). Measurement of clinical pain. In A. K. Jacox (Ed.), *Pain: A source book for nurses and other health professionals* (pp. 107-137). Boston: Little, Brown.

Stickler, G. B., & Murphy, D. B. (1979). Recurrent abdominal pain. *American Journal of Diseases of Children, 133,* 486-489.

Stoddard, F. J. (1982). Coping with pain: A developmental approach to the treatment of burned children. *American Journal of Psychiatry, 139,* 736-740.

Stone, R. J., & Barbero, G. J. (1970). Recurrent abdominal pain in childhood. *Pediatrics, 45,* 732-738.

Stroebel, C. F., & Glueck, B. C. (1976). Psychophysiological rationale for the application of biofeedback in the alleviation of pain. In M. Weisenberg & B. Tursky (Eds.), *Pain: New perspectives in therapy and research* (pp. 75–81). New York: Plenum Press.

Sullivan, D. B. (1982). The pediatric rheumatology clinic. In J. T. Cassidy (Ed.), *Textbook of pediatric rheumatology* (pp. 615–629). New York: Wiley.

Susman, E. J., Hersh, S. P., Nannis, E. D., Strope, B. E., Woodruff, P. J., Pizzo, P. A., & Levine, A. S. (1982). Conceptions of cancer: The perspectives of child and adolescent patients and their families. *Journal of Pediatric Psychology, 7,* 253–261.

Sutow, W. W., Vietti, I. J., & Fernbach, D. J. (Eds.). (1977). *Clinical pediatric oncology* (2nd ed.). St. Louis: C. V. Mosby.

Swafford, L. I., & Allan, D. (1968). Pain relief in the pediatric patient. *Medical Clinics of North America, 52,* 131–136.

Sweet, W. H., & Poletti, C. E. (1984). Operations in the brain stem and spinal canal, with an appendix on open cordotomy. In P. D. Wall & R. Melzack (Eds.), *Textbook of pain* (pp. 615–631). Edinburgh: Churchill Livingstone.

Szyfelbein, S. K., & Osgood, P. F. (1984). The assessment of analgesia by self-reports of pain in burned children. *Pain* (Suppl. 2), S27.

Szyfelbein, S. K., Osgood, P. F., Atchison, N. E., & Carr, D. B. (1987). Variations in plasma beta-endorphin and cortisol levels in acutely burned children. *Pain* (Suppl. 4), S234.

Szyfelbein, S. K., Osgood, P. F., & Carr, D. B. (1985). The assessment of pain and plasma β-endorphin immunoactivity in burned children. *Pain, 22,* 173–182.

Tainter, M. L. (1948). Pain. *Annals of the New York Academy of Sciences, 59,* 3–11.

Takagi, H. (1982). Critical review of pain relieving procedures including acupuncture. In H. Yoshida et al. (Eds.), *Advances in pharmacology and therapeutics: Ser. II. CNS pharmacology. Vol. 1. Neuropeptides* (pp. 79–92). Elmsford, NY: Pergamon Press.

Talbert, L. M., Kraybill, E. N., & Potter, H. D. (1976). Adrenal cortical response to circumcision in the neonate. *Obstetrics and Gynecology, 48,* 208–210.

Tappan, F. (1984). Massage. In P. D. Wall & R. Melzack (Eds.), *Textbook of pain* (pp. 735–740). Edinburgh: Churchill Livingstone.

Tasker, R. R. (1984). Stereotaxic surgery. In P. D. Wall & R. Melzack (Eds.), *Textbook of pain* (pp. 639–655). Edinburgh: Churchill Livingstone.

Teghtsoonian, M. (1980). Children's scales of length and loudness: A developmental application of cross-modal matching. *Journal of Experimental Child Psychology, 30,* 290–307.

Tennes, K., & Carter, D. (1973). Plasma cortisol levels and behavioral states in early infancy. *Psychosomatic Medicine, 35,* 121–128.

Terenius, L. Y. (1978). Endogenous peptides and analgesia. *Annual Review of Pharmacology and Toxicology, 18,* 189–204.

Terenius, L. Y. (1984). The endogenous opioids and other central peptides. In P. D. Wall & R. Melzack (Eds.), *Textbook of pain* (pp. 133–141). Edinburgh: Churchill Livingstone.

Terenius, L. Y. (1985). Families of opioid peptides and classes of opioid receptors. In H. L. Fields, R. Dubner, & F. Cervero (Eds.), *Advances in pain research and therapy* (Vol. 9, pp. 463–477). New York: Raven Press.

Tesler, M., Savedra, M., Ward, J., Holzemer, W., & Wilkie, D. (1988). Children's language of pain. In R. Dubner, G. F. Gebhart, & M. R. Bond (Eds.), *Pain research and clinical management* (Vol. 3, pp. 348–352). Amsterdam: Elsevier.

Tesler, M., Ward, J., Savedra, M., Wegner, C., & Gibbons, P. (1983). Developing an instrument for eliciting children's description of pain. *Perceptual and Motor Skills, 56,* 315–321.

Tesler, M. D., Wegner, C., Savedra, M., Gibbons, P. T., & Ward, J. A. (1981). Coping strategies of children in pain. *Issues in Comprehensive Pediatric Nursing, 5,* 351–359.

Thomas, R., & Holbrook, T. (1987). Sickle cell disease: Ways to reduce morbidity and mortality. *Postgraduate Medicine, 81,* 265–280.

Thompson, K. F. (1976). A clinical view of the effectiveness of hypnosis in pain control. In

M. Weisenberg & B. Tursky (Eds.), *Pain: New perspectives in therapy and research* (pp. 67-74). New York: Plenum Press.

Thompson, K. L., & Varni, J. W. (1986). A developmental cognitive-biobehavioral approach to pediatric pain assessment. *Pain, 25,* 283-296.

Thompson, K. L., Varni, J. W., & Hanson, V. (1987). Comprehensive assessment of pain in juvenile rheumatoid arthritis: An empirical model. *Journal of Pediatric Psychology, 12,* 241-255.

Thompson, S. C. (1981). Will it hurt less if I can control it? A complex answer to a simple question. *Psychological Bulletin, 90,* 89-101.

Tondare, A. S., & Nadkarni, A. V. (1982). Femoral nerve block for fractured shaft of femur. *Canadian Anaesthetists' Society Journal, 29,* 270-271.

Tritt, S. G., & Esses, L. M. (1988). Psychological adaptation of siblings of children with chronic medical illnesses. *American Journal of Orthopsychiatry, 58,* 211-220.

Truby, H., & Lind, J. (1965). Cry sounds of the newborn infant. *Acta Paediatrica Scandinavica, 163,* 7-59.

Turk, D. C. (1978). Cognitive behavioral techniques in the management of pain. In J. P. Foreyt & D. P. Rathjen (Eds.), *Cognitive behavior therapy* (pp. 199-232). New York: Plenum Press.

Turk, D. C., & Meichenbaum, D. (1984). A cognitive-behavioral approach to pain management. In P. D. Wall & R. Melzack (Eds.), *Textbook of pain* (pp. 787-794). Edinburgh: Churchill Livingstone.

Turk, D. C., Meichenbaum, D., & Berman, W. H. (1979). Application of biofeedback for the regulation of pain: A critical review. *Psychological Bulletin, 86,* 1322-1338.

Turk, D. C., Meichenbaum, D., & Genest, M. (Eds.). (1983). *Pain and behavioral medicine: A cognitive-behavioral perspective.* New York: Guilford Press.

Turnbull, I. M. (1984). Brain stimulation. In P. D. Wall & R. Melzack (Eds.), *Textbook of pain* (pp. 706-714). Edinburgh: Churchill Livingstone.

Turner, J. A., & Chapman, C. R. (1982). Psychological interventions for chronic pain: A critical review. *Pain, 12,* 1-46.

Twycross, R. G. (1978). Pain and analgesics. *Current Medical Research and Opinion, 5,* 497-505.

Twycross, R. G. (1979). The Brompton cocktail. In J. J. Bonica & V. Ventafridda (Eds.), *Advances in pain research and therapy* (Vol. 2, pp. 291-300). New York: Raven Press.

Twycross, R. G. (1984). Narcotics. In P. D. Wall & R. Melzack (Eds.), *Textbook of pain* (pp. 514-525). Edinburgh: Churchill Livingstone.

Ty, T. C., Melzack, R., & Wall, P. D. (1984). Acute trauma. In P. D. Wall & R. Melzack (Eds.), *Textbook of pain* (pp. 209-214). Edinburgh: Churchill Livingstone.

Tyler, D. C. (1987). Patient controlled analgesia in adolescents. *Pain* (Suppl. 4), S236.

Ungerer, J. A., Morgan, B., Chaitow, J., & Champion, G. D. (1988). Psychosocial functioning in children and young adults with juvenile arthritis. *Pediatrics, 81,* 195-202.

Unruh, A., McGrath, P., Cunningham, S. J., & Humphreys, P. (1983). Children's drawings of their pain. *Pain, 17,* 385-392.

Vahlquist, B., & Hackzell, G. (1949). Migraine of early onset. A study of 31 cases in which the disease first appeared between 1 and 4 years of age. *Acta Paediatrica (Uppsala), 38,* 622.

Vane, J. R. (1971). Inhibition of prostaglandin synthesis as a mechanism of action for aspirin-like drugs. *Nature: New Biology, 231,* 232-235.

Varni, J. W. (1981a). Behavioral medicine in hemophilia arthritic pain management: Two case studies. *Archives of Physical Medicine and Rehabilitation, 62,* 183-192.

Varni, J. W. (1981b). Self-regulation techniques in the management of chronic arthritic pain in hemophilia. *Behavior Therapy, 12,* 185-194.

Varni, J. W. (1984). Pediatric pain: A biobehavioral perspective. *Behavior Therapist, 7,* 23-25.

Varni, J. W., Gilbert, A., & Dietrich, S. L. (1981). Behavioral medicine in pain and analgesia management for the hemophilic child with Factor VIII inhibitor. *Pain, 11,* 121-126.

Varni, J. W., & Jay, S. M. (1984). Biobehavioral factors in juvenile rheumatoid arthritis: Implications for research and practice. *Clinical Psychology Review, 4,* 543-560.

Varni, J. W., Katz, E. R., & Dash, J. (1982). Behavioral and neurochemical aspects of pediatric pain. In

D. C. Russo & J. W. Varni (Eds.), *Behavioral pediatrics: Research and practice* (pp. 177–224). New York: Plenum Press.

Varni, J. W., Thompson, K. L., & Hanson, V. (1987). The Varni/Thompson Pediatric Pain Questionnaire: I. Chronic musculoskeletal pain in juvenile rheumatoid arthritis. *Pain, 28,* 27–38.

Ventafridda, V., Spoldi, E., Caraceni, A., Tamburini, M., & DeConno, F. (1986). The importance of continuous subcutaneous morphine administration for cancer pain control. *Pain Clinic, 1,* 47–55.

Vernon, D. T. A. (1974). Modeling and birth order in responses to painful stimuli. *Journal of Personality and Social Psychology, 29,* 794–799.

Verrill, P. (1984). Sympathetic ganglioni lesions. In P. D. Wall & R. Melzack (Eds.), *Textbook of pain* (pp. 581–589). Edinburgh: Churchill Livingstone.

Vichinsky, E., & Lubin, B. H. (1987). Suggested guidelines for the treatment of children with sickle cell anemia. *Hematology/Oncology Clinics of North America, 1,* 483–501.

Vincent, C. A., & Richardson, P. H. (1986). The evaluation of therapeutic acupuncture: Concepts and methods. *Pain, 24,* 1–13.

von Graffenried, B., Adler, R., Abt, K., Nuesch, E., & Spiegel, R. (1978). The influence of anxiety and pain sensitivity on experimental pain in man. *Pain, 4,* 253–263.

Wagner, M. M. (1984). The pain of burns. In P. D. Wall & R. Melzack (Eds.), *Textbook of pain* (pp. 304–306). Edinburgh: Churchill Livingstone.

Wakeman, R. J., & Kaplan, J. Z. (1978). An experimental study of hypnosis in painful burns. *American Journal of Clinical Hypnosis, 21,* 3–12.

Wall, P. D. (1967). The laminar organisation of dorsal horn and effects of descending impulses. *Journal of Physiology, 188,* 403–423.

Wall, P. D. (1978). The gate control theory of pain mechanisms: A re-examination and re-statement. *Brain, 101,* 1–18.

Wall, P. D. (1980). The role of substantia gelatinosa as a gate control. In J. J. Bonica (Ed.), *Pain* (pp. 205–231). New York: Raven Press.

Wall, P. D. (1984a). Introduction. In P. D. Wall & R. Melzack (Eds.), *Textbook of pain* (pp. 1–16). Edinburgh: Churchill Livingstone.

Wall, P. D. (1984b). The dorsal horn. In P. D. Wall & R. Melzack (Eds.), *Textbook of pain* (pp. 80–87). Edinburgh: Churchill Livingstone.

Wall, P. D. (1984c). Mechanisms of acute and chronic pain. In L. Kruger & J. C. Liebeskind (Eds.), *Advances in pain research and therapy* (Vol. 6, pp. 95–104). New York: Raven Press.

Wall, P. D. (1985). Cancer pain: Neurogenic mechanisms. In H. L. Fields, R. Dubner, & F. Cervero (Eds.), *Advances in pain research and therapy* (Vol. 9, pp. 575–587). New York: Raven Press.

Wall, P. D. (1988). Stability and instability of central pain mechanisms. In R. Dubner, G. F. Gebhart, & M. R. Bond (Eds.), *Pain research and clinical management* (Vol. 3, pp. 13–24). Amsterdam: Elsevier.

Wall, P. D., & R. Melzack, R. (Eds.). (1984). *Textbook of pain.* Edinburgh: Churchill Livingstone.

Wall, P. D., & Sweet, W. H. (1967). Temporary abolition of pain in man. *Science, 155,* 108–109.

Wang, W. C., Parker, L. J., George, S. L., Harber, J. R., Presbury, G. J., & Wilimas, J. A. (1985). Transcutaneous electric nerve stimulation (TENS) treatment of sickle cell painful crises. *Blood, 66* (Suppl. 1), 67a.

Waranch, H. R., & Keenan, D. M. (1985). Behavioral treatment of children with recurrent headaches. *Journal of Behavior Therapy and Experimental Psychiatry, 16,* 31–38.

Wasz-Hockert, O., Lind, J., Vuorenkoski, V., Partanen, T., & Valanne, E. (1968). The infant cry: A spectographic and auditory analysis. *Clinics in Developmental Medicine, 29,* 9–42.

Wasz-Hockert, O., Partanen, T., Vuorenkoski, V., Valanne, E., & Michelsson, K. (1964). Effect of training on ability to identify preverbal vocalizations. *Developmental Medicine and Child Neurology, 6,* 393–396.

Watkins, L. R., & Mayer, D. J. (1982). Organization of endogenous opiate and nonopiate pain control systems. *Science, 216,* 1185–1192.

Weber, E., Roth, K. A., & Barchas, J. D. (1981). Colocalisation of α-neoendorphin and dynorphin immunoreactivity in hypothalamic neurons. *Biochemical and Biophysical Research Communications, 103*, 951–958.

Weinstein, D. J. (1976). Imagery and relaxation with a burn patient. *Behaviour Research and Therapy, 14*, 481.

Weinstein, S., & Sersen, E. A. (1961). Phantoms in cases of congenital absence of limbs. *Neurology, 11*, 905–911.

Weisenberg, M. (1977). Pain and pain control. *Psychological Bulletin, 84*, 1008–1041.

Weisenberg, M. (1980). Understanding pain phenomena. In S. Rachman (Ed.), *Contributions to medical psychology* (Vol. 2, pp. 79–111). Oxford: Pergamon Press.

Weisenberg, M. (1984). Cognitive aspects of pain. In P. D. Wall & R. Melzack (Eds.), *Textbook of pain* (pp. 162–172). Edinburgh: Churchill Livingstone.

Weisenberg, M. (1987). Psychological intervention for the control of pain. *Behaviour Research and Therapy, 25*, 301–312.

Weisenberg, M., & Tursky, B. (Eds.). (1976). *Pain: New perspectives in therapy and research.* New York: Plenum Press.

Wells, P. (1984). Movement education and limitation of movement. In P. D. Wall & R. Melzack (Eds.), *Textbook of pain* (pp. 741–750). Edinburgh: Churchill Livingstone.

Werder, D. S., & Sargent, J. D. (1984). A study of childhood headache using biofeedback as a treatment alternative. *Headache, 24*, 122–126.

White, J. C., & Sweet, W. H. (1955). *Pain: Its mechanisms and neurosurgical control.* Springfield, IL: Charles C Thomas.

White, J. C., & Sweet, W. H. (1969). *Pain and the neurosurgeon.* Springfield, IL: Charles C Thomas.

Whitten, C. F., & Fischhoff, J. (1974). Psychosocial effects of sickle cell disease. *Archives of Internal Medicine, 133*, 681–689.

Wiener, J. M. (1970a). Reaction of the family to the fatal illness of a child. In B. Schoenberg, A. C. Carr, D. Peretz, & A. H. Kutscher (Eds.), *Loss and grief: Psychological management in medical practice* (pp. 88–101). New York: Columbia University Press.

Wiener, J. M. (1970b). Response of medical personnel to the fatal illness of a child. In B. Schoenberg, A. C. Carr, D. Peretz, & A. H. Kutscher (Eds.), *Loss and grief: Psychological management in medical practice* (pp. 102–115). New York: Columbia University Press.

Wiley, F. M., & Rhein, M. (1977). Challenges of pain management: One terminally ill adolescent. *Pediatric Nursing, 3*, 26–27.

Wilkinson, V. A. (1981). Juvenile chronic arthritis in adolescence: Facing the reality. *International Rehabilitation Medicine, 3*, 11–17.

Willer, J.-C., Roby, A., Boulu, P., & Boureau, F. (1982). Comparative effects of electroacupuncture and transcutaneous nerve stimulation on the human blink reflex. *Pain, 14*, 267–278.

Williamson, D. A., Monguillot, J. E., Jarrell, M. P., Cohen, R. A., Pratt, J. M., & Blouin, D. C. (1984). Relaxation for the treatment of headache. *Behavior Modification, 8*, 407–424.

Williamson, P. S., & Williamson, M. L. (1983). Physiologic stress reduction by a local anesthetic during newborn circumcision. *Pediatrics, 71*, 36–40.

Willis, W. D. (1984). The origin and destination of pathways involved in pain transmission. In P. D. Wall & R. Melzack (Eds.), *Textbook of pain* (pp. 88–99). Edinburgh: Churchill Livingstone.

Willis, W. D. (1985). *The pain system: The neural basis of nociceptive transmission in the mammalian nervous system.* Basel: Karger.

Willis, W. D., & Coggeshall, R. E. (1978). *Sensory mechanisms of the spinal cord.* New York: Wiley.

Willis, W. D., Haber, L. H., & Martin, R. F. (1977). Inhibition of spinothalamic tract cells and interneurons by brain stem stimulation in the monkey. *Journal of Neurophysiology, 40*, 968–981.

Willoughby, M., & Siegel, S. E. (1982). *Pediatrics: Vol. 1. Hematology–oncology.* London: Butterworths Scientific.

Wolff, B. B. (1980). Measurement of human pain. In J. J. Bonica (Ed.), *Pain* (pp. 173–184). New York: Raven Press.

Wolff, B. B., & Jarvik, M. E. (1965). Quantitative measures of deep somatic pain: Further studies with hypertonic saline. *Clinical Science, 28*, 43-56.

Wolff, P. H. (1969). The natural history of crying and other vocalizations in early infancy. In B. Foss (Ed.), *Determinants of behaviour* (Vol. 4, pp. 81-109). London: Methuen.

Wolpe, J. (1982). *The practice of behavior therapy.* Elmsford, NY: Pergamon Press.

Womack, W. M., Smith, M. S., & Chen, A. C. N. (1988). Behavioral management of childhood headache: A pilot study and case history report. *Pain, 32*, 279-283.

Wood, B., Boyle, J. T., Watkins, J. B., Nogueira, J., Zimand, E., & Carroll, L. (1988). Sibling psychological status and style as related to the disease of their chronically ill brothers and sisters: Implications for models of biopsychosocial interaction. *Journal of Developmental and Behavioral Pediatrics, 9*, 66-72.

Wood, K. M. (1984). Peripheral nerve and root chemical lesions. In P. D. Wall & R. Melzack (Eds.), *Textbook of pain* (pp. 577-580). Edinburgh: Churchill Livingstone.

Woodrow, K. M., Friedman, G. D., Siegelaub, A. B., & Collen, M. F. (1972). Pain tolerance: Differences according to age, sex, and race. *Psychosomatic Medicine, 34*, 548-556.

Woolf, C. .J. (1984). Transcutaneous and implanted nerve stimulation. In P. D. Wall & R. Melzack (Eds.), *Textbook of pain* (pp. 679-690). Edinburgh: Churchill Livingstone.

Wyllie, W. G., & Schlesinger, B. (1933). The periodic group of disorders in childhood. *British Journal of Children's Diseases, 30*, 1-21.

Yaffe, S. J. (Ed.). (1980). *Pediatric pharmacology: Therapeutic principles in practice.* New York: Grune & Stratton.

Yaksh, T. L. (1981). Spinal opiate analgesia: Characteristics and principles of action. *Pain, 11*, 293-346.

Yaksh, T. L., & Rudy, T. A. (1976). Analgesia mediated by a direct spinal action of narcotics. *Science, 192*, 1357-1358.

Yaster, M. (1987). Analgesia and anesthesia in neonates. *Journal of Pediatrics, 111*, 394-396.

Yurt, R. W., & Pruitt, B. A., Jr. (1983). Burns. In J. Umbreit (Ed.), *Physical disabilities and health impairments: An introduction* (pp. 175-184). Columbus, OH: Charles E. Merrill.

Yutang, L. (Ed.). (1942). *The wisdom of India.* New York: Random House.

Zborowski, M. (1962). Cultural components in responses to pain. *Journal of Social Issues, 8*, 16-30.

Zeltzer, L. K. (1980). The adolescent with cancer. In J. Kellerman (Ed.), *Psychological aspects of childhood cancer* (pp. 70-99). Springfield, IL: Charles C Thomas.

Zeltzer, L. (1986). Commentary on "Clinical approach to recurrent abdominal pain in children." *Journal of Developmental and Behavioral Pediatrics, 7*, 62-63.

Zeltzer, L., Dash, J., & Holland, J. P. (1979). Hypnotically induced pain control in sickle cell anemia. *Pediatrics, 64*, 533-536.

Zeltzer, L., Kellerman, J., Ellenberg, L., Dash, J., & Rigler, D. (1980). Psychologic effects of illness in adolescence: II. Impact of illness in adolescents—crucial issues and coping styles. *Journal of Pediatrics, 97*, 132-138.

Zeltzer, L., & LeBaron, S. (1982). Hypnosis and nonhypnotic techniques for reduction of pain and anxiety during painful procedures in children and adolescents with cancer. *Journal of Pediatrics, 101*, 1032-1035.

Zimmermann, M. (1980). Physiological mechanisms of chronic pain. In H. W. Kosterlitz & L. Y. Terenius (Eds.), *Pain and society* (pp. 283-298). Weinheim, West Germany: Verlag Chemie.

Zotterman, Y. (1933). Studies in the peripheral nervous mechanism of pain. *Acta Medica Scandinavica, 80*, 185-242.

Index